PRACTICAL JOINT ASSESSMENT
UPPER QUADRANT
A Sports Medicine Manual

PRACTICAL JOINT ASSESSMENT
UPPER QUADRANT
A Sports Medicine Manual

Anne Hartley, **B.P.H.E., Dip A.T.M., C.A.T.(C)**
Professer Sheridan College of Applied
Arts and Technology
The Sports Injury Management Program
Oakville, Ontario
Canada

Second Edition

with 266 illustrations

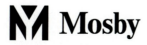 **Mosby**

St. Louis Baltimore Berlin Boston Carlsbad Chicago London Madrid
Naples New York Philadelphia Sydney Tokyo Toronto

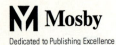
Mosby
Dedicated to Publishing Excellence

Executive Editor: Martha Sasser
Associate Developmental Editor: Kellie F. White
Project Manager: Carol Sullivan Wiseman
Production Editor: Florence Achenbach
Designer: Betty Schulz
Manufacturing Supervisor: Karen Lewis
Cover Art: Rip Kastaris

SECOND EDITION
Copyright © 1995 Mosby–Year Book, Inc.

Previous edition copyrighted 1990

Printed in the United States of America
Composition by Digital Prepress, Inc.
Printing by Von Hoffmann Press, Inc.

Mosby–Year Book, Inc.
11830 Westline Industrial Drive
St. Louis, MO 63146

Library of Congress Cataloging-in-Publication Data

Hartley, Anne
    Practical joint assessment: upper quadrant: a sports medicine manual/ Anne Hartley, -- 2nd ed.
        p.   cm.
    First ed. published in 1 v.
    Companion v. to: Practical joint assessment: lower quadrant, 2nd ed. 1994.
    Includes bibliographical references and index.
    ISBN 0-8151-4237-4
    1. Joints Examination.   2. Joints—Wounds and injuries-
-Diagnosis.   3. Sports injuries—Diagnosis   I. Title.
    [DNLM: 1. Joints—physiology.   2. Muscles--physiology.
3. Athletic Injuries—diagnosis.   4. Physical Examination—methods.
5. Sports Medicine.   WE 300 H332pd 1994]
RD97.H374   1994
617.4′72—dc20
DNLM/DLC   94-11608
for Library of Congress   CIP

94 95 96 97 98   /   9 8 7 6 5 4 3 2 1

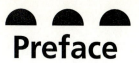

Preface

This manual was originally written for the students in Sports Injury Management Program in athletic therapy at Sheridan College in Oakville, Ontario, and for the Certification Candidates of the Canadian Athletic Therapist Association. The manual is designed to give a hands-on approach to the assessment of the joints of the body. Each chapter is divided into these sections: history, observations, functional tests, special tests, accessory tests, and palpations. On one side of the page the instructions are outlined and on the opposing side of the page are the possible interpretations of the patient's responses or results. It allows the reader to develop a systematic and thorough approach to assessing musculoskeletal disorders. Line drawings throughout the manual help to clarify hand placements or body positions for testing, as well as depicting anatomical structures and mechanisms of injury.

The upper and lower quadrant practical assessment manuals are useful clinical tools for all therapists, physicians, osteopaths, chiropractors, or other allied health professionals with a basic understanding in sports medicine. They are especially valuable for instructors and students in sports medicine or orthopaedics. The hands-on practical nature of the manuals allows the students to progress at their own pace.

Wherever possible, I have attempted to recognize the originators of the assessment techniques in my references and bibliography. However, in the course of twenty years of clinical experiences, the origins of some techniques have faded from memory. To any of the originators that I have inadvertently overlooked, please accept my sincere apologies.

ACKNOWLEDGMENTS

I would like to acknowledge and sincerely thank:

Mark Hartley, my husband, for his patience, encouragement, and time during this lengthy undertaking. Any valuable time lost will be regained.

Paul and **Dean Hartley**, my children, who allowed for maternity leave time and afternoon naps when most of my writing was accomplished. Heavens knows what more I could write by having another.

Alfred Chalmers, my father, for his advice and financial expertise in helping to develop, market, and originally publish these manuals.

Janet Chandler, my good friend and computer specialist, who never complained even when called on to rush things. Her advice was invaluable and her ideas on layout paramount.

Sheridan College of Applied Arts and Technology for providing the classroom and clinical environment in which to learn.

The Sports Injury Management students who kept me challenged and motivated daily. Most of their questions are still unanswered.

My college program colleagues who encouraged and humored me.

My medical illustrators, **Beverley Ransom** and **Susan Leopold**, who can work magic with a pen.

Anne Hartley

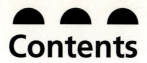

Contents

Introduction

GUIDELINES FOR USE OF THIS TEXT

The plan given in this text is a menu for assessing a joint. The order of the functional testing routine should be varied according to the history and observations recorded.

Not all of the tests may be necessary for each assessment. It will depend on your findings as you progress.

The left column is the guide for questions, instructions for hand placements, and general instructions. The right column presents the different interpretations of the findings and directs the assessor to possible damaged structures.

The interpretation section is designed to gear your thinking toward all the alternatives and allow the different possibilities to be incorporated into your assessment procedures.

Never rush your interpretation. Always rule out other possible conditions and structures.

Record all the limited joint ranges, end-feels, and painful movements, because these are the keys to determining the condition. But more importantly, these are the keys to help determine how to design an effective rehabilitation program.

GENERAL ASSESSMENT GUIDELINES

Always observe and functionally assess the joints bilaterally,

Begin with the uninjured limb first, then repeat the test on the injured limb. Compare ranges of motion, end feel, and muscular strength.

It may be necessary to retest the normal or injured site more than once, Differences in mobility can be very small (2 to 10 mm) yet very significant.

Try to arrange your testing so that the most painful test is last. This ensures that the condition will not be aggravated by your testing procedure or make the athlete apprehensive.

Your testing should be influenced by the history and observations to rule out needless testing, but you must be thorough enough to rule out all other possible injured structures, the possibility of multiple injuries, and visceral, vascular, or systemic conditions.

Always support the injured limb securely to gain the athlete's confidence and prevent further injury. If the injury is inflamed or swollen, it may be necessary to elevate the area while taking the history and between tests.

Rule out the joint above and below, especially if the history or observations suggest other joint involvement.

A scan of the entire quadrant may be necessary if the onset of the problem is insidious, if the pain is diffuse and nonspecific, or, if during testing, several joints or body parts seem to be implicated.

It may be necessary to analyze the entire quadrant's kinetic chain because any weak link can lead to dysfunction, or conversely, dysfunction can alter the normal kinetic chain.

Be aware of *radicular pain syndromes* in which the spinal nerves or nerve roots are irritated. The *radicular referred pain* is lancinating and travels down the limb in narrow bands. With radicular pain syndromes there are definite segmental neurological signs that include: dermatome numbness or paresthesia, myotome weakness, and/or reflex changes.

Be aware of somatic pain syndromes in which the source of pain comes from one or more of the musculoskeletal elements around the spine (ligament, muscle, intervertebral disc, facet joint). These syndromes have somatic referred pain that does not involve the nerve root or have neurological changes (i.e., reflexes, paresthesia). Somatic referred pain is a dull, achy pain that is perceived in an area separate from the primary source of dysfunction or pain.

Be aware that systematic disorders, visceral injuries or disease, circulatory conditions, neural disorders, and others can also affect muscle and joint function and can also refer pain.

As described above, pain is not always perceived

at the point of origin. To determine the lesion site and structure, functional structure testing must be done *before* palpation. Palpation of the painful site before functional testing not only prejudices the testing but the primary lesion may be missed.

Ask the athlete the location of the pain, nature of the pain, and any difference in the pain during the testing procedure.

Active Tests

During your active tests, the athlete should be asked to move the joint through as much range as possible. If the active range is full, an overpressure may be applied to determine the end feel of the joint. This test is important because it indicates the athlete's willingness to move the joint, as well as the range of motion of the joint and the strength of the surrounding structures.

Passive Tests

These tests are designed to test the inert structures.

During your passive tests, you move the joint until an end feel or end range is felt.

The type of end feel at the end of the range of motion is important because it assists in determining the condition, the structure at fault, and the severity of the injury. Cyriax defines six end feels.

1. **Bone-to-bone** is an abrupt hard sensation when one bone engages with another bone. This can be a normal or an abnormal end feel.
   - normal (e.g., elbow extension)
   - abnormal (e.g., when the boney end feel occurs before the end of the joint range). This can indicate an osteophyte or abnormal boney development.
2. **Spasm** is a vibrant twang as the muscles around the joint spasm to arrest movement. A knee extension with hamstring spasm is one example. This is an abnormal end feel and it is contraindicated to force the joint through more range to mobilize or manipulate. It can indicate acute or subacute capsulitis or severe ligamentous injury.
3. **Capsular feel** is a firm arrest of movement with some give to it (i.e., stretching leather). This can be normal or an abnormal end feel.
   - normal (e.g., glenohumeral lateral rotation)
   - abnormal (e.g., talocrural plantar flexion with joint effusion)

This can indicate chronic joint effusion, arthritis, or capsular scarring.

4. **Springy block** causes the joint to rebound at the end of range due to an internal articular derangement catching between the joint surfaces. This is an abnormal end feel. A knee extension with a meniscal tear or an elbow extension with a bone chip are two examples. This can indicate an intra-articular loose body.
5. **Tissue approximation** is range limited because of tissue compression. This is a normal end feel. A knee flexion with the lower leg against the posterior thigh is one example. Elbow flexion with the lower arm against the biceps muscle is another example.
6. **Empty end feel** occurs when considerable pain stops the movement before the end of range is met. There is no tissue resistance, yet the athlete arrests movement due to pain. This is an abnormal end feel. Acute bursitis, extra-articular abscess, or neoplasm can be suspected. Extreme apprehension or fear of pain by the athlete may also cause this end feel.

Not mentioned by Cyriax, but commonly found, is a normal **tissue stretch end feel**. This is due to a muscular, ligamentous, or fascial stretch (i.e., hip flexion with hamstring stretch).

Do **not** force the joint if the athlete is unwilling to move it due to pain or muscle spasm, but attempt to determine the range and what is limiting the range.

Record the quality of the motion and the presence of painful arc, crepitus, and snapping or popping that occurs during the passive movement. Also record the type and quality of the end feel.

Resisted Tests

During your resisted tests, do **not** allow joint movement. The best testing position of the joint is usually in mid-range or neutral position (resting position). Your hand placements must stabilize the joint and prevent joint movement. It may be necessary to stabilize the body part above or below the joint being tested.

Instruct the athlete to build up to a strong contraction gradually and then relax gradually as you resist, to prevent overpowering or underpowering the muscle group that you are testing.

The athlete should contract the muscles strongly. If the contraction appears weak, repeat the test. Make sure that the weakness is not from unwillingness, fear, or lack of comprehension. With this test, you are looking for strength or weakness and a pain-free or painful contraction.

The contraction may be repeated several times if the therapist suspects that there is a neural or circulatory insufficiency to the muscle that will display pain or weakness with repetitions.

Position yourself at a mechanical advantage over the limb that you are testing.

Resist more distally on the limb for better leverage with very strong athletes.

If you have determined that the injury is in a contractile tissue, specialize your testing for the muscle involved. Test the inner, middle, and outer ranges, if possible, to determine what part of the range is limited by pain or weakness.

Weakness may also be due to nerve involvement, vascular insufficiency, disuse atrophy, stretch weakness, apprehension, pain, or fatigue.

It may be necessary to position the limb so gravity assists the muscle if there is considerable weakness (Grades 1 and 2).

The strength can be graded and recorded on a scale from 0 to 5.

0 = no contraction felt
1 = muscle can be felt to tighten but cannot produce movement
2 = produces movement with gravity eliminated but cannot function against gravity
3 = can raise against gravity
4 = can raise against outside moderate resistance, as well as against gravity
5 = can overcome a great amount of maximal resistance, as well as gravity.

Record the strength and whether it is painful or pain free. Record the weakness for inner, middle, or outer range of the joint. Record the muscle or muscles causing the weakness.

Special Tests

The special tests are uniquely designed to test a specific anatomical structure for dysfunction.

Accessory Movements (Joint Play Tests)

Most joints have very small but precise joint movements that are not controlled by muscles. These movements are important for normal articular cartilage nutrition, for pain-free range of motion, and for the muscles to work through their full range. If these small joint play movements are decreased (hypomobile), increased (hypermobile), or lost, dysfunction will develop.

The therapist must test these accessory movements with the athlete relaxed and in a comfortable position. A small amount of traction is needed to open the joint space and the joint must be in its resting or loose-packed position (muscles, ligaments, capsule lax). The grip should be close to the joint surface with one hand on each side of the joint. One hand must stabilize one bone while the other hand gently moves the opposite bone in the desired direction. It must be determined if the joint play movement seems normal, hypermobile, or hypomobile compared to the other side. Often these movements are very small (about 1/8 of an inch). The accessory movements should be assessed whenever the active and passive range is limited, yet resisted tests are full. Record the degree of joint play movement (hypomobility, normal, or hypermobility) if the movement elicits pain. This helps in assessing the joint and in designing the rehabilitation program.

For each joint described in the assessment book, the close-packed, resting or loose-packed positions, and capsular patterns are given. The reasons for their inclusion are described next.

Close-packed Joint Positions

- The *close-packed positions* for the joints occur when the joint surfaces fit together tightly (maximally congruent).
- The joint, ligament, and capsule are taut and often twisted to cause firm approximation of the articular cartilage involved.
- The closer the joint is toward its close-packed position, the greater the joint restriction.
- According to Kaltenborn, when in the close-packed position, the joint surfaces cannot be separated by traction.
- This joint position is not indicated for most joint assessments, especially for joint accessory movement or joint play movement tests.
- On occasion some joints may be locked in the close-packed position while more proximal or distal joints are tested (i.e., lock PIP joints while testing DIP joints of the hand).
- When direct trauma or overstretch forces are applied to a joint in its close-packed position,

the joint structures have no joint play, or give, and therefore have more serious injuries associated with them (fractures, maximal internal derangements).

- In close-packed position, the capsule and ligaments are already taut; therefore they are more susceptible to sprain or tear, depending on the external forces involved.
- The articular cartilages (and menisci in some cases) of each joint are tightly bound; therefore, in the case of close-packed position, boney or articular cartilage damage is more likely.

Resting or Loose-packed Joint Positions

- The *resting* or *loose-packed position* is the position where the joint and its surrounding structures are under the least stress.
- The joint capsule and surrounding ligaments are lax while the articular cartilages (and menisci in some joints) that make up the joint have some space between them.
- This is the position that the joint will assume if there is intracapsular swelling or joint effusion and it is often in the joint's midrange.
- It is important to learn this position for each joint because:
  1. It is the ideal position to test the accessory or joint play movements for that joint.
  2. It is a good position in which to place the joint to allow it to rest from stress.
  3. It can indicate to the therapist the presence of joint swelling.
  4. It is an ideal position in which to place the joint to ensure stress reduction in an acute joint injury or when immobilizing the joint.

Capsular Patterns (Cyriax)

- A *capsular pattern* is the limitation of active and passive movements in characteristic proportions for each joint.
- It is a total joint reaction that occurs only in synovial joints.
- It is characterized by an abrupt muscle spasm end feel stopping the joint motion during active and passive motion at the exact same ranges.
- The limitations in ranges can be progressively more restrictive with eventual capsular and ligamentous adhesion formation, osteophyte development, and even eventual joint fusion.
- In early capsular patterns, the restriction may

appear in only one range (the one with eventual greatest restriction if not rehabilitated) and later progress to more ranges.
- The capsular pattern does not indicate the injured structure. Further testing, as well as a thorough history and observations, is needed to help determine the lesion site.
- These capsular patterns are important to learn because they can confuse your joint testing interpretation due to their combination of restrictions if you are not aware of the capsular patterns. If the pattern progresses, there are serious consequences because of the multiplane restriction. They require gentle testing and rehabilitation to regain normal joint function.

Palpations in General

Palpations are a very important part of the assessment and should confirm your functional testing results. They are always carried out *bilaterally*. The injured anatomical structure should be palpated its entire length. This ensures that avulsions or partial tears can be recognized. Any temperature changes, abnormal contours, thickening, swelling, nodules, or any other palpable difference from the contralateral limb should be documented and may need further investigation.

When palpating, begin superficially and attempt to palpate each layer of tissue (i.e., from skin to fat, to fascia, to muscle, to bone) to the deepest underlying structures. It is best to visualize anatomically the structures that are being palpated as the lesion site is being examined. The entire surface of the hand should touch the injured area, although the finger pads may probe for smaller structures. Do *not* use the tips of the fingers or use *too* much force. Very careful and thorough palpations are needed to determine the lesion site, the extent of the injury, the stage of healing (inflamed-hotter than opposite side), the depth of the lesion, and potential complications.

Palpation of Myofascial Trigger Points

In the palpation section for each muscle the myofascial trigger point locations are given, as well as the areas of somatic referred pain. This information is taken from Janet Travell and David Simons' work in this area and their book (*Myofascial Pain and Dysfunction—The Trigger Point Manual*). This is important in determining the structure at fault and in realizing that the areas of referred pain may be remote from the lesion site.

According to Travell's and Simons', a myofascial "active" trigger point has several characteristics:

- It is a hyper-irritable spot within a tight band of skeletal muscle.
- When compressed, it can cause referred pain, an autonomic response, a local muscle twitch or "jump sign" (intense, quick body movement).
- The referred pain can be from a low-grade dull ache to a severe incapacitating pain.
- The referred pain follows specific patterns for each muscle.
- It is caused by acute overload, overwork, fatigue, chilling, or gross trauma.
- Passive or active stretching of the involved muscle increases the pain.
- Resisted maximal contraction force of the muscle involved will be weakened.

PERSONAL MEDICAL HISTORY

The athlete's personal medical history is important to obtain before getting the history of the injury. Many athletes have previous injuries of medical conditions that are important to the new injury and its rehabilitation.

These facts help to develop a rapport with the athlete and determine their immediate concerns and expectations. During the history-taking:

- Keep the questions simple.
- Ask relevant questions in a natural progression.
- Listen attentively and clarify inconsistencies.
- Encourage cooperation and confidence.
- Remain professional at all times.

The necessary facts are:

Athlete's Name
- Introduce yourself at this time.

Age
- Many conditions develop at a certain age. Age is important because of the vulnerability of the epiphyseal plates in a growing athlete.

Address
- An address is important in case further correspondence is necessary (i.e., medical or legal).

Telephone
- A phone number is important in case an appointment needs to be changed or a follow-up is necessary.

Occupation
- Occupation can indicate time spent in certain postures (i.e., sitting, standing), and lifting or repetitive movement patterns.

Sport
- Level of competition (intramural, local, national, international, professional, recreational).
- Warm up – cool down.
- Years in sport.
- Type of training (i.e., frequency, duration).
- Position (i.e., forward, defense).

Previous Injuries
- Injury to the same quadrant or relevant information from a previous injury.
- Injury with resulting adaptations.

Previous Surgery
- Any previous surgery can cause scar tissue or postural adaptations, which may predispose the athlete to injury or problems.

Family Background
- History of similar problem that runs in the family.

Pre-existing Medical Condition(s)
- Certain conditions can affect the nature or extent of injury (i.e., hemophilia, rheumatoid arthritis, diabetes, ankylosing spondylitis).
- Certain conditions can affect healing rates (diabetes, hemophilia).

Previous Surgery
- Any previous surgery can cause scar tissue or postural adaptations, which may predispose the athlete to injury or problems.

Medication Being Taken
- Certain medications can affect the testing or mask symptoms (i.e., anti-inflammatory medication, pain killers, muscle relaxants, insulin).

CHAPTER 1
Temporomandibular Assessment

The temporomandibular joint can not be viewed in isolation.

Dysfunction of this joint can be a result of a problem anywhere along the kinetic chain, which includes:

- Cranium position in relation to the cervical vertebrae
- cranial bones
- cervical spine
- mandible
- maxilla
- hyoid bone
- shoulder girdle
- teeth and the dentoalveolar joints (joints of the teeth)

Temporomandibular joint problems often coexist with upper cervical joint dysfunction and shoulder girdle postural problems (Grieve G). Temporomandibular joint (TMJ) dysfunction can cause a variety of symptoms in the cervical region, cranium, dentition, face, throat, and even ears. Because of these symptoms, it is very difficult to determine the exact site of the problem. Therefore other head, neck, and shoulder problems may need to be ruled out. To rule out other pathologic conditions, it may be necessary to consult a dentist, physician, otolaryngologist, or orthopedic surgeon before a final diagnosis can be determined.

Temporomandibular dysfunction can affect the masticatory muscles or tendons, joint structures, dental tissue, or periodontal ligaments. A problem with any of these structures will cause pain and/or dysfunction in the others, making it difficult to determine which tissue is at the root of the problem.

The temporomandibular joint is the articulation between the mandibular condylar process, the mandibular fossa, and the articular eminence of the cranium bilaterally. The temporal articular surface is usually less than 2.5 cm long. In the horizontal plane, the condyles are on an oblique axis with the disc attached by a ligament to the joint (Rocabado M). The strongest ligamentous attachments are on the medial side (medio disco ligament [Tanaki ligament]). From a functional standpoint, the two temporomandibular joints work together and one joint cannot be moved independently. Therefore dysfunction on one side will alter the opposite side and eventually there will be problems bilaterally.

Dual temporomandibular problems are frequently seen in x-rays where degenerative arthritis has shortened a condyle on one side, causing disc displacement on the other side. This is frequently seen as a result of the arthritic side becoming less mobile and the opposite temporomandibular ligaments stretching to compensate.

The growth site of the mandible is different from the growth site of other bones because it is located in part of the articular surface. Any trauma or disease that affects the articular surface of a growing individual can affect mandibular growth, maxilla growth, and even cranial development.

The temporomandibular joint is unique because its function is directly related to the dentition and the contacting tooth surfaces. Problems with occlusion can directly influence the temporomandibular joints and vice versa.

The periodontal ligament surrounds the teeth and their roots and is therefore made up of a large amount of tissue. This tissue has many receptors that relay enormous amounts of afferent messages to the central nervous system (CNS) (via the reticular and limbic systems). Biting with the teeth meeting in slightly different places will alter the impulses to the CNS and in turn will alter the messages to the musculature. Everyone has habitual functional patterns of mandibular and tongue movements that have a direct effect on the surrounding musculature and, in turn, on the temporomandibular joints. Even minor dental work, or a change in these oral patterns, can influence the CNS and the temporomandibular joints.

Temporomandibular joints consist of an upper and a lower joint cavity. The articular surfaces of

Upper Quadrant

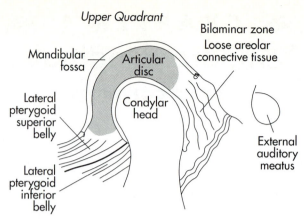

Fig. 1-1 Anatomy of the temporomandibular joint.

the joints are covered with a collagen fibrocartilage rather than the hyaline cartilage in most joints of the body.

The meniscus or articular disc in the temporomandibular joint also consists of pliable collagen (Fig. 1-1). This pliability allows stabilization of the condyle in the articular eminence, even though the articular surface changes during forward condylar translation. Shaped like a biconcave oval plate, the meniscus is thicker posteriorly than anteriorly. This prevents it from moving too far anteriorly and helps it move backward when the joint is compressed. The meniscus itself can translate forward as far as 2 cm anteriorly. The posterior attachment of the meniscus is made up of loose areolar connective tissue called the bilaminar zone, which allows forward mobility. Anteriorly, the disc is attached to the superior and inferior portions of the lateral pterygoid muscle; contraction of the superior lateral pterygoid moves the disc anteriorly. Posteriorly, the disc movements are checkreined by the loose periarticular connective tissue that allows the disc to move forward with the lateral pterygoid contraction; but when the muscle relaxes, the posterior elastic tissue pulls the disc posteriorly like a rubber band.

The disc is highly innervated and vascularized on the anterior and posterior edges. It is avascular and non-innervated in the midportion (Rocabado M).

The temporomandibular joint has no capsule on the medial half of the anterior aspect. Unfortunately this allows hypertranslation of the condyle, which can lead to a great deal of temporomandibular joint pathology.

The temporomandibular joint is innervated by primary articular nerves and accessory intramuscular branches. The posterior, posterolateral, posteromedial, and lateral capsule of the joint are innervated by primary articular nerves from the auriculotemporal nerves; the anterior and anterolateral capsule are innervated by the accessory articular nerves. The deep temporal nerve branches supply the medial capsule. Because branches of the auriculotemporal nerve supply the tragus, external acoustic meatus, and tympanic membrane, temporomandibular dysfunction is often associated with hearing problems, tinnitus, vertigo, etc. Temporalis and masseter muscle spasm can occur also with temporomandibular dysfunction. Part of the reason for this spasm may be because these muscles are also innervated by the auriculotemporal (superficial branches) and deep temporal nerve (posterior branch) respectively.

The sphenoid and hyoid bones can also be affected by the temporomandibular joint and vice versa. The great wings of the sphenoid bone join into the pterygoid plates that serve as attachments for the medial and lateral pterygoid muscles. These muscles directly effect the TMJ because they move the mandible during protrusion and lateral excursions. The hyoid bone is a horseshoe-shaped bone that is level with C3 and acts as an attachment for the supra- and infra-hyoid muscles. These muscles, and therefore the hyoid position, have a direct effect on the mandible and an indirect effect on the TMJ.

The loose-packed (or resting) position for the temporomandibular joint is with the jaw slightly open. According to Rocabado, the loose-packed position is any position that is not in an anterior or posterior close-packed position (see his definition of close-packed position). The close-packed position is with the jaw tightly closed. According to

Rocabado, the temporomandibular joint has two close-packed positions:

- maximal retrusion where the condyle cannot go further back and the ligaments are taut
- maximal anterior position of the condyle with maximal mouth opening

The capsular pattern for the TMJ is with limited jaw opening.

Most temporomandibular joint problems are associated with an emotional factor. They seem to occur more often in women aged 17 to 25 with their own teeth or in middle-aged women with dentures.

In summary, the temporomandibular joint has several unique features that are important to consider when determining joint problems. These features include:

- a wide variety of symptoms
- many structures and tissues affected by temporomandibular dysfunction
- two temporomandibular joints directly affecting the function of one another
- a mandibular growth center located on the joints articular surface
- movement patterns that affect dental occlusion and periodontal afferent messages
- articular surfaces covered by dense, avascular collagen fibrocartilage (not hyaline)
- no capsule on the medial anterior half of the joint
- a fibrocartilaginous disc interposed between the upper and lower articulating surfaces of the joint

ASSESSMENT

INTERPRETATION

HISTORY

Mechanism of Injury

Unlike other joints of the body, there is rarely a singular mechanism of injury. Only occasionally does injury occur as one traumatic incident (i.e., a direct blow or whiplash). Usually there are multiple factors that cause low-grade microtrauma over a long period of time. The multiple causes of temporomandibular joint dysfunction are usually a combination of the following:

- malocclusion
- muscular imbalances
- muscular overload
- psychologic or emotional factors
- dental or oral habits (i.e., bruxism, clenching)
- postural and work-related habits (i.e., singing, excessive phone use)
- intracapsular diseases (i.e., infections, rheumatoid arthritis, psoriatic arthritis, gout, synovial chondromatosis, osteoarthritis, steroid necrosis, metastatic tumors)
- developmental abnormalities (hypermobility, hypomobility, condylar hypoplasia, condylar hyperplasia, condylar tumors, agenesis)
- partial or total absence of the temporomandibular joint

Because of these multiple causes or factors, the history must include questions related to all of these factors and their combinations.

ASSESSMENT   INTERPRETATION

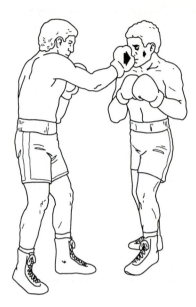

Fig. 1-2 Direct trauma can drive the mandible backward, causing temporomandibular injuries.

Direct Trauma
Was there direct trauma to the mandible?

Mild Force
Contusion
Synovitis

Severe Force
Subluxation
Dislocation
Fracture
- mandible (see Fig. 1-3)
- maxilla
- zygoma

Even a mild force causing a contusion to the soft tissue can affect the temporomandibular joint and cause:
- edema
- loosening of the disc or meniscal attachment
- joint effusion or synovitis
- temporomandibular capsule and ligament sprain or partial tear

A severe force can cause subluxation or dislocation of the joint, or a severe joint synovitis.

1. Subluxation—The most common subluxations occur when the teeth are closed and the mandible is forced backward (blow on the chin) against the posterior soft tissue of the joint, causing the temporomandibular ligament and capsule to be sprained or torn (Fig. 1-2).

2. Dislocation—Temporomandibular joint dislocation is more common in the athlete with joint hypermobility or previous subluxations. This hypermobility can be congenital or occur as a result of the joint being opened too wide or held open too long or the chin receiving a direct blow during mouth opening. This can lead to anterior joint dislocation. After dislocation the mandibular condyle comes to rest anterior to the articular eminence of the fossa and is held there by muscle spasm of the mastication muscles. This anterior dislocation can be unilateral or

ASSESSMENT

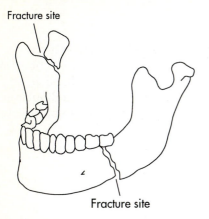

Fracture site

Fracture site

Fig. 1-3 Fractured mandible from a direct blow.

INTERPRETATION

bilateral. With the unilateral dislocation the mandible deviates to the side opposite the dislocation toward the uninjured side. With the bilateral dislocation the chin protrudes forward. A unilateral dislocation is usually the result of a side blow to the open mouth.

3. Fracture—A mandibular fracture is more common than a maxillary fracture and occurs in the following:
- subchondral area
- body
- angle
- symphysis
- tooth bearing area
- condyle
- condylar neck

Because of the curved structure of the mandibular arch, fractures can occur at two sites. Therefore it is important to look for a second fracture, usually on the contralateral side (Fig. 1-3).

When the mandible is traumatized with a direct blow, the force is dissipated over the entire curve of the bone. If the force is severe, the bone will fracture. Mandibular fractures account for approximately 10% of maxillofacial fractures in sports-related accidents.

A fracture of the condylar process can occur from a direct blow mechanism (uncommon) or from falling and striking the mandible against a hard surface. The fracture is usually accompanied by a sprain or tear of the temporomandibular joint capsule, ligaments, or its disc.

The superior maxilla can be fractured but this is rare. These fractures usually occur from a direct blow in contact sports such as rugby, football, ice hockey, field hockey, and boxing. Irregularity and tenderness can be felt along its border under the eye. One half of the cheek may be numb, and there may be double vision and malocclusion. Edema may occlude the airway at the soft palate and hemorrhage can block the nasal cavity. Therefore this type of fracture can be very serious.

Fracture of zygomatic bone or arch can occur when compressed inwardly resulting from a direct blow during a contact sport. This fracture can compress the zygoma.

Indirect Trauma

Whiplash

Was there a history of whiplash or neck injury? (Fig. 1-4)

With the sudden overextension of the neck that occurs with the whiplash mechanism, the supra- and infra-hyoid muscles can not lengthen eccentrically quickly enough. These hyoid muscles then pull the condyles forward, which can result in:
- temporomandibular joint (TMJ) capsular sprain, subluxation, or dislocation (there is no capsule on the anterior medial half of the TMJ to prevent this)

ASSESSMENT

INTERPRETATION

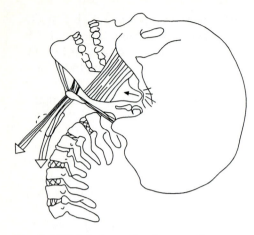

Fig. 1-4 Whiplash mechanism can damage the temporomandibular joint.

- lateral pterygoid strain
- temporomandibular joint synovitis
- posterior meniscal attachment sprain or attenuation

Often the mouth flies open, evoking a stretch reaction from the masseter muscle. Cervical traction during rehabilitation for whiplash cervical problems can add to temporomandibular joint dysfunction and pain because traction causes compressive forces on the temporomandibular joint.

Dental History
Malocclusion
(Fig. 1-5)

CLASS I

CLASS II
- Division 1
- Division 2

CLASS III

Is there an occlusion problem?

During normal occlusion, teeth should close maximally and in good alignment (centric occlusion). The mandibular teeth are posterior to the corresponding maxillary teeth by a distance of one half the width of the bicuspid. Normal occlusion allows the teeth to fit together with cusps and fossae occluding stably.

Absent or abnormally positioned teeth can displace the mandible, which disturbs the balance between the teeth, temporomandibular joints, and musculature. A lack of posterior teeth from tooth loss, dental restoration work, or underoccluded teeth result in increased mandibular elevation activity and excessive TMJ loading.

Malocclusion problems may be the most common cause of temporomandibular joint dysfunction and pain. Malocclusion patterns are categorized into three classes according to the relationship between the upper first and lower first molars.

CLASS I

The first molar relationship is normal but there are tooth irregularities elsewhere.

CLASS II, DIVISION **1**

The lower first molar is posterior to the upper first molar, causing mandibular retrusion. It may be caused by an anterior maxilla or a posterior mandible.

CLASS II, DIVISION **2**

The lower first molar is posterior to the upper first molar but greater than Division 1, causing a large overbite.

CLASS III

The lower first molar is anterior to the upper first molar,

ASSESSMENT

INTERPRETATION

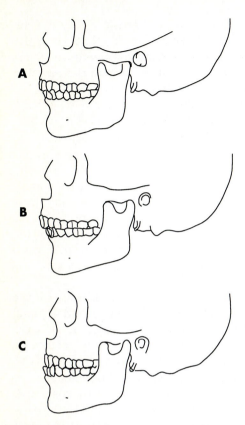

Fig. 1-5 Malocclusion. **A,** Overbite Class II, division 1. **B,** Overbite Class II, division 2. **C,** Underbite Class III.

causing an underbite with mandibular protrusion. The maxilla may be shifted posteriorly or the mandible anteriorly.

Malocclusion of any of the above can lead to temporomandibular disc problems, muscle imbalances, and joint deterioration. Individuals with Class II malocclusion are more prone to muscle and joint dysfunction of their temporomandibular joints than individuals with Class I or Class III malocclusion problems. The disc can also be damaged with the Class II or posterior-superior position of the condyle, which displaces the disc anteriorly. When the disc sits anteriorly, its posterior attachments become stretched, leading to eventual reciprocal clicking and locking. Malocclusion problems, primarily Class II, can result in the following temporomandibular pathology:

- disc damage and stretching of its posterior attachment
- muscle spasm and imbalances
- posterior capsule sprains or capsulitis
- joint dysfunction
- alteration of mandibular growth (in the youth)

Loss of Teeth

Was a tooth knocked out and not replaced? (Fig. 1-6)

Malocclusion causing boney, muscle, and temporomandibular joint problems.

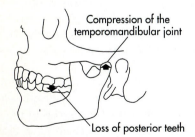

Compression of the temporomandibular joint

Loss of posterior teeth

Fig. 1-6 Loss of posterior teeth causes decrease in vertical dimension of mandible.

Malocclusion can result when the athlete loses teeth that are posterior to the first premolars without replacement (Fig. 1-6). At jaw closing, a fulcrum is created at the premolars with the mandibular elevator muscles working posteriorly to the fulcrum, creating a force that drives the condyle up to close pack the temporomandibular joints. With the lack of posterior teeth support, the TMJ will degenerate and the anterior, upper teeth will wear and become hypermobile as the occlusal load is shifted forward.

Malocclusion can affect the development of the head and neck condylar formation of the mandible in a young athlete.

An individual with malocclusion will adapt to the problem by using different oral musculature or contracting the muscles at the incorrect time. This can lead to muscle dysfunction, imbalance, and muscle spasm. An individual with an occlusion problem caused by a toothache or a poor filling can reflexly avoid closing on that tooth cusp. This can lead to severe temporomandibular joint symptoms and muscular dysfunction.

Another type of malocclusion causing temporomandibular

ASSESSMENT

INTERPRETATION

symptoms involves loss of the vertical dimension (VD 3) of the jaw (vertical dimension is the distance from the bottom of the nose to the tip of the chin). If the teeth are chipped or too short this will lead to excessive temporomandibular joint compression and shortening of the muscles of mastication.

Bite

Is there an overbite or off-center bite?

An off-center bite can originate from, or cause overwork to, the muscles on one side of the jaw. The temporomandibular joint on the shortened side is compressed while the opposite temporomandibular joint is extended. To maintain joint stability, the lateral and medial pterygoid muscles on one side must overwork, leading to muscle fatigue and/or spasm. This will eventually lead to TMJ disc dysfunction. Excessive wear of the teeth and bruxism also can result from uneven occlusion forces.

Dental Work

Has there been much recent dental work?

If the athlete has had substantial dental work lately, or if the mouth is held open for dental work for a long period of time, reactive temporomandibular synovitis can develop.

Anesthetic

Has a general anesthetic been given recently?

Positions for a general anesthetic with maximal jaw opening can also stretch or tear the posterior attachment of the disc.

Dental, Jaw, and Oral Habits

Is or was the patient a thumb or finger sucker?

Is the patient a gum chewer, pipe smoker, or jaw clencher?

On which side of the mouth does the patient most often chew?

Does the patient grind teeth (bruxism)?

Is the patient a mouth or a nose breather?

Does the patient have frequent colds, allergies, or adenoid problems?

What is normally the position of the patient's tongue?

Thumb or finger sucking will affect the palate and jaw formation of a child. The mandibular development can be affected until the age of 20 when jaw development is complete.

Gum chewing, pipe smoking, jaw clenching, or tooth grinding (bruxism) can cause several progressive temporomandibular problems, including:
- muscle imbalance
- joint compression, synovitis, and edema
- disc damage

Lengthy or excessive chewing strengthens the mandibular elevator, the retractor, and lateral deviator muscles during clenching and grinding but this causes several problems. A muscular imbalance between the elevators and depressors develops, as well as repeated ischemia and fatigue in the involved muscles. This repeated compression also leads to microtrauma of the temporomandibular joints.

The lateral pterygoid muscles often work overtime under a great load (Fig. 1-7). This muscle becomes fatigued and loses the fine motor coordination necessary to adjust the speed of the disc movement with the speed of the condylar forward movement. As a result, disc damage can also occur.

Chewing on one side more than the other causes muscle imbalances bilaterally, which also leads to uneven temporo-

ASSESSMENT

INTERPRETATION

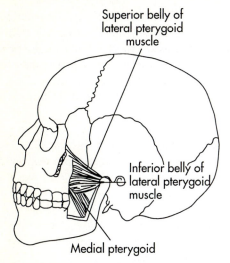

Fig. 1-7 Lateral view of the pterygoid muscles of the temporomandibular joint. Medial and lateral pterygoid muscles.

mandibular joint wear. Grinding or clenching of the teeth also causes abnormal tongue positions.

An athlete who breathes through the mouth rather than through the nose may have a problem with allergies or frequent colds, which in turn makes nose breathing difficult. Breathing with the mouth open results in the tongue moving forward and downward to the floor of the mouth. The weight of the tongue and open jaw puts more weight forward. As a result, the suboccipital muscles are forced to overwork. To allow better air flow, the athlete will extend the neck and move the head forward. This will eventually lead to a forward head posture and cervical dysfunction.

In young children, the tongue must rest against the palate for normal palate development. Tongue position affects the equilibrium of the temporomandibular joint and its muscles. At rest, the tongue should lay against the back of the upper incisors, with the middle one third of the tongue resting on the roof of the mouth and the posterior one third of the tongue forming a 45° angle between the hard palate and the pharynx. During swallowing, the tongue should move up and back with the lips closed. If this tongue position or swallowing pattern is altered, the normal temporomandibular joint and cervical spine kinetic chain is altered, resulting in problems.

Postural Habits

In what position does the athlete hold his/her head during sitting and standing?

If the athlete habitually has a forward head position or excessive midcervical lordosis, the jaw forward position contributes to muscle imbalances of the flexor and extensor muscles of the head and neck. The tonic neck reflex (TNF) plays a primary role in an individual's ability to achieve correct head-neck posture. There is an interrelationship with the vestibular and ocular systems with the TNF. If the tonic neck reflexes or cervical proprioceptive afferents are injured (i.e., whiplash, trauma) or overused (daily posture, sports activities), they may lose their ability to position the head and neck. A forward head posture is often assumed and TMJ dysfunction results.

Job- or Sport-related Habits

Does one's job or sport require a specific head, neck, or jaw position?

Does the sport require an intraoral device or chin strap?

Certain sports or occupations predispose the temporomandibular joint to extra stress:
- singers spend a great deal of time with the mouth open
- telephone receptionists spend all day talking
- shot putters compress the jaw on one side before the throw
- weight lifters clench the teeth before a lift
- boxers' jaws are a target for punches

Certain jaw and neck postures required for sports or occupations also stress the temporomandibular joint:
- violinists tilt and lean the head forward over the violin
- freestyle swimmers repeatedly turn the head and neck

ASSESSMENT

INTERPRETATION

Certain sports require intraoral devices that can cause malocclusion or TMJ stress. Ice hockey, football, and boxing, for example, use oral mouthguards that protect the teeth. These devices should be examined to ensure that they do not alter occlusion or load the temporomandibular joints. Chin straps should also be examined to ensure that they are not too tight and do not compress the temporomandibular joints.

Systemic Factors

Are there any systemic factors that could be related to this problem?

The following conditions may lead to temporomandibular synovitis:
- viral infections
- measles
- mumps
- infectious mononucleosis
- bacterial infections from chronic otitis
- a local lesion
- a sinus infection
- septicemia

The following inflammatory systemic diseases can also lead to temporomandibular joint problems:
- rheumatoid arthritis
- ankylosing spondylitis
- psoriatic arthritis
- osteoarthritis (arthrosis)
- gout

Congenital, Genetic, or Abnormal Developmental Factors

Are there any congenital or genetic factors possibly related to the temporomandibular joint dysfunction?

TMJ Ankylosis

Ankylosis (joint motion consolidation) can result from trauma, rheumatoid arthritis, or congenital problems (i.e., facial deformities).

TMJ Condylar Hypoplasia (Fig. 1-8) and Hyperplasia

Postnatal congenital problems such as overdevelopment (hyperplasia) or underdevelopment (hypoplasia) of a condyle will lead to unequal forces in the temporomandibular joints.

Unilateral condylar hypoplasia (unilateral condylar growth arrest) can be congenital or post-traumatic. Facial asymmetry is grossly affected and a Class II malocclusion occurs. On the involved side, the face will be fuller with a shortened condylar body; while on the uninvolved side, the face will be flatter and the mandibular body elongated. The involved side will have a ramus with a reduced vertical height and the mandibular neck may lean posteriorly.

ASSESSMENT   INTERPRETATION

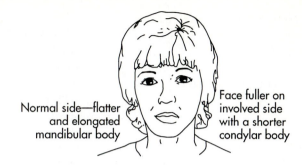

Normal side—flatter and elongated mandibular body

Face fuller on involved side with a shorter condylar body

Fig. 1-8 Unilateral condylar hypoplasia.

With unilateral condylar hyperplasia (unilateral condylar enlargement or condylar neck enlargement) the mandible becomes rounded on the lower border and displaced away from the maxilla with a Class I or Class II malocclusion. This is probably due to a continuation of growth in the subchondral growth center. It results in the body of the mandible displacing downward and laterally.

TMJ Rheumatoid Arthritis

Rheumatoid arthritis of the temporomandibular joints is characterized by intermittent pain, swelling, and limitation of jaw opening. Fifty percent of rheumatoid arthritis sufferers will eventually have temporomandibular joint involvement. With the condylar destruction, they will develop an anterior open bite.

TMJ Hypermobility

Hypermobility of the temporomandibular joints can occur when the joint is stretched by trauma, although some individuals are born with a greater degree of mobility in these joints. The capsule and ligaments are lax and allow greater jaw opening. Jaw subluxations, dislocations, and resulting disc damage are a more common cause of hypermobility in athletes.

TMJ Osteoarthritis

Osteoarthritis is the degeneration of the temporomandibular joint occurring in individuals over 40 years of age (this is twice as common in women). There is degenerative loss of articular cartilage leading to secondary inflammation of the capsular tissue. The joint space narrows with spur formation and marginal lipping of the joint. There is often erosion of the condylar head, articular eminence, and fossa. Some causes of this degenerative process include: repetitive overloading, internal derangement, anterior placed disc, and prolonged loss of posterior teeth.

ASSESSMENT

INTERPRETATION

Temporomandibular Overload

Are the temporomandibular joints overloaded?

Are there psychological or emotional factors affecting the athlete?

Overload problems are usually related to emotional stress. Stress leads to excessive musculature activity; the lateral pterygoid is particularly overworked. A raised muscular activity level may be found in several of the muscle groups, not only around the TMJ but also around the cervical spine and cranium. For example, emotional tension causing the masseter and temporalis to contract can tilt the head forward, and, as a result, the suboccipitals and suprahyoids are forced to contract to keep the head level.

Bruxism (grinding the teeth) for a long period of time will overstrengthen the jaw elevators. Repeated overload leads to microtrauma and an inflammation reaction in the capsule, the loose peripheral parts of the disc, and the lateral pterygoid insertion. The overfatigued lateral pterygoid's ability to move the disc harmoniously during jaw movements can be upset and result in disc displacement. Repeated inflammation results from microtrauma with the condyle in a forward and downward displaced position, resulting in further joint dysfunction.

If the temporomandibular joint is overloaded when malocclusion exists, joint dysfunction occurs more readily. There is usually an interplay of several factors, including:

- malocclusion
- emotional stress
- muscle imbalance
- previous trauma
- oral habits
- joint hypomobility or hypermobility
- poor posture

Pain
Location

What is the location of the pain?

Local Pain

Any traumatic, degenerative, mechanical derangement or inflammatory lesion can contribute to or cause the temporomandibular pain. Specific local pain at the temporomandibular joint is not always present, although on palpation there is usually point tenderness on the lateral or posterior part of the joint. Because there is so much referred pain, the athlete may seek medical help for head, cervical, shoulder, ear, or dental problems.

An acute temporomandibular synovitis will have the typical hot joint pain and exquisite point tenderness (especially related to TMJ movements).

ASSESSMENT

INTERPRETATION

Referred Pain from the TMJ (Fig. 1-9)

1. Headache, eye pain
2. Facial pain
3. Cervical pain
4. Ear pain
5. Shoulder pain
6. Dental pain (tooth soreness, toothache)

1. Retro-orbital, temporal, and occipital headache pain are the most common complaints of temporomandibular joint sufferers. There may be local pain right over the joint but this is not as frequent as retro-orbital discomfort.
2. Facial pain in the maxillae and muscles of mastication is very common. Pain or point tenderness at the temples, occiput, zygomatic arch, ramus, and angle of the jaw can also occur.
3. Cervical pain, especially felt in the cervical and head extensors, also occurs with specific trigger points in the sternocleidomastoid and the trapezius muscles.
4. Ear pain or stuffiness is often indicated.
5. Shoulder pain may occasionally be present due to nerve compression or entrapment from muscle spasm. This is usually caused by muscle spasms of the scalenes, causing entrapment of the long thoracic nerve, or trapezius spasm, affecting the suprascapular nerve. The mandible is attached to both the cranium and the shoulder girdle and any positional change of either can be manifested in positional changes of the mandible (Rocabado M). Positional changes of the mandible can lead to TMJ dysfunction and pain.
6. Dental pain referred from the TMJ is usually the result of a malocclusion problem.

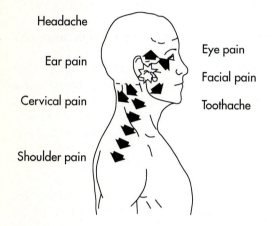

Headache

Ear pain

Cervical pain

Shoulder pain

Eye pain

Facial pain

Toothache

Fig. 1-9 Referred pain from the TMJ.

Pain Referred to the TMJ and Dentition

According to Travell and Simons, muscle trigger points can refer pain to the dentition and TMJ. These include the following muscles:

- temporalis muscle refers pain into the maxillary teeth and the temporal area of the head.
- medial pterygoid refers pain inside the mouth.
- lateral pterygoid refers pain deep into the TMJ and the maxillary sinus.
- masseter muscle refers pain to the lower jaw, molars, and surrounding gums and to the maxilla, over the eyebrow, TMJ, and ear areas.

Pain can also be referred from the following:

- Trigeminal neuralgia can refer shocking or burning pain unilaterally to one side of the face.
- Facial neuralgia may refer continuous facial pain unilaterally or bilaterally.
- Odontogenic pain from the teeth may project into the maxilla, mandible, or TMJ.
- Sinus infection can project pain into the teeth, head, or TMJ.
- Ear pain or infection can spread into the TMJ or surrounding muscles.

ASSESSMENT   INTERPRETATION

Description
Can the athlete describe the pain?

Persistent Pain

The athlete with persistent TMJ pain, especially headache, becomes irritable and anxious. Persistent pain is usually caused by a major occlusion problem or severe arthritic changes in the joint.

Intermittent Pain
When does the pain occur?

Intermittent discomfort usually results from aggravating the temporomandibular joint with:
• an emotional situation with bruxism or jaw clenching
• an acute synovitis due to a traumatic blow, overstretch, infection, or postdental work

Aggravating Factors
When does the pain occur?

WITH STRESS

When pain increases at time of stress, malocclusion, bruxism, clenching, muscle spasm, and emotional factors may be involved.

AFTER EATING

If there is pain after eating, malocclusion or local joint problems could be at fault.

WITH YAWNING

Pain with yawning is linked to an anterior disc displacement that causes pain when the mouth is wide open.

Swelling

Location
Where is the swelling?

Intracapsular

Intracapsular swelling occurs with synovitis and its many causes.

Extracapsular

Fracture sites have local point tenderness and swelling. Soft tissue damage resulting from direct trauma, muscle overuse, or muscle strains causes extracapsular swelling.

ASSESSMENT

INTERPRETATION

Sensation

Ear symptoms

Are there ear symptoms?
- Ear stuffiness
- Tinnitus
- Hearing loss
- Hearing sensitivity
- Dizziness

The muscles of mastication are innervated by the same nerves as the tensor tympani and tensor palatini. This may explain the ear symptoms caused by temporomandibular joint dysfunction. If the tensor muscles go into spasm, it may lead to tinnitus, hearing problems, and a sensation of ear stuffiness. There is also a reflex arc with sympathetic nerve fibers. The fibers originate in the temporomandibular joint and end up in the cochlea. This could also explain the dizziness and tinnitus.

Throat, Tongue, or Palate Symptoms

Are there any symptoms in the throat, tongue, or palate?

Occasionally, symptoms involving the throat, tongue, and palate occur. These include swallowing difficulty (feeling of globus) and burning or numbness of the throat, tongue, or palate.

A forward head posture can cause an altered swallowing sequence, termed an *anterior tongue thrust*. Symptoms with this tongue thrust are difficulty swallowing, scratching sensations in the throat, and shortness of breath.

Grinding or Crepitus

Is there grinding or crepitus during jaw movements?

Grinding or crepitus in the joint surfaces usually indicates the beginning of degenerative arthritis and is heard mostly on condylar translation.

Grating or Cracking

Is there grating or cracking?

Grating or cracking indicates advanced degenerative arthritis and occurs during opening and closing.

Clicking and Popping (Rocabado M)

Does the temporomandibular joint click or pop?

Clicking is the first sign of TMJ dysfunction. These sounds are associated with meniscus-condyle disharmony (Fig. 1-10).

The opening click occurs when the condyle moves beneath the thickened posterior band of the disc and falls into its normal position in the concave articular surface beneath the disc. A click occurring early in jaw opening indicates a small degree of anterior disc displacement; a click occurring near maximal opening signals further anterior displacement.

The closing (or reciprocal) click occurs near the end of the closing movement as the condyle slips behind the posterior edge of the band of the disc, leaving the disc displaced anteriorly and medially. Clicks are classified as early, intermediate, or late, depending on when the click occurs during opening. Therefore the closing click results in disc displacement and the opening click occurs as the disc snaps back into its normal position. This clicking worsens with time as the posterior disc ligamentous attachments get further stretched and damaged. With the stretching of its posterior attachments the disc advances forward and medially until full disc dislocation occurs.

ASSESSMENT   INTERPRETATION

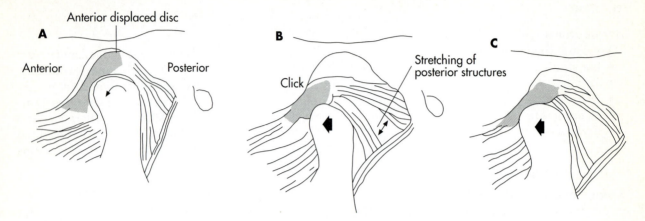

Fig. 1-10 Mandibular depression mechanics. **A,** Condyle rotates, allowing jaw opening. **B,** Attempts to open wider are blocked by the anterior displaced disc—it overrides the thickness of the disc material and clicks. **C,** The condyle is now free to open the mouth wider.

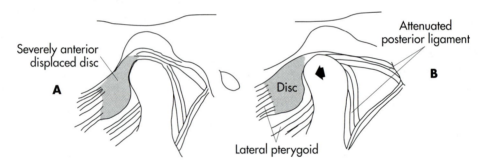

Fig. 1-11 TMJ locking. **A,** Resting position. **B,** Anterior displaced disc blocks forward translation.

Function

Locking (Fig. 1-11)

Does the joint lock?

What is the degree of disability?

Are there chronic or sudden episodes of disability?

Does the patient have problems relating to daily function?

With disc dislocation, the disc lodges anterior and medial to the mandibular condyle and mechanically blocks jaw opening. The posterior attachment of the disc will be stretched excessively or torn. In a close-locked condition, the joint can only rotate, and no anterior translation occurs because the disc will jam between the condyle and the articular eminence. The individual will be able to open his/her jaw only 25 mm and the joint will *not* click.

On occasion, the joint can dislocate when both the condyles and discs are anterior to the articular eminence. The patient is unable to fully close the jaw.

In both cases, normal articular nutrition of the joint can not occur due to the restricted range and the loss of the cushioning effect of the disc.

ASSESSMENT

INTERPRETATION

The result is joint degenerative disease if normal mechanics and movement are not restored.

The progression of TMJ dysfunction is:

- clicking on jaw opening
- clicking on jaw closing (reciprocal clicking)
- inability to fully open jaw (closed-lock)
- inability to close—if problem bilateral
- crepitus and grating with partial jaw opening
- limited opening with TMJ fusion (arthrosis)

Degree of Disability

The functional ability of the joint is rarely limited until the degree of joint degeneration is significant. Ongoing pain from chronic temporomandibular joint dysfunction is the problem.

Chronic or Sudden Disability

Chronic long term problems usually mean that there is significant joint dysfunction with resulting muscle imbalances or malocclusion. Sudden episodes usually indicate a joint subluxation or early disc problems. Many sudden acute temporomandibular joint episodes follow a long dental appointment, yawning, or changes in occlusion (i.e., insertion of dental appliance, root canal work).

Daily Functions

Problems with eating, sleeping, or talking usually indicate an acute joint problem. These problems are usually of short duration. However, if they are ongoing, a significant temporomandibular problem probably exists.

Particulars

Has the family physician, dentist, neurologist, osteopath, orthopedic surgeon, otolaryngologist, orthodontist, physiotherapist, physical therapist, chiropractor, or psychiatrist been consulted?

What was the diagnosis?

Are there x-rays?

Were there prescriptions given?

Was there previous treatment and physiotherapy?

Are there any signs of depression, anxiety, or tension?

Any previous dental history, physician's diagnosis, prescriptions, oral splints, and orthodontal work should be recorded.

Repeated trauma, dislocations, or dysfunction are important to record, including dates of reoccurrence and length of disability.

Note what treatments or rehabilitation techniques proved helpful.

If signs of anxiety or tension are seen during the history-taking, discussion of emotional status may be necessary because of the strong connection between dysfunction of the temporomandibular joint and emotional stress.

OBSERVATIONS

The walking and standing posture should be observed during the athlete's

ASSESSMENT INTERPRETATION

entrance and throughout the history-taking.

Sitting

Anterior View
Head and Cervical Alignment

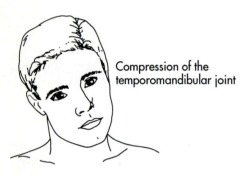

Compression of the temporomandibular joint

Fig. 1-12 Cervical side bending with unilateral TMJ compression, anterior view.

When the head is held in a relaxed upright posture, the opposing teeth do not contact each other (interocclusal clearance). This mandibular resting position should have no muscle contractions and the temporomandibular joint is in equilibrium between the tonus of the muscles and gravity. This relaxed position allows the muscles and joint structures to rest and, if necessary, repair themselves.

If the interocclusal clearance is decreased or nonexistent, there is constant muscular tension and temporomandibular joint compression. Altered head or neck positions affect this occlusion (Fig. 1-12). For example, if the neck is sidebent to the left, maximal occlusion occurs on the right with more temporomandibular joint compression on this side. If the neck is sidebent and rotated to the same side, maximal occlusion occurs on this side.

Jaw Position and Temporomandibular Joint Symmetry

If the ramus is tilted and there is a history of recent trauma, unilateral temporomandibular joint dislocation is possible.

A more prominent temporomandibular joint on either side can also indicate dislocation or a local contusion or fracture. If a fracture is suspected, view the contour of the jaw.

With a facial fracture, the bite is usually malaligned; there is facial asymmetry and altered speech, vision, or sense of smell.

With a mandibular fracture, there is loss of occlusion, bleeding around the teeth, asymmetry to the jaw alignment, decreased jaw opening, or malocclusion.

Observe any local redness, edema, ecchymosis, or deformity.

Anterior View
Facial Features (Facial Dimension Measurements)
VERTICAL DISTANCES (FIG. 1-13)

VD 1 = distance from the hair line or top of the forehead to the top of the nasal bone

VD 2 = distance from the top of the nasal bone to the base of the nose

VD 3 = distance from the base of the nose to the inferior midline of the chin

These three distances should be equal; if they are not equal, there is a structural problem that can add problems to the temporomandibular joint. A loss in the lowest vertical dimension (VD 3) is associated with temporomandibular compression and dysfunction. In young children, VD 3 will normally be shorter.

ASSESSMENT   INTERPRETATION

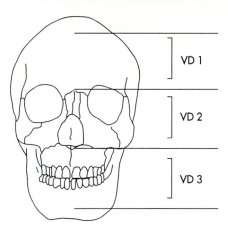

Fig. 1-13 Facial dimension measurements—vertical distances (VD), anterior view.

VERTICAL ALIGNMENT

Imaginary lines through the pupils (bipupilar plane), the nostrils (otic plane), and the center of the mouth (transverse occlusal plane) should be parallel to each other and the ground. Mechanoreceptors in the upper cervical and mandible react to changes in the cranial, cervical, and mandibular posture to keep these planes parallel (Rocabado M). If these lines are not parallel, there may be a structural growth problem. Unilateral agenesis or unilateral mandibular growth will cause uneven lines and a long face on one side and a shorter face on the other side.

Unilateral condylar hypoplasia (a growth arrest of a congenital or traumatic nature) will also affect these lines. This condition causes condylar deformity, a short ramus, short body of the mandible, and face fullness on the affected side.

Unilateral condylar hyperplasia (enlargement of a condyle) will also cause asymmetry and malocclusion. The condylar neck or body can be affected and the affected side is elongated.

Condylar tumors also cause asymmetry.

Facial Features
FACIAL SYMMETRY

Measurements bilaterally from the angle of the ramus to the center of the chin should be equal, unless condylar hypoplasia or hyperplasia exists (Fig. 1-14).

Measurements from the temporomandibular joints to the center of the chin should also be equal, unless there is a growth difference (Fig. 1-14).

LIP POSITION

When the athlete folds back the upper and lower lips the frenulums should line up.

In the resting position, the lower lip should cover one

ASSESSMENT   INTERPRETATION

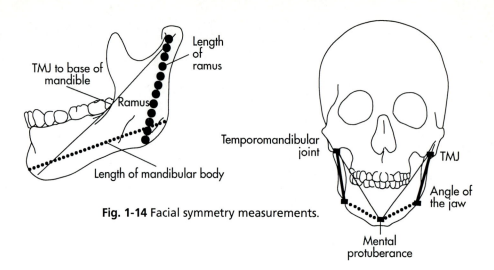

Fig. 1-14 Facial symmetry measurements.

fourth of the top teeth and the top lip should cover three fourths of the top teeth.

ORAL CAVITY

The tongue should be observed for size and resting position.

A small tongue (microglossia) will not exert pressure against the teeth and may cause poor development of the roof of the mouth.

A large tongue (macroglossia) may prevent occlusion of the front incisors and cause an open bite, especially if the child is a tongue thruster or thumb sucker.

DENTAL CONDITION

Any missing teeth, dentures, braces, retainers, or spacers should be noted.

The incisors should line up and any crossbite should be noted.

FACIAL MUSCLE DEVELOPMENT

The muscles on each side of the face must be equal in development.

Chewing on one side or injury to one temporomandibular joint may lead to a muscle imbalance between sides of the face.

Overdevelopment of the mandibular elevators from jaw clenching or overwork can be seen in the muscle development of the masseters and temporalis muscles.

HYOID POSITION

Position of the hyoid is determined mainly by the cervical spine curvature and cranial posture; this position is influenced by the tension of the muscles, ligaments, and fascia attached to it

ASSESSMENT   INTERPRETATION

above and below (Grieve G). A forward head posture places the lower cervical spine in flexion with increased activity of the anterior neck muscles. In particular, longus capitis and longus colli increase tension on the hyoid bone (Rocabado M). With the hyoid pulled downward the mandible is pulled down and back (in relation to the maxilla), causing occlusion and swallowing problems.

STERNOCLEIDOMASTOID MUSCLE

Hypertonus in the sternocleidomastoid is a key sign that the mandible shoulder girdle area and cervical spine are not functioning harmoniously.

SHOULDER GIRDLE

The mandible is attached to the cranium and the shoulder girdle. Any alteration in the shoulder girdle will influence the mandible, cervical spine, and cranium.

A forward shoulder and head posture can lead to cranial vertebral and cranial mandibular dysfunction.

Lateral View
Head and Neck Position

The position of the head, cervical spine, and temporomandibular joint, and the occlusion of the teeth are all interrelated.

A change in the head position changes the occlusion and temporomandibular joint position.

A balance between the flexors and extensors of the head and neck is essential for normal occlusion and mastication and vice versa (Fig. 1-15, *A*).

A forward head or excessive cervical lordosis is common and leads to head, neck, and temporomandibular joint pain and dysfunction (Fig. 1-15, *B*).

Jaw Position

Class II (Division 1 and 2) and Class III malocclusion can be seen from a lateral view.

The maxilla:
- protrudes slightly with a Class II, Division 1
- protrudes excessively with a Class II, Division 2
- recedes with a Class III

Top View (from above)
Facial Symmetry

The symmetry can be observed from a different angle by looking down the front of the face from above.

A fractured zygomatic arch is more readily seen if one arch is more depressed than the other (cheek flattening).

ASSESSMENT   INTERPRETATION

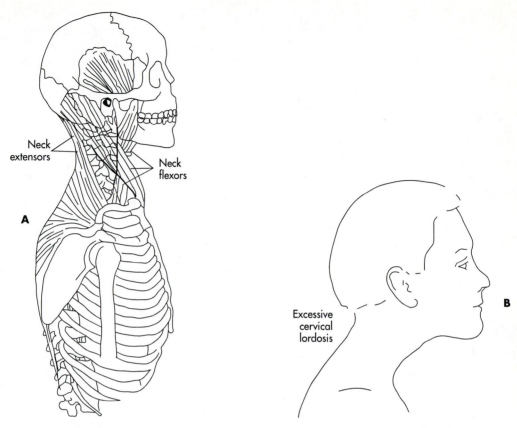

Fig. 1-15 A, Muscle balance of the head and neck. **B,** Forward head posture.

Talking

During the history-taking, the athlete's jaw movements during speech should be observed for the following:
- pain
- jaw deviations
- amount of jaw opening
- emotional status of the athlete

During the history-taking, the athlete's jaw movements during speech should be observed. An anterior dislocated disc can also block jaw opening. If the condition is in an acute state, jaw opening may be reduced. Deviations during jaw opening or closing from a temporomandibular joint synovitis or muscle imbalance should be noted. Anxiety and rushed or tense speech should also be noted.

Oral Habits

Watch for abnormal oral habits such as:
- jaw clenching
- unusual tongue positions
- abnormal resting jaw position
- mouth or nose breathing

Any abnormal tongue, jaw, or tooth positions should be noted because they may be caused by bad oral habits, developmental problems, or joint dysfunction.

ASSESSMENT   INTERPRETATION

SUMMARY OF TESTS

FUNCTIONAL TESTS

Rule Out
    Cervical spine
    Neurological dysfunction
    Auditory dysfunction
    Systemic problem
    Cranial sacral problem
Tests in Sitting
    Active mandible depression
    Resisted mandible depression
    Active mandible elevation
    Resisted mandible elevation
    Passive mandible elevation and
      depression
    Active mandible lateral excursions
    Resisted mandible lateral excur-
      sions
    Passive mandible lateral excur-
      sions
    Active mandible protrusion
    Resisted mandible protrusion
    Active mandible retrusion
    Resisted mandible retrusion
    Passive mandible retrusion

SPECIAL TESTS

    Jaw reflex
    Chvostek test
    Sensation tests

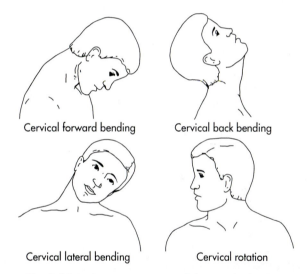

Cervical forward bending   Cervical back bending

Cervical lateral bending   Cervical rotation

Fig. 1-16 Active movements of the cervical spine.

Rule Out

Cervical Spine

Throughout the history and observations, cervical dysfunction should be ruled out. If unsure whether the cervical spine is involved, active functional tests of cervical forward bending, backward bending, lateral bending, and rotation should be done (Fig. 1-16).

Cervical spine problems, especially the upper cervical vertebrae, can refer pain to the head and temporomandibular area and cause some of the same symptoms (i.e., dizziness, tinnitus, and headaches). Cervical rotation toward the injured temporomandibular joint may be limited because of spasm of the sternocleidomastoid or scalenes muscles.

ASSESSMENT

INTERPRETATION

Neurological Dysfunction

If the headaches, facial pain, or eye pain do not seem to fit a TMJ referred pain (see history-referred pain) pattern, then a neurologist may be consulted.

Migraine sufferers can experience altered visual sensations and have some of the same problems with headaches and dizziness. There may be neural problems with the trigeminal or facial nerves, causing facial pain or weakness.

Auditory Dysfunction

If the ear symptoms seem to be more specific than a referred TMJ pain, consultation with an otolaryngologist may be necessary.

Problems with the ear can be referred to the temporomandibular joint and vice versa because of their shared neural supply and close proximity.

Systemic Problem

If a systemic problem is indicated in the history, a consultation with the family physician is necessary.

A viral infection (i.e., mumps, rheumatoid arthritis) can mimic temporomandibular joint problems. A systemic disease such as rheumatoid arthritis can also affect the TMJ. The family physician can rule out these systemic problems.

Cranial Sacral Problem

If a cranial sacral problem is suspected in the history, a consultation with an osteopath or cranial sacral specialist is necessary.

If the athlete has any of the following history or symptoms, a cranial sacral assessment and treatment may also be necessary:
- previous significant head injury
- previous head harness device for orthodontal correction
- difficult birth or delivery (forceps)
- hyperactivity
- headaches
- decreased cranial sacral rhythm

Tests in Sitting

Active Mandible Depression (mouth opening) (Fig. 1-17)

Ask the athlete to open his or her mouth as wide as possible. The athlete then attempts to put two knuckles, or three fingers vertically, between the widest part of his or her upper and lower incisors.

With a clear ruler, measure the range of motion and amount of lateral devia-

First, the two condylar heads rotate around a horizontal axis with most of the motion occurring between the articular disc and condyle in the lower part of the joint (Fig. 1-18). Then there is a gliding and translatory motion of the condyles moving anterior and inferior. At the same time, the meniscus slides forward and down the articular eminence. The forward sliding motion of the meniscus is stopped by fibroelastic tissue attached to the meniscus and temporal bone posteriorly.

ASSESSMENT   INTERPRETATION

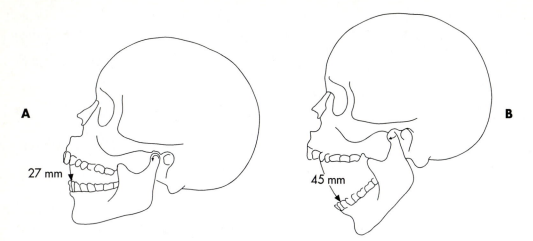

Fig. 1-17 Active mandible depression. **A,** The mandibular condyle rotates against the surface of the disc for the initial 27 mm of opening. **B,** After the 27 mm, the condyle translates forward and allows 45 mm of jaw opening.

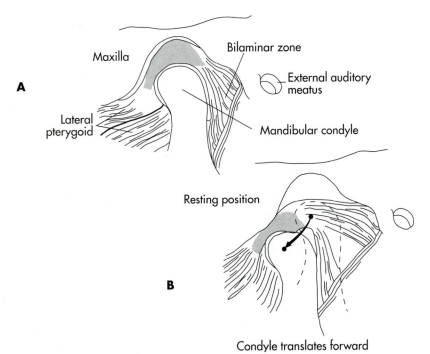

Fig. 1-18 Normal mandibular condyle rotation and forward translation. **A,** Resting position. **B,** The mandibular condyle rotates and translates forward.

ASSESSMENT

tion during opening. Hold the ruler perpendicular to the mandible in line with a lower incisor and upper incisor. Measure the movement of the lower incisor from the occluded position to full mandible depression. Record if the lower mandible deviates during opening.

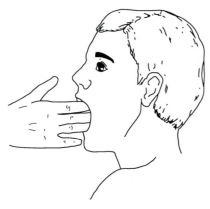

Fig. 1-19 Active mandible depression, maximal opening.

Hypermobility

Hypomobility

INTERPRETATION

Pain, weakness, or limitation of range can be caused by the muscles or their nerve supply. The prime movers and their nerve supply are:

- Lateral pterygoid—anterior trunk of the mandibular nerve
- Digastric—mylohyoid branch of the inferior alveolar nerve and the facial nerve
- Geniohyoid—first cervical nerve through the hypoglossal nerve
- Mylohyoid—mylohyoid branch of the inferior alveolar nerve.

The two bellies of the lateral pterygoid function antagonistically.

The large inferior belly contracts on mouth opening; the superior belly contracts on mouth closing.

The lateral pterygoid (inferior portion) pulls the meniscus forward to cushion rotation of the condyle on mandibular depression.

The geniohyoid and mylohyoid only depress the mandible against resistance and when the hyoid is fixed.

To initiate mandible depression there must be relaxation of the masticatory muscles.

The athlete should be able to put at least two knuckles or three fingers between the upper and lower incisors for normal jaw opening (Fig. 1-19).

The interincisal distance should be 35 to 50 mm when measured from the ridge of the upper incisors to the lower incisors. This is the total range, but a functional range is 40 mm according to Rocabado. To complete the 40 mm of functional range, 25 mm is rotational and 15 mm occurs with the anterior and inferior translational glide. The lateral pterygoid is mainly responsible for the translation movement.

If the athlete has temporomandibular joint hypermobility, he or she may be able to insert three knuckles (or four fingers) between the incisors. Mastication cannot operate efficiently if mandibular laxity exists. There is laxity of the capsule, ligaments, and posterior disc attachment to allow this excessive joint mobility. Joint hypermobility is often characterized by large anterior translation at the beginning of opening when rotation should be occurring. This can cause, or be the result of, muscle imbalances.

If the joints are hypomobile the athlete may not be able to insert two knuckles (or three fingers) (Fig. 1-19).

ASSESSMENT

INTERPRETATION

The opening should be measured in millimeters.

A close-locked meniscus problem limits the mandibular opening to about 25 to 30 mm in the acute phase.

The locking or close-locked meniscal problem can be the result of:

- shortening of the periarticular connective tissue (response to trauma)
- an anterior disc displacement

The mandibular opening may also be limited by an infected tooth or temporomandibular synovitis.

Noises

There may be a click on mouth opening as the condyle moves under the disc. This is a sign of an anterior medial displaced disc (from trauma or malocclusion).

A grinding noise during the translation of the condyle is a sign of degenerative joint arthritis.

Deviations

With normal mandible opening the arc of movement is smooth and coordinated, with both temporomandibular joints working synchronously. Using the center point between the upper two incisors and the center point between the lower incisors as reference points the line of opening should remain perpendicular. The midline relationship between the incisors should remain constant throughout opening.

If the jaw deviates, it is important to note where in the opening cycle this occurs and to measure the deviation with a clear ruler.

Some deviations are:

- With intracapsular edema or posterior capsulitis of the temporomandibular joint, the mandible deviates toward the affected side in maximal opening and toward the opposite side during rest.
- Spasm of the lateral pterygoid causes early deviation on the opposite side.
- Restriction and deviation to the opposite side at maximal opening indicates an anteriorly displaced disc.
- A muscle imbalance can cause deviation in the middle or late part of the opening cycle.
- A restricted joint capsule can cause limited opening and deviation toward the affected side.
- A "C" type deviation on opening implicates hypomobility toward the side of deviation (Fig. 1-20).
- An "S" type deviation is probably a result of a muscle imbalance.

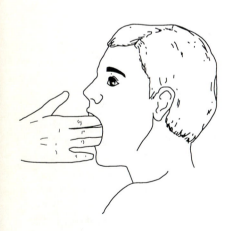

Fig. 1-20 Mandibular deviation due to hypomobility.

ASSESSMENT

INTERPRETATION

Resisted Mandible Depression

Ask the athlete to open his or her mouth 1 to 2 cm. Push the underside of the mandible upward while the athlete attempts to keep the mouth open. Place one hand behind the athlete's head to prevent head movement. The contraction by the athlete and the therapist's resistance must be a gradual, gentle force.

Pain and/or weakness can be caused by an injury to the muscles or their nerve supply (see Active Mandible Depression).

Lateral pterygoid and hyoids should be strong in comparison to the elevators.

An athlete whose jaw clenches may have weaker mandible depressors.

These muscles are very important to test because imbalance problems cause temporomandibular joint problems or results from temporomandibular joint dysfunction.

Active Mandible Elevation (mouth closing)

Ask the athlete to close his or her mouth from the fully open position.

Initially, the condyles glide backward then rotate on the menisci that are restrained by the lateral pterygoids.

The inferior head of the lateral pterygoids relaxes while the superior head contracts, allowing the menisci and condyles to move backward over the temporal bone.

Pain, weakness, or limitation of range can come from the muscles and their nerve supply. The prime movers are:
- Masseter—branch of the anterior trunk of the mandibular nerve
- Temporalis—deep temporal branches of the anterior trunk of the mandibular nerve
- Medial pterygoid on both sides—a branch of the mandibular nerve
- Lateral pterygoid (superior belly)—anterior trunk of the mandibular nerve

The superior belly contracts while the inferior belly relaxes. A click during closing indicates an anterior displaced meniscus. An athlete with rheumatoid arthritis may not be able to bring the incisors into occlusion and may develop an anteriorly open bite caused by the destruction of the condylar surfaces and progressive loss of height of the rami.

Resisted Mandible Elevation (Fig. 1-21)

Ask the athlete to open the mouth 1 to 2 cm. Apply downward force on the incisal edges of the athlete's lower teeth.

Instruct the athlete to attempt to elevate the jaw.

The test must be isometric.

Place other hand behind the athlete's head to prevent head movement.

Build a gradual contraction.

Pain and/or weakness can be caused by an injury to the muscles or their nerve supply (see Active Mandible Elevation).

If the athlete is a boxer, clencher, or overworks these muscles, he or she may be in spasm or elicit pain.

The strength of the elevators can easily overcome the therapist's resistance, so a careful graded contraction must be done.

Overwork in these muscles often causes ischemia and fatigue, weakness, and pain.

ASSESSMENT   INTERPRETATION

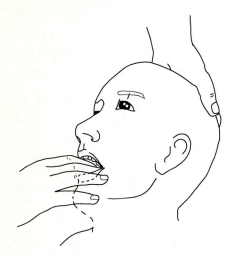

Fig. 1-21 Resisted mandible elevation.

Passive Mandible Elevation and Depression

With the athlete's jaw totally relaxed and the athlete leaning forward slightly, hold his or her chin between the thumb and fingers. Tap the jaw open and closed. Either the athlete or therapist can elevate and depress the mandible passively, depending on the athlete's ability to relax.

The athlete reports which teeth make contact first on closing.

When the athlete taps his or her teeth together, all teeth should meet simultaneously. High cusps or fillings that contact first cause the jaw to rotate toward the opposite side, compressing the temporomandibular joint. This high spot may not be symptomatic unless the individual is overusing the masticatory muscles. A dentist should be consulted if there are any cusps or fillings that are meeting prematurely.

Active Mandible Lateral Excursions (Deviations)

Ask the athlete to open his or her jaw slightly and then move it into right and left lateral excursions. Measure these with a clear ruler.

Lateral excursion to the right occurs when the left mandibular condyle and meniscus slide downward medially and anteriorly along the articular eminence. At the same time, the right condyle moves downward, laterally, and posteriorly while staying in the fossa. The anterior mandible deviates to the right. Pain, weakness, or limitation of range can come from the muscles or their nerve supply.

Ipsilateral Side

The prime movers are:
- Temporalis, posterior fibers—anterior trunk of mandibular nerve
- Digastric, anterior belly (right and left)—mylohyoid branch of the inferior alveolar nerve
- Geniohyoid (right and left)—first cervical spinal nerve through hypoglossal nerve
- Mylohyoid—mylohyoid branch of the inferior alveolar nerve

ASSESSMENT   INTERPRETATION

Contralateral Side

The prime movers are:
- Lateral pterygoid—anterior trunk of mandibular nerve
- Medial pterygoid—branch of the mandibular nerve

The middle part of the temporalis is also active with some slight contractions of the digastric, mylohyoid, and geniohyoid to stabilize the hyoid during the mandible movements (Grieve G).

Pain, weakness, or limitation of range can be caused by:
- joint capsule pathology
- an anterior displaced disc
- coronoid impingement

Using the line between the two incisors above and below as a reference point, measure maximal right and left excursion with a clear ruler. Excursion to the right with right temporomandibular joint pain indicates intracapsular joint problems. If excursion to the right causes left temporomandibular joint pain, capsular, ligamentous, or muscular structures on the left side are involved.

Resisted Mandible Lateral Excursions (Deviations) (Fig. 1-22)

Ask the athlete to open slightly his or her jaw and then resist lateral excursion to each side. With the other hand, stabilize the head. Be careful not to put your hand over the injured temporomandibular joint during the resistance.

Pain and/or weakness can be caused by an injury to the muscles or their nerve supply (see Active Mandible Lateral Excursions). A weak lateral pterygoid might not be obvious on resisted mandible depression but is evident with resisted excursion when compared bilaterally.

Problems with the lateral pterygoid or medial pterygoid cause pain or weakness on the contralateral side.

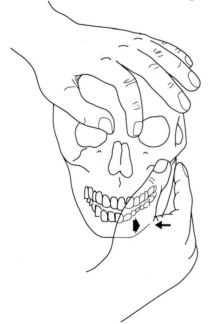

Fig. 1-22 Resisted mandible lateral excursion.

ASSESSMENT

INTERPRETATION

Passive Mandible Lateral Excursions (Deviations)

Ask the athlete to open slightly his or her mouth. Passively move the mandible laterally until an end feel is reached in each direction. The athlete must be relaxed. If he or she is not relaxed, then it may be done in a supine position.

A temporomandibular ligament sprain causes pain on the side away from the direction of movement.

Excessive range is caused by a ligamentous tear.

Range should be equal on each side in the normal temporomandibular joint.

When the meniscus becomes dislocated anteriorly it jams the temporomandibular joint. Lateral excursion is limited to the opposite side. Therefore if the right meniscus is dislocated, lateral excursion is limited to the left.

Active Mandible Protrusion

Ask the athlete to open slightly his or her mouth and protrude the lower jaw as far as possible. Measure the protrusion from where the teeth are in maximum contact to the end of the protrusion (in millimeters).

The average amount of movement is 5 mm (Trott P). The lower teeth are drawn forward over the upper teeth by both lateral pterygoids. The condyles and menisci move forward and downward along the articular eminences without rotation of the condyles. The elevating muscles contract to prevent the jaw from opening further during protrusion. Pain, weakness, or limitation of range can be caused by an injury to the muscles or their nerve supply.

The prime movers (see Fig. 1-17) are:
- Lateral pterygoids—anterior trunk of the mandibular nerve
- Medial pterygoids—branch of the mandibular nerve

The accessory movers are:
- Middle temporalis
- Masseter
- Digastric
- Geniohyoid

Pain at the end of range or limitation can be caused by:
- a joint capsule sprain or tear
- synovitis
- a displaced meniscus

Resisted Mandible Protrusion

Ask the athlete to open his or her mouth and protrude the mandible slightly.

Support the occiput and attempt to push the jaw posteriorly as the athlete resists.

This tests the lateral and medial pterygoids, not the suprahyoid muscles. It can confirm a suspected weakness from the resisted mandible depression in the lateral pterygoid.

Active Mandible Retrusion

Ask the athlete to open slightly his or her mouth and then have the athlete actively retract the mandible as far as possible.

The mandible is drawn backward by the deep portion of the masseter muscles and by the posterior fibers of the temporalis muscle. The digastric and geniohyoid contract to maintain the mandible position. Pain, weakness, or limitation of range can be caused by the muscles or their nerve supply.

ASSESSMENT   INTERPRETATION

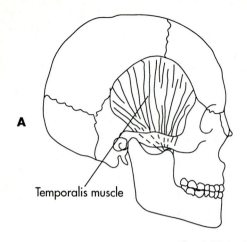 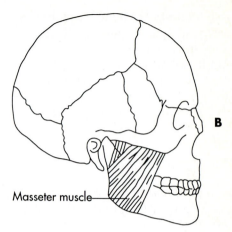

Temporalis muscle

Masseter muscle

Fig. 1-23 Active mandible retrusion muscles.

The prime movers (Fig. 1-23) are:
- Masseter—branch of the anterior trunk of the mandibular nerve
- Temporalis—deep temporal branch of the anterior trunk of the mandibular nerve

The accessory movers are:
- Digastric
- Geniohyoid

Any intracapsular injury causes pain at the end of active retrusion.

Resisted Mandible Retrusion

Ask the athlete to open slightly his or her mouth.

Place fingers on the lingual surfaces of the athlete's lower anterior teeth, attempting to pull the mandible forward while the athlete resists (use gauze to protect the fingers).

This mainly tests the temporalis and masseter muscles for weakness or pain.

Passive Mandible Retrusion

With the athlete relaxed, push the mandible backward gently until an end feel is reached.

Backward movement of the mandible is limited by the lateral mandibular ligament. A sprain or tear of this ligament elicits pain and muscle spasm.

When the temporomandibular joint ligament is taut, the condyle is supported by the disc (when it is not displaced). If the disc is displaced anteriorly, retrusion triggers muscle spasm and pain.

Retrusion also stresses the posterior and lateral parts of the temporomandibular capsule. Any previous subluxation or dislocation damages the capsule, and then this retrusion causes pain.

TMJ capsulitis or synovitis is also painful with retrusion.

ASSESSMENT
INTERPRETATION

SPECIAL TESTS

Jaw Reflex

Place two fingers over the athlete's chin with his or her mouth slightly open (jaw relaxed). Tap your fingers with a reflex hammer. The athlete's mouth should close.

This tests the stretch reflexes of the masseter and temporalis muscles. If there is a diminished or no response, there is pathologic damage to the fifth cranial nerve. If the response is excessive, there is an upper motor lesion.

Chvostek Test

Tap the area of the parotid gland over the masseter muscle to elicit a response from the facial nerve. The athlete's jaw should be closed and the athlete relaxed.

If the facial muscles contract with a muscle twitch, the athlete is low in blood calcium. This is a test of the seventh cranial nerve (facial nerve).

Sensation Tests (Fig. 1-24)

Test the cutaneous nerve supply of the face, scalp, and neck if a neural deficit or neural problem is suspected.

Prick the skin over the areas of the cutaneous nerve supply with a pin while the athlete closes his or her eyes.

Have the athlete report any sharp or dull sensations and location of the area being stimulated.

Any neurological deficit or hypersensitivity should be referred to a neurologist. Neuritis of the trigeminal (maxillary) or facial nerve can result in pain or loss of sensation. A Class II, Division 2, malocclusion can subject the facial nerve to compression resulting from the posterior position of the condylar head.

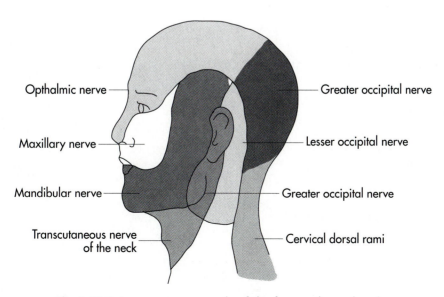

Opthalmic nerve

Maxillary nerve

Mandibular nerve

Transcutaneous nerve of the neck

Greater occipital nerve

Lesser occipital nerve

Greater occipital nerve

Cervical dorsal rami

Fig. 1-24 Cutaneous nerve supply of the face, scalp, and neck.

ASSESSMENT   INTERPRETATION

PALPATION

Palpate areas for point tenderness, temperature differences, swelling, adhesions, calcium deposits, muscle spasms, and muscle tears (Fig. 1-25). Palpate for muscle tenderness, lesions, and myofascial trigger points.

According to Janet Travell, trigger points in muscle are activated directly by overuse, overload, trauma, or chilling and are activated indirectly by visceral disease, other trigger points, arthritic joints, or emotional distress. Myofascial pain is referred from trigger points that have patterns and locations for each muscle. Trigger points are hyperactive spots, usually in a skeletal muscle or the muscle's fascia, that are acutely tender on palpation and evoke a muscle twitch. These points can evoke autonomic responses (i.e., sweating, pilomotor activity, and local vasoconstriction). Palpations should be done with the athlete in the supine position. Always compare bilaterally.

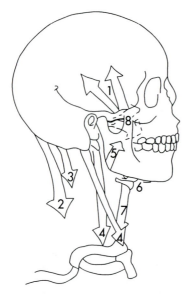

1. Temporalis
2. Trapezius
3. Suboccipital muscles
4. Sternocleidomastoid
5. Masseter
6. Suprahyoid muscles
7. Infrahyoid muscles
8. Lateral pterygoid

Fig. 1-25 Muscle locations and their lines of pull.

Lateral Aspect

Boney

Palpate the bones of the skull for tenderness, deformity, and symmetry (see Fig. 1-27).

Temporal Bone (including mastoid process)

Palpate for any irregularities, especially if the area has had direct trauma. Palpate along the zygomatic process of the temporal bone for any irregularities and compare bilaterally.

ASSESSMENT

INTERPRETATION

Zygomatic Bone

Any fracture or deformity of the zygomatic bone can affect the temporomandibular joint function.

Maxilla

Palpate for fracture and boney symmetry.

Mandible
- coronoid process
- styloid process
- body
- ramus
- angle

Palpate the coronoid process, styloid process, body, ramus, and angle of the jaw for any growth irregularities, asymmetry, and suspected fracture sites. When the mandible fractures, it often fractures at two different sites.

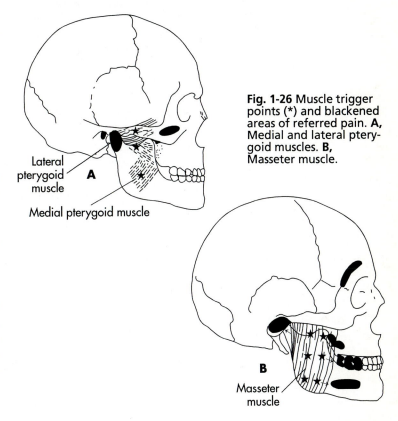

Fig. 1-26 Muscle trigger points (*) and blackened areas of referred pain. **A,** Medial and lateral pterygoid muscles. **B,** Masseter muscle.

Lateral pterygoid muscle

Medial pterygoid muscle

Masseter muscle

Soft Tissue (see Fig. 1-25)

Because of the muscle spasm and overuse of the masticatory muscles, temporomandibular patients often develop active myofascial trigger points and related pain. The masticatory muscles consist of the following:

Masseter (see Fig. 1-26, B)

The masseter should be palpated from the angle of the jaw to the zygomatic arch and may be palpated more easily if the athlete clenches his or her teeth.

Bruxers or clenchers may have fatigue or spasming of this muscle.

Individuals with masseter tenderness often have sternocleidomastoid and mylohyoid muscle tenderness and cervical spine pain.

Masseter myofascial trigger points can develop in several locations in the muscle. These points refer pain into the mandible, maxilla, upper and lower teeth, and the ear and temporomandibular joint area.

This muscle is often very tender when bruxism is indicated in the history.

Temporalis (see Fig. 1-23, A)

Superficial to the muscle are the skin, the temporal vessels, the auriculotemporal nerve, the temporal branches of the facial nerve, and other pain sensitive tissue. Temporalis should be fully palpated.

The temporalis muscle is made up of three portions: anterior, middle and posterior fibers. The anterior fibers run vertically and their action is mainly to elevate and/or position the mandible. Pain in these fibers often elicit headache pain. The middle fibers run obliquely and act to stabilize the mandible. The posterior fibers on the chewing side cause lateral and vertical movements, whereas the opposite side posterior fibers permit retrusion of the jaw during mouth closing. These fibers are

ASSESSMENT   INTERPRETATION

often tender in the athlete with an overbite. Palpation is most effective with the athlete clenching his or her teeth. If there is point tenderness or spasm, determine if it is greater on one side. Overuse of the masticators will make this tender.

Temporalis myofascial trigger points can develop anywhere along the lower third of the muscle. The referred pain caused by overactivity of these points can refer pain throughout the temple, along the eyebrow, or in the upper teeth.

Medial Pterygoid (Fig. 1-26, A; see Fig. 1-7)

Palpate the medial pterygoid externally on the anterior edge of the ramus and intraorally to the lower medial surfaces of the ramus and angle of the mandible.

Individuals with medial pterygoid muscle tenderness will often have tenderness in the masseter and hyoid muscles. Tenderness here is often associated with the symptoms of dizziness. Myofascial trigger points in the medial pterygoid muscle can refer pain inside the mouth, in the temporomandibular joint area, and on the mandible and throat, and also cause a feeling of stuffiness in the ear.

Lateral Pterygoid (Fig. 1-27; see Fig. 1-7)

Palpate the lateral pterygoid intraorally for spasm or tenderness. Use the index finger to palpate this muscle behind the last molar toward the neck of the mandible. Have the athlete open and close slightly his or her mouth and feel the muscle.

If the temporomandibular joint has been subluxed or dislocated this muscle may go into spasm and cause temporomandibular joint discomfort. The superior head originates from the infratemporal surface of the greater wing of the sphenoid bone and inserts into the disc and neck of the mandibular condyle. The inferior head arises from the lateral surface of the lateral pterygoid plate and inserts into the neck of the mandibular condyle.

Individuals with lateral pterygoid tenderness often have digastric muscle tenderness as well. Myofascial trigger points in the lateral pterygoid can refer pain deeply into the temporomandibular joint itself and the maxillary sinus just below the orbit.

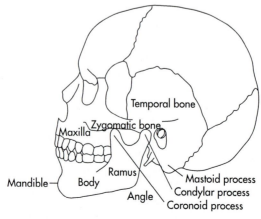

Fig. 1-27 Boney palpations around the temporomandibular joint.

ASSESSMENT

INTERPRETATION

Suprahyoid and Infrahyoid

Palpate the supra- and infra-hyoid muscles under the mandible. It may be necessary to gently move the trachea or esophagus aside a short way while palpating.

Individuals who overuse the mandible elevators may also have pain due to fatigue of these muscles.

The suprahyoid muscles include:

- digastric
- stylohyoid
- mylohyoid
- geniohyoid

These muscles control the hyoid bone and the floor of the mouth. They often become shortened or spasmed with poor posture or injury. According to Travell and Simons, the digastric trigger points, located midbelly, can refer pain into the head and occasionally the lower four incisors.

The infrahyoid muscles include:

- sternohyoid
- sternothyroid
- thyrohyoid
- omohyoid

These muscles are antagonists to the suprahyoid group and also control the hyoid bone. These muscles often show stretch weakness from a forward head posture. It may be necessary to gently move the esophagus aside a short way while palpating these muscles. Muscle spasm is common in these muscles after a hyperextension or whiplash injury.

Facial Muscles

The facial muscles can be palpated for any painful trigger points.

The jaw elevators are often overdeveloped compared to the jaw depressors. The muscles on one side of the face may be more developed than the other side if this group is overworked or if there has been a growth disturbance on one side.

Cervical Spine Flexors and Extensors

Palpate the cervical spine flexors and extensors for spasm, especially if there is cervical or headache pain. Compare each side if pain or spasm is located.

Trapezius

Trapezius may be spasmed or have a trigger point. This spasm may be present to prevent head movements and the resulting temporomandibular joint movements. Trigger points may be stimulated by the muscle spasm associated with temporomandibular joint dysfunction. The upper fibers of trapezius trigger points refer pain unilaterally along the posterolateral neck and head. The middle fibers of trapezius have a trigger point on the midscapular border of the muscle. Pain is referred toward the spinous process of C7 and T1. A trigger point can sometimes be found distal to the acromion causing pain to the acromion process or top of the shoulder. The lower fibers of

ASSESSMENT

INTERPRETATION

trapezius have a trigger point midbelly that can refer pain to the cervical paraspinal area, mastoid process, and acromion. It can also refer tenderness to the suprascapular area. A trigger point over the scapula and below the scapular spine can refer a burning pain along the scapula's vertebral border.

Sternocleidomastoid

There are myofascial trigger points in the sternal and clavicular portions of the sternocleidomastoid muscle. Active trigger points are found along the length of the sternal portion of the muscle. These refer pain around the eye, into the occipital region of the head, auditory canal, and the throat (during swallowing). Active trigger points in the deeper clavicular portion refer pain to the frontal area, ear, cheek, and molar teeth.

Suboccipital Muscles

Myofascial trigger points in the major and minor rectus capitis and superior and inferior obliquus capitis can refer headaches deeply in the head.

Temporomandibular Ligament

The temporomandibular ligament strengthens the anterolateral part of the temporomandibular joint capsule (from zygomatic process of the temporal bone to the mandibular condyle). The inner horizontal fibers are tender if the mandible has been forced posteriorly. The outer oblique fibers assist in moving the condyle forward when the jaw is opened.

Sphenomandibular Ligament

The sphenomandibular ligament connects the spines of the sphenoid with the inner aspect of the lower ramus of the mandible. It is not palpable.

Stylomandibular Ligament

The stylomandibular ligament is actually a specialized band of the cervical fascia that runs from the styloid process of the temporal bone to the mandibular angle. It can be palpated for point tenderness.

Temporomandibular Joint Palpations

Externally

Palpate the temporomandibular joints in front of the ears bilaterally and ask the athlete to open and close his or her jaw a couple of times (Fig. 1-28). The therapist can listen to joint sounds with a stethoscope, noting any crepitus, clicking, or grating.

Palpate for smoothly articulating condyles, tenderness, swelling, and temperature.

Clicking or snapping is caused by an anterior displaced meniscus.

Grinding or cracking can come from degenerative arthritic changes in the joint.

Marked swelling of the joint can come from a joint subluxation, dislocation, synovitis, or capsulitis.

ASSESSMENT   INTERPRETATION

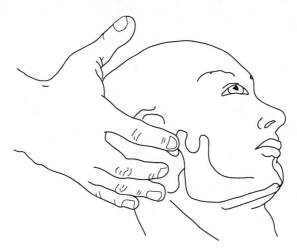

Fig. 1-28 Temporomandibular joint, external palpations.

An increased temperature of the joint comes from an infection or acute synovitis.

Determine if one temporomandibular joint is more point tender than the other.

Posterior and lateral aspects of the joint are point tender when there is capsular inflammation.

Synovitis can come from:
- subluxation or dislocation of the joint
- anterior disc displacement
- systemic disease
- infection

An inability to palpate condylar protrusion suggests a blockage to normal translation. Anterior disc displacement can prevent this normal forward movement.

Internally

To palpate internally, place the tips of the little fingers in the athlete's external ear canals bilaterally. Ask the athlete to open and close his or her jaw a couple of times. Apply pressure anteriorly.

Palpate for pressure against the finger when the condyle moves. Determine if the condyles move synchronously or if one condyle moves farther or sooner. Palpation of the posterior aspect of the joint in this way is very important because joint synovitis is usually localized in the posterior joint space. Pain on condylar palpation is also a sign of joint dysfunction. Palpate for crepitus, clicking, and grating.

BIBLIOGRAPHY

Anderson JE: Grant's Atlas of anatomy, ed 7, Baltimore, 1980, Williams & Wilkins.

Atkinson TA et al: The evaluation of facial , head, neck and temporomandibular joint patients, 1982.

Babcock JK: Sheridan College Medical Lecture Series: "Dental and Temporomandibular Joint Injuries" April 1986, 1987.

Cyriax J: Textbook of orthopaedic medicine: diagnosis of soft tissue lesions, vol 1, London, 1978, Bailliere Tindall.

Farrar WB and McCarty WL: The TMJ dilemma, J Alabama Dent Assoc 63:19, 1979.

Friedman MH and Weisberg J: Application of orthopaedic principles in evaluation of the temporo
mandibular joint, Phys Ther 62(5):597, 1982.

Gould JA and Davies GJ: Orthopaedic and sports physical therapy, Toronto, 1985, Mosby.

Grieve G: Common vertebral joint problems, New York,
Churchill Livingstone, 1988.

Grieve G: Modern manual therapy of the vertebral column, New York, 1986, Churchill Livingstone.

Helland MM: Anatomy and function of the temporomandibular joint, J Orthop Sports Phys Ther 145, 1980.

Hoppenfeld S: Physical examination of the spine and
extremities, New York, 1976, Appleton-Century
Crofts.

Kessler RM and Hertling O: Management of common
musculoskeletal disorders: physical therapy principles
and methods, New York, 1983, Harper & Row.

Kraus SL (ed.): TMJ disorders: management of the craniomandibular complex, New York, 1988, Churchill
Livingstone.

Libin B: The cranial mechanism: its relationship to craniomandibular function, J Prosthet Dent 58(5):632,
1987.

Magee DJ: Orthopaedics: conditions, assessments, and
treatment, vol II, Alberta, 1979, University of Alberta
Publishing.

O'Donaghue D: Treatment of injuries to athletes,
Toronto, 1984, WB Saunders .

Peterson L and Renstrom P: Sports injuries year book.
Chicago, 1986.

Rocabado M: Arthrokinematics of the temporomandibular joints (article and seminar), Nov 26-27, 1989.

Rocabado M: "Diagnosis and treatment of abnormal
craniocervical and craniomandibular mechanics,"
Rocabado Institute, 1981, lecture and handout.

Russel J: CATA Credit Seminar Lecture, Halifax.

Solberg WK and Clark GT: Temporomandibular joint
problems, Chicago, 1980, Quintessence Publishing Co,
Inc.

Torg J: Athletic injuries to the head, neck, and face,
Philadelphia, 1982, Lea & Febiger.

Travell J and Simons D: Myofacial pain and dysfunction:
the trigger point manual, 1983, Williams & Wilkins.

Trott PH: Examination of the temporomandibular joint.
In Grieve G: Modern manual therapy of the vertebral
column, New York, Churchill Livingstone, pg 691,
1986.

Upledger JE and Vredevoogd JD: Craniosacral therapy,
Seattle, 1986, Eastland Press.

Upledger JE: Craniosacral therapy II: beyond the dura,
Seattle, 1987, Eastland Press.

Warwick R and Williams PL: Grays anatomy, ed 35,
London, 1978, Longman.

Cervical Spine Assessment

Examining the cervical spine requires a thorough neurological and arthrological scan of the spine and entire upper quadrant. The temporomandibular joint, upper thoracic spine, costovertebral joints, costotransverse joints, first rib, rib cage, and shoulder complex also have a large influence on the cervical spine and should be ruled out when assessing cervical pathologic conditions. Because of the frequent occurrence of motor vehicle accidents, the athlete must always be questioned regarding a previous accident or whiplash injury. If there has been a previous whiplash to the cervical spine, there is usually scar tissue and dysfunction that will affect the testing. It is also important to determine the emotional status of the athlete in the general history because stress or increased muscle tension can make testing more difficult and may alter the results.

The joints of the cervical spine include the atlanto-occipital joint (O-C1 or A-O joint), atlanto-axial joint (C1-C2 or A-A joint), and the lower cervical joints (C3-C7), (including the facet joints, and the uncus joints [uncovertebral joints of Von Lushka]).

The cervical spine has several functions:
1. It gives support and stability to the skull.
2. It allows a full range of motion for the head.
3. It houses and protects the spinal cord, the nerve roots, and the vertebral artery.
4. The cervicocranial junction and its muscles are important in maintaining equilibrium with very fine and precise coordinated muscle activity to position the head in space.

The neck requires a great deal of flexibility, yet must provide adequate protection to the spinal cord. A high level of proprioceptive responsiveness is provided by the richly innervated cervical musculature and connective tissue around the cervical vertebral synovial joints. Abnormalities in the afferent joint receptors in the cervical spine caused by degenerative changes or trauma can dramatically reduce postural control and equilibrium.

The neck and shoulder complex is strongly influenced by the limbic system. Increased muscle spasm and muscle tone resulting from impaired function of the limbic system is common in the cervical musculature. Tension, stress, or fear can result in hyperactivity of the neck and shoulder musculature and influence the mechanics of the entire upper quadrant.

Temporomandibular joint injury or faulty mechanics can lead to myofascial trigger points and referred pain into the neck musculature. Problems with visual acuity can result in changes in head carriage. The individual may tilt, rotate, or move the head forward to assist in focusing. This can lead to cervical muscle fatigue and imbalances. Problems with hearing can also alter the head position with the individual turning the stronger ear toward sounds. This can lead to altered cervical spine mechanics and muscle imbalances. The cervical nerve roots are most affected by osteophytes of the uncus or facet joints rather than by acute disc prolapses.

The most common cervical pathologic condition is spondylosis.

The cervical vertebrae according to Kapandji are made up of two anatomically and functionally distinct segments:
1. The superior or suboccipital cervical segment contains the first vertebra (atlas) and the second vertebra (axis). Some researchers label the occiput, atlas, and axis as the cranioverte-bral region.
2. The inferior cervical segment stretches from the inferior surface of the axis to the superior surface of T1.

SUPERIOR OR SUBOCCIPITAL CERVICAL SEGMENT

The atlanto-occipital joint (occiput and C1) allows about 18° of flexion and extension, 5° of lateral bending, and 3° or less of axial rotation.

The atlanto-axial joint (C1-C2) allows about 47° of axial rotation in each direction, 13° of flexion and extension, and 4° or less of lateral bending.

Axial rotation between the atlas and axis results in contralateral side bending between the atlas and occiput. Worth and Selkirk and Kapandji determined that axial rotation to the left resulted in translation of the occiput to the left in relation to the atlas (approximately 2 to 3 mm). This large degree of C1-C2 rotation can cause stress on the vertebral artery, with symptoms of vertigo, nausea, tinnitus, and visual disturbances. The axis (C2) is a transitional vertebra between the occipital-atlanto-axial complex and the lower cervical spine.

INFERIOR CERVICAL SEGMENT (C3-C7)

Most of the range of motion of flexion and extension occurs in the central cervical vertebrae. Most flexion occurs around C5-C6 and most extension occurs at C6-C7. The movement of side bending occurs close to the head, especially C2-C3 and C3-C4. Studies have shown that 50% of the cervical rotation occurs at C1-C2 with the remainder in the lower segment, mainly at C2-C3, C3-C4, and C4-C5. Each lower segment rotates 8° to 10° in either direction.

The cervical discs are more fibrous and herniate less frequently than in the lumbar spine. The greater the height of the intervertebral disc, the greater the degree of cervical range of motion. Therefore, as the discs degenerate, the ranges decrease.

FACET JOINTS

The cervical facet joints are involved in some weight bearing and resist torsion less than in the lumbar spine. The facet joints are a common source of pain in the cervical spine and can refer pain into the upper limb. Normally facet joint dysfunction is unilateral and two or three joints can be involved.

Acute facet locking (wry neck) commonly occurs following a sudden unguarded neck movement. The cervical spine is locked in side bending to the opposite side. The cause of this locking may be impaction of synovial villi or meniscoids between the facet joint surface.

The resting or loose-packed position for the cervical facet joints is midway between flexion and extension. The close-packed position for the cervical facet joints is extension. The capsular pattern for the atlanto-occipital joint is extension and side bending, equally restricted. The capsular pattern for the remainder of the cervical spine is side bending and rotation, equally limited, then extension.

UNCUS, UNCOVERTEBRAL (VON LUSCHKA) JOINTS

These joints are formed between the uncinate processes (the superior and inferior lateral edges of the vertebral bodies) of the C3-C7 vertebral bodies. It is controversial as to whether these are true joints, since some researchers believe they are the result of disc degeneration. These joints are affected by degenerative change especially from flexion and extension shear forces. Defects appear here more commonly than in the facet joints. These degenerative changes and their boney outgrowths may affect the nerve root, vertebral artery, sympathetic rami, and intervertebral discs.

ON SITE CERVICAL EMERGENCIES

Injuries to the cervical spine can be the most serious and life threatening of athletic injuries. Careful assessment and proper immobilization and transportation are essential. It is important to be extremely cautious and conservative when assessing the cervical injury.

If there is significant force to injure the cervical spine, there is also enough force to cause a head injury and vice versa. Always assume that there is a head and neck injury until proven otherwise. A concussion analysis should be carried out at the time of injury and proper medical attention with follow-up given if a concussion is suspected.

Signs of cerebral concussion include:
- alteration or momentary loss of consciousness (mild concussion)
- total loss of consciousness (the longer the period, the more severe the concussion)
- slight or temporary memory loss, especially retrograde amnesia (mild to moderate concussion)
- total memory loss of recent events (moderate to severe concussion)
- disturbance of vision or equilibrium (mild to moderate concussion)
- tinnitus or ringing in the ears (mild to moderate concussion)
- headache, nausea, or confusion (mild to severe concussion)
- fluid from the nose or ears (severe concussion)
- unequal pupil dilation (severe concussion)

Signs of a significant cervical spine injury with potential cord damage include:
- localized neck pain and muscle spasm
- dermatomal numbness or paresthesia (abnor-

mal sensations: i.e., pins and needles, burning)
- myotomal or motor weakness or paralysis
- athlete apprehension on moving the head or neck

If there are any signs of a significant cerebral concussion or a cervical spine injury, it is imperative that the therapist stabilize the athlete's head and neck and call for immediate emergency assistance. There should be no attempt to move the head or neck for further assessment or remove an athlete's helmet. Only qualified medical personnel should transport the athlete. If the extent of injury is questionable, be conservative and safe.

GENERAL INSTRUCTIONS FOR CERVICAL FUNCTIONAL TESTING

All acute traumatic cervical spine injuries should be x-rayed to rule out fracture before the neck is assessed. Elderly athletes with osteoarthritic or osteoporotic changes should also be x-rayed before assessment. If the athlete develops nystagmus or other vertebrobasilar symptoms during the testing, stop the testing until further medical investigation can be done.

The active movements are done through the full range. Give clear instructions on the desired head or neck motion and, if necessary, demonstrate the movement. If the range is pain free, an overpressure can be done. An overpressure in back bending is *not* recommended because of the pain or possible damage from the forced spinous process approximation and facet pressure. The range of motion of the head does not necessarily indicate the cervical range. Judge the range in the superior and inferior cervical segments separately.

Resisted tests require a fine orchestration of muscle work between you and the athlete. Conduct all resisted tests with the head and neck in neutral or resting position. The test involves a pure isometric contraction with no head or neck movement. Your instructions must be clear to the athlete. The athlete should gradually build to a strong contraction against your gradual resistance. Neither party should overpower the other. The contraction should then gradually relax to prevent stress to the cervical joints on release. If the resisted test is not carried out properly, a whiplash effect may occur.

Prevent this by positioning one hand in the direction of resistance and the other opposite the force. The resisted tests may aggravate an acute facet joint or a herniated disc so they should *not* always be carried out. The passive tests should be done in the supine position and the athlete must be comfortable and confident that you will not overstretch or move the joint too quickly. If the athlete is not relaxed, the muscles around the neck will be held tight and passive testing will be ineffective and difficult. A pillow under the head above the shoulders and a pillow under the knees will help achieve relaxation. Position your hands under the neck and head by depressing the pillow.

The special tests need to be done to rule out or confirm the suspected condition. Pain in the cervical region and along its dermatomes can come from many locations (i.e., temporomandibular joint, brachial plexus, cervical rib). Therefore the rule-outs are very important. Palpations are also very important because of muscle spasm, myofascial trigger points, ligamentous tenderness, facet tenderness, and skin reactions caused by cervical pathologic conditions.

The cervical movements are complex and involve combinations rather than pure movement patterns. The following are some examples of the complexities of cervical spine movement:

1. Pure side bending does not occur but is associated with extension, rotation, and translation.
2. In the typical cervical vertebrae C2 to T1, the vertebrae side bend and rotate in the same directions.
3. At the atlanto-occipital joint the vertebrae side bend and rotate in opposite directions to keep the head vertical.
4. The shape of the articular facets prevent pure rotation or pure side bending.
5. The head positions are controlled by the movements of the upper vertebrae that, by antagonistic and synergistic action, give the appearance of pure movements.

These coupling movements and complex patterns are beyond the scope of this manual. For simplicity, the cervical movements have been described as pure movements.

ASSESSMENT   INTERPRETATION

HISTORY

Mechanism of Injury

Direct Trauma

Direct blows to the anterior, posterior, or lateral aspect of the neck can be serious, depending on the force of the blow, the object involved, and the cervical spine position. For example, contact with a puck, softball, or baseball moving at full speed can be serious. Contact with an opposing player's stick, arm, knee, or elbow is fairly common in contact sports and results in mild to moderate injury. In football, piling on, late hits, and hitting "on the numbers" can cause serious head and neck injuries.

Posterior Aspect
Was there direct trauma to the back of the neck?

The posterior aspect of the neck is protected by strong musculature such as the trapezius and the erector spinae muscles. Extra protection to the area is often incorporated in the shoulder pads or a neck roll.

Contusion
Posterior musculature (Fig. 2-1)

Contusions to the posterior cervical musculature occur sometimes in sport. The resulting muscle spasms make it difficult to determine if underlying pathologic conditions exist.

Fracture
Spinous processes

A blow to the posterior spinous processes can fracture them. If the blow is received with the neck in forward bending position, the muscle and ligament tension can cause a fracture anywhere from the base to the tip of the spinous process.

Transitory Paralysis

A blow on the neck occasionally causes transitory paralysis from the trauma directly to the cord. Sensation usually returns quickly. Paralysis from direct trauma occurs rarely and it is seldom permanent.

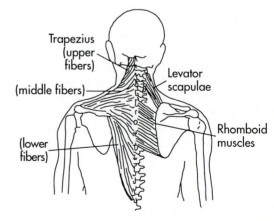

Fig. 2-1 Posterior cervical musculature.

ASSESSMENT   # INTERPRETATION

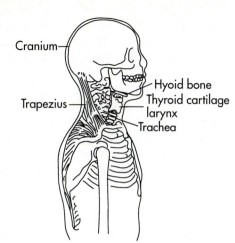

Fig. 2-2 Structures of the anterior neck that can be traumatized. Lateral view.

Anterior Aspect

Anterior neck and throat (Fig. 2-2)
- larynx
- trachea
- thyroid cartilage
- hyoid bone

The anterior aspect of the neck has very poor muscular protection. Most protective equipment does not cover this area.

Contusion to the front of the neck (larynx and/or trachea) can result in severe athlete distress (see Fig. 2-56). Distress is caused by an inability to breath or talk and a fear of asphyxiation. The spasm in the area usually subsides and breathing and speech return quickly. If the laryngospasm persists, there may be a developing hematoma in the larynx, trachea, or cervical musculature. Send the athlete to the hospital immediately, because this is a medical emergency. In some cases, edema or hemorrhage develop slowly after trauma; therefore the athlete should be monitored.

On occasion, the thyroid cartilage, hyoid bone, or trachea may be compressed or fractured by direct trauma (i.e., hockey stick or puck, foot in martial arts).

A cervical rib syndrome can develop from a direct blow just above the clavicle.

Instruct the athlete to protect the neck by tucking the chin in when a blow is imminent or by using throat protectors. Hockey goalies and baseball catchers wear specially designed neck protection because of this vulnerability.

Lateral Aspect

Lateral aspect of the neck
- brachial plexus
- long thoracic nerve
- common carotid artery

The musculature on the lateral aspect does not afford much protection for the cervical spine but a neck roll can help. Direct trauma to the side of the neck can damage the brachial plexus or transverse processes of the cervical spine with related neural symptoms into the arm or shoulder. The symptoms do not usually persist unless there is significant damage to the plexus or process.

The cervical facet joints can be sprained if the cervical spine is side bent with the trauma.

A direct blow to the side of the neck close to the base of the

ASSESSMENT

INTERPRETATION

cervical vertebrae can impinge the long thoracic nerve that serves the serratus anterior. The nerve injury can cause motor weakness or even paralysis of the serratus anterior. This causes winging of the scapula and an inability to fully abduct the shoulder.

Occasionally, the common carotid artery can be contused or damaged by a direct force. The direct blow may compress the vessel or contuse it against the cervical vertebrae, causing acute spasm or thrombosis. Fortunately, this injury is not common because the carotid artery is well protected by the sternocleido-mastoid and suprahyoid muscles.

Direct Axial Compression

Head-on type collision with the top or crown of a football or hockey helmet.

Epidemiological study as well as biomechanical and cine-matographic analysis, have determined that cervical spine quad-riplegia in football results from direct compression in head-on collisions. Force is not absorbed or dissipated by the surrounding musculature and goes directly through the spine. Axial loading of the cervical spine occurs when the neck is slightly flexed (approximately 30°) so that the cervical lordosis is straightened. The impact can damage:

- intervertebral discs (vertebral end-plate fracture, rupture, herniation)
- the vertebral body (central depression fracture)
- surrounding ligaments (sprain or rupture)
- facet joints (sublux or fracture)

According to Torg, Wiesal, and Rothman, vertebral body fractures are classified in five types:

1. simple wedge compression fracture without ligamentous or boney disruption (most common)
2. comminuted burst fracture of the vertebral body without displacement
3. comminuted burst fracture of the vertebral body with displacement into the vertebral canal (usually with neurological involvement)
4. comminuted burst fracture of the vertebral body with posterior instability resulting in quadriplegia
5. comminuted burst fracture of the vertebral body associated with a neural arch fracture

An axial load on the head causes the occiput to drive the atlas down on to the axis that can cause a burst fracture of the ring of the atlas, called a "Jefferson fracture." The occipital condyles are driven into the atlas, causing the ring to fracture (usually in four parts) (Fig. 2-3).

This axial load can also cause posterior arch fracture to the atlas, which is more common than the burst fracture. Injuries from axial loading usually occur at the level of the third and fourth cervical vertebrae. Once maximal vertical compression is reached the spine will be forced into flexion or rotation that causes:

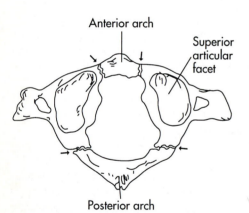

Fig. 2-3 First cervical vertebra (atlas)—Jefferson "burst fracture." Four fracture sites (*arrows*).

ASSESSMENT

INTERPRETATION

- fracture (teardrop fracture-dislocation, usually resulting in cord damage)
- anterior subluxation of C3 over C4 (after tearing of the interspinous ligament)
- unilateral or bilateral facet dislocation

This injury occurs most often in recreational diving, gymnastics, rugby, wrestling, tackle football, trampolining, and hockey. Axial compression of this sort can occur with a direct blow that compresses the cervical spine, or when the head is fixed and the trunk is still moving so that the cervical spine is compressed between the head and trunk. This occurs in hockey when the athlete is pushed from behind into the boards. Tator sites this as one of the major mechanisms in hockey for damage to the cervical spine and spinal cord.

Head tackling, butting, "forehead hitting the numbers," and spearing in football also lead to these injuries. The resulting cervical fractures and dislocations can lead to quadriplegia, partial paralysis, or death. High school football players are most vulnerable because of immature epiphyses, immature ligamentous and cartilaginous structures, and weak musculature in the cervical spine (Tator et al.). In football, offensive linemen have the highest frequency of cervical injuries, followed by defensive linemen, then running backs.

Overstretch
Cervical joints

For simplicity, the overstretch mechanisms are divided into cervical forward bending, back bending, rotation, and lateral bending. Usually the cervical injury involves combinations of these movements, such as forward bending with slight rotation.

Cervical Forward Bending (Hyperflexion)
Was the neck forced into excessive forward bending (hyperflexion)? (Fig. 2-4; see Fig. 2-6)

Excessive cervical forward bending (hyperflexion) can cause a sprain, strain, subluxation, dislocation, or fracture. Protective muscle spasm and associated pain make it difficult to determine which of the cervical structures is injured. The mechanism is not actually a pure hyperflexion but a combination of compression and flexion or flexion and rotation. Major stress occurs at C5-C6 level where the mobile cervical vertebrae join the less mobile vertebrae of C7 and T1. This forward bending mechanism of injury occurs frequently in sports such as diving (into shallow water), trampolining, rugby, football, and ice hockey.

Diving into shallow water is the leading cause of sports-related spinal cord injuries in Canada, according to Tator and Edmonds. An inexperienced diver can sustain either a hyperflexion or vertical compression injury from diving into shallow water or striking a submerged object. There is a high incidence of resulting paraplegia or quadriplegia, especially if the water depth is 5 feet or less. A vertical compression fracture of the fifth cervical vertebra is the most common result. Damage to C5 or

ASSESSMENT

INTERPRETATION

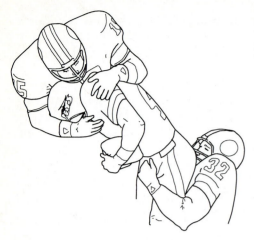

Fig. 2-4 Cervical excessive forward bending.

both C1 and C5 are usually stable fractures. If immobilized, transported, and reduced properly, injury can be held to only transitory paralysis. Damage to C5 and C2, however, is more likely to cause quadriplegia or death respectively. Another danger is when the vertical load fractures the vertebral body and a piece of the posterior vertebral body damages or transects the cord.

Motor sports (motorcycle, dirt bike, and minibike riding) are the second leading cause of spinal cord injuries, followed by hockey. The normal mechanism of a cervical injury in ice hockey involves collision of the helmet and head into the boards with axial loading of the slightly flexed neck. Most often the player was checked from behind into the boards with the helmet striking the boards and the cervical spine in slight flexion. This situation causes a high incidence of spinal cord damage and paralysis.

Trampolines and minitrampolines have caused a high incidence of paraplegia or quadriplegia, especially during somersault maneuvers. Other causes of spinal cord injuries from excessive cervical forward bending include water skiing, snow skiing, tobogganing, and football.

Forward bending with cervical compression (Figs. 2-5 and 2-6)

The worst injuries to the cervical spine occur with forced forward bending and compression. The head makes contact with an object (hockey boards or football opponent) with the cervical spine in a full forward bent position. The neck can stand less force in this position than in an extended position. Most of these injuries cause damage to the middle or lower cervical region and involve C4-C7. According to Kapandji, during forward bending the upper vertebral body tilts and slides anteriorly, the disc nucleus pulposus moves posteriorly, and the movement is checked mainly by the ligaments.

Excessive forward bending can injure the ligamentum nuchae and the interspinous ligaments because the cervical bodies move together and the spinous processes move apart. The ligamentum nuchae, the ligamenta flava, and the interspinous ligaments can sprain but if the force continues they can tear centrally or from one of the processes. If these tear, the flexion force

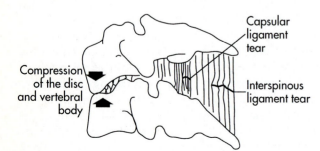

Compression of the disc and vertebral body

Capsular ligament tear

Interspinous ligament tear

Fig. 2-5 Structures of the cervical spine damaged with excessive forward bending.

ASSESSMENT

INTERPRETATION

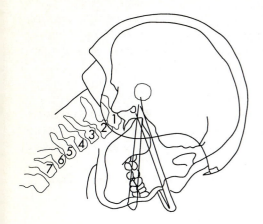

 Fig. 2-6 Cervical excessive forward bending with cervical compression.

carries on to the laminal and articular ligaments. These ligaments can sprain or tear along with the capsular ligaments, or an avulsion of the tip of the spinous process can also occur. As the flexion force progresses, the superior articulations can sublux forward and then spontaneously reduce.

The ligaments that can be damaged with this subluxation include:

- posterior longitudinal ligament
- capsular ligaments of the joint between the articular processes
- ligamenta flava
- interspinous ligament
- ligamentum nuchae

With this subluxation, if the ligamentous support is torn, trauma to the spinal cord can occur.

With a subluxation or dislocation the neural arch can fracture at the pars interarticularis or on the lamina.

On occasion, the forward bending and compression can sublux or dislocate the first cervical vertebra. Atlanto-axial lesions occur more frequently in a forward bending overstretch than back bending.

A forward bending mechanism can cause:

- an anterior shear of C1. The transverse ligament of C1 can tear, leaving the dens in the neurocanal with resulting atlanto-axial subluxation or dislocation and potential paralysis or death. If the ligament does not tear, the joint may be relocated or spontaneously reduced.
- the dens to fracture through the base or just below the level of the superior articular process or through the tip where the alar ligaments attach.
- the cervical bodies to fracture.
- a wedge-shaped or teardrop fracture that is a chip off the anterior lip of C5.
- the disc between C5 and C6 to be expelled posteriorly into the spinal canal.

ASSESSMENT   INTERPRETATION

- the entire vertebral body (in extreme cases) to crumble, with the posterior segment splitting off and displacing posterolaterally into the cord. The dangerous aspect of such a fracture is not the anterior chip but the posterior margin of the vertebral body that can displace backward and possibly damage the spinal cord.

When an athlete falls on the back of the head and the cervical spine bends forward, the odontoid process or dens may fracture. The odontoid fracture can occur at the tip of the dens, base of the dens (where it joins the body of the axis), or into the body of the axis. The forces in the cranium are transmitted to the odontoid.

Forward Bending with Rotation

Forward bending and rotation forces can rupture the intervertebral disc or the joints and ligaments of the atlanto-occipital or atlanto-axial complex. The combined motion can cause the inferior articular facet of the upper vertebrae to become displaced upward and over the superior articular facet of the lower vertebrae. This causes a unilateral dislocation of the joint that can compress the cervical nerve root and stretch or tear the joint capsule and ligaments.

The athlete may experience a clicking sound as the facets override and the head may appear locked to one side. This can occur to both sides or include a pedicle fracture if the force was significant.

Bilateral facet dislocations are unstable and almost always are associated with neurological involvement (quadriplegia).

Athletes who frequently experience cervical neuropraxia have developmental or congenital reasons for these problems:
- cervical stenosis
- cervical ligament instability
- cervical boney irregularities

According to Torg et al., an athlete who experiences transient quadriplegia with weakness or a complete absence of motor function in all four limbs for a short period of time (5 to 10 minutes) has either a congenital fusion or developmental cervical stenosis.

Cervical Back Bending (Hyperextension)

Was the neck forced into excessive back bending? (Figs. 2-7 and 2-8)

This movement occurs frequently in contact or collision sports. Examples include:
- a football player whose face mask is grabbed and pulled backward
- A football player who is "clotheslined" by his opponent (the defensive player outstretches his arm while the offensive player hits the arm at the neck or head, forcing hyperextension of the neck)
- a hockey player who is hit hard from behind so that the head is thrown backward

ASSESSMENT

INTERPRETATION

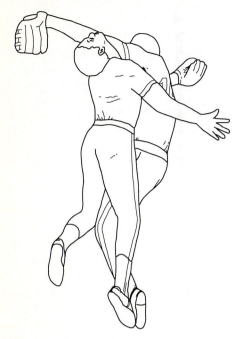

Fig. 2-7 Cervical excessive back bending (hyperextension).

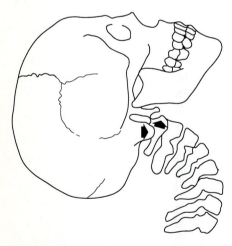

Fig. 2-8 Head and cervical spine hyperextension that can compromise the vertebral artery.

- a wrestler in a bridge (head on the mat and back and neck hyperextended)

The anterior muscles of the neck are weaker than the posterior muscles and not a great deal of force is needed to overextend the cervical spine.

If the athlete was unprepared for the cervical hyperextension, the anterior musculature contraction to protect the cervical spine may be delayed and the stresses are thrown onto the passive inert structures.

Cervical back bending (hyperextension) is limited by the tension in the anterior longitudinal ligament, the anterior fibers of the annulus fibrosis of the intervertebral disc, and by the impact of the cervical facet joints and spinous processes.

These injuries usually involve C5-C6 and are serious because they may have associated spinal cord or root damage and posterior element fracture or dislocation.

An athlete with neurapraxia following this mechanism can have congenital or developmental reasons for it such as:

- cervical stenosis
- cervical instability
- herniation of nucleus pulposus
- cervical boney abnormalities (fusion, incomplete arch)

Athletes with cervical spinal stenosis are especially at risk from a hyperextension mechanism. This stenosis may be developmental or the result of spondylosis or degenerative disease. Excessive back bending can injure many cervical structures:

- The anterior longitudinal ligament can sprain, tear, or avulse a fragment of the vertebral body.
- The sternocleidomastoid muscle can be strained.
- The spinous process can fracture if the anterior longitudinal ligament remains intact.
- If the anterior longitudinal ligament tears, the joint can sublux or dislocate.
- The indentation of ligamentum flavum can impinge the spinal cord and narrow the canal by up to 30% of its width.
- With a subluxation or dislocation, the disc may be ruptured and the posterior longitudinal ligament may tear.
- The facets may dislocate or fracture.
- With a full dislocation, the upper vertebra can displace backward over the vertebra beneath it.
- A fracture between the articular facets of C2 can occur.
- If C3 remains flexed and the upper cervical vertebrae are hyperextended over C3, the arch of the axis can fracture with or without subluxation of C2 over C3.
- The lamina may fracture along with an anterior superior chip off the vertebral body.
- A fracture and/or dislocation can cause spinal cord damage but usually the spinous process fracture allows the vertebrae to move back in place so that the cord is not damaged.

ASSESSMENT

INTERPRETATION

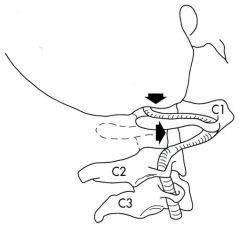

Fig. 2-9 Vertebral artery compression from head hyperextension.

- The first cervical vertebra on the dens process of the second can fracture and anteriorly dislocate. This can lead to cord damage or death.

The vertebral artery passing through the foramen transversarium or over the laminae of the atlas beneath the occipital condyles can be impinged with a head hyperextension (see Fig. 2-8). The artery can be compressed between the occipital condyles and the flattened atlas laminae (Fig. 2-9). Vertebral artery problems can cause tinnitus and vertigo.

A central cervical cord injury can occur with this overstretch from the buckling of the ligamentum flavum or the laminae pressing into the posterior surface of the cord.

Cervical Back Bending and Rotation

With excessive back bending and rotation, a facet can override posteriorly with pinching of the nerve roots on the involved side. The lower cervical nerve roots are susceptible to injury because of the angulated course of the rootlets to reach their relevant foramen. These forces may produce vertebral artery ischemia or thrombosis with a tingling in the limbs or momentary feeling of paralysis. This is the most common mechanism of nerve root injury at C5-C6, C6-C7, or C7-T1.

Whiplash

Was the neck forced into back bending then forward bending (whiplash)? (Fig. 2-10)

The athlete is hit from behind; the head remains still while the body accelerates forward. The cervical spine is forced into excessive back bending that can be coupled with rotation (depending on head position). The head then rebounds forward. The same damage of excessive back bending and forward bending (as mentioned previously) can occur.

The whiplash mechanism can subject the brain to a contrecoup phenomenon (the brain moves forward and backward in the cranium and trauma to the cortex or cerebellum can result). A full concussion evaluation should be done if a whiplash mechanism occurs.

ASSESSMENT   INTERPRETATION

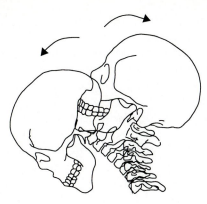

Fig. 2-10 Whiplash mechanism. Cervical back bending then forward bending.

Damage to the temporomandibular joint (TMJ) during hyperextension with the mouth open can also occur and the TMJ should always be examined when there has been a whiplash mechanism (see Chapter 1).

Pharyngeal and retropharyngeal hematomas or hemorrhage of the muscular layers of the esophagus can also occur from the hyperextended position.

Symptoms may also develop in the thoracic or lumbar spine, depending on the forces involved and the degree of damage.

Cervical Rotation (Fig. 2-11)

Was the neck twisted into excessive rotation?

Facet and nerve root injuries are more common with a rotational overstretch of the cervical spine. Wrestling, football, and rugby cause vigorous rotational forces to the neck. Rarely is the rotational force a pure movement. It is often associated with a forward bending, back bending, or side bending component as well. The cervical over-rotation is coupled with lateral flexion to the same side as the rotation.

As the rotary forces increase, facet joint structures can be injured in the following sequence:

- The articular capsular ligaments can sprain with resulting capsular effusion.
- The capsular ligaments can be torn.
- The joint can sublux (unilateral) with a spontaneous reduction.
- The joint can sublux and may not relocate (this will also pull the vertebral body forward).
- The joint may dislocate with the inferior articular facet displaced upward and forward over the superior articular facet of the vertebra below.
- The articular process or even the pedicle on the opposite side can be fractured.

During over-rotation of the cervical spine the internal carotid artery can be compressed against the C1 tubercle, causing a vasospasm or thrombosis. The vertebral artery can also be occluded by over-rotation in several ways:

- Bands of deep cervical fascia that cross the artery can constrict it during cervical rotation.

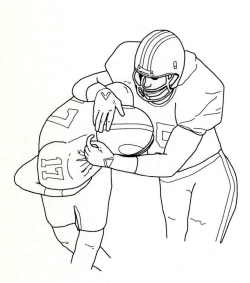

Fig. 2-11 Cervical rotation.

ASSESSMENT

INTERPRETATION

- The great amount of rotation at C1-C2 level can stretch and occlude the artery.
- Laterally projecting osteophytes from the uncus joints can occlude the artery with cervical spine rotation.

The nerve root can be impinged from a rotary force because rotation reduces the size of the foramen for the nerve root to pass through. If a sudden twist causes nerve impingement with nerve root pain or paresthesia, it should subside quickly.

Reoccurring nerve root pain with neck rotation can suggest a disc lesion, osteophyte impingement, or hypermobile cervical vertebrae.

Quick, Unguarded Movement

Was the neck twisted quickly in an unguarded movement?

If an athlete quickly turns the head or has it quickly turned during sport, the cervical facet joint may appear to lock, causing a torticollis or wry neck (side bending away from the involved side with slight flexion). This occurs in children, young adults, and in the hypermobile athlete, often at the C2-C3 or C3-C4 level. It is described by different researchers as a condition caused by impaction of a synovial villus (meniscoid structure) between the surfaces of a cervical facet joint. There is articular pillar point tenderness with a sharp pain on movement of the involved facet joint.

Cervical Side Bending (with some associated rotation)

Was the neck forced into excessive side bending?

The normal mechanism of injury occurs when a player's body is tackled form one side and the head and neck are quickly side bent toward that side. This occurs frequently in hockey, wrestling, and football. There is compression of the structures on one side and tension on the opposite side.

Excessive side bending may cause a fracture through the pedicle, vertebral foramen, or facet joint on one side with ligamentous sprain or ruptures on the opposite side.

Damage to the brachial plexus or cervical plexus can occur if the cervical region is side bent and rotated in one direction while the other arm is pulled in the opposite direction (Fig. 2-12). This commonly occurs in football when the player holds the head side bent away from the side of injury and the involved shoulder is driven downward or backward while tackling or blocking an opposing player. "Burners" occur more frequently in defensive players than offensive players and more in the game than practice situations. Players often describe the resulting sensation as a "burner" or "stinger" with the sharp pain radiating from the shoulder into the arm and hand. The brachial plexus usually suffers only a mild neuropraxia (temporary loss of motor and sensory function for a few minutes to several hours but with a complete recovery within 12 hours). There may be an associated diminished deep tendon reflex if the nerve root or roots is/are also stretched. The most prominent weakness

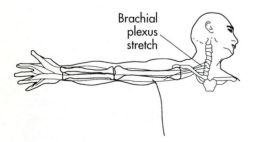

Brachial plexus stretch

Fig. 2-12 Excessive cervical side bending with brachial plexus stretch.

ASSESSMENT   INTERPRETATION

occurs in the deltoid, biceps, supraspinatus, and/or infraspinatus.

With severe forces, the upper trunk of the brachial plexus can be damaged (axonotmesis) with sensory and motor loss beyond 12 hours lasting up to 3 weeks and full recovery only after 6 months. On occasion, the upper trunk of the brachial plexus can be damaged so severely (neurotmesis) that the athlete will never recover full motor and sensory function.

Impingement or overstretch of a nerve root causing neuropraxia can also occur when an athlete's head is quickly side bent.

Moderate stretching of a nerve root causes temporary impairment of conduction more on motor fibers than sensory fibers.

An athlete involved in contact sports with repeated cervical nerve root neuropraxia may have an underlying cervical stenosis (decreased anteroposterior diameter of the cervical spinal canal). Repeated cervical nerve root neuropraxia also occurs in athletes with a congenital cervical fusion, cervical instability, or a protrusion of an intervertebral disc with an associated stenosis. Because of the severity of stenosis problems, these episodes must be further evaluated.

Irreparable damage can occur if traction of the plexus or nerve root causes axon damage and scarring.

With significant side bending and axial rotation the facet joints can sublux or dislocate with or without a fracture.

A unilateral dislocation usually has no neurological deficit.

Insidious Onset

Is the athlete unable to determine the mechanism of injury or the cause of the neck discomfort?

The athlete's daily head carriage position may subject the neck to undue stress and contribute to degenerative changes (see observations for cervical position and its interpretation). An athlete with true postural pain complains of a dull ache after prolonged training or working. The pain may be generalized in the cervical area or referred into the arms. He or she may not have a mechanism of injury or previous trauma.

A faulty compensatory cervical posture may be the result of a more distal alignment pathology (i.e., leg-length difference, pelvic rotation, unilateral pronation, unilateral femoral anteversion, shoulder girdle dysfunction). It may be necessary to rule out the upper and lower quadrant if the cervical posture appears to be in a compensatory position.

Daily Activities or Postures

Is the mouth habitually open?
Is the head in a forward posture?
Does the athlete rotate the cervical spine repeatedly during the sporting event or at work?
Does the athlete repeatedly extend

If the mouth is habitually open, the weight of the mandible causes a continual forward force that pulls the cervical spine into excessive lordosis (Fig. 2-13). The mouth is often open in an athlete who is unable to breathe through the nose, due to allergies or nasal problems. When the chin is tucked in toward the neck the cervical lordotic curve is reduced and there is less

ASSESSMENT   # INTERPRETATION

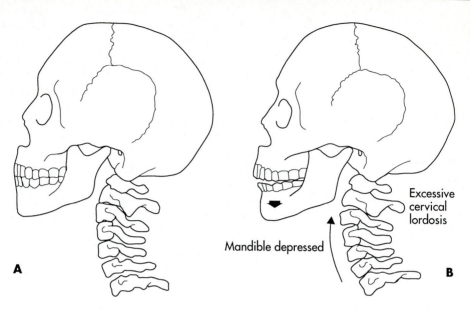

Fig. 2-13 Daily head carriage—lateral aspect of the cervical spine. **A,** Normal posture. **B,** Excessive cervical lordosis with jaw opening.

the neck during the sporting event or at work?

Does the athlete repeatedly side bend the neck during sporting events or at work?

Does the athlete's daily activities or occupation require lifting or prolonged static postures?

Occupation

stress on the posterior cervical segment. With the mouth open and the mandible down, the cervical suboccipital muscles contract continuously to keep the head balanced. This open mouth position will eventually lead to muscle imbalances of the entire upper quadrant with a typical forward head posture.

Repeated cervical rotation to one side can lead to facet irritation, ligament sprain, or intervertebral disc wear. Certain sports involve repeated motion to one side:

- Pistol shooters and archers rotate the head to one side only.
- Skaters usually turn the head in one direction for jumps and turns.

Certain occupations, such as dentistry, assembly line work, and telephone reception, also lead to repeated one-sided head rotation. Repeated neck extension can lead to impingement of the facet joints and nerve roots, anterior ligament stretch, or disc degeneration. Examples of these are found in sports such as high jumping (neck and back arch position over the bar), gymnastics (neck arch posture), and wrestling (bridge position). These problems also occur in occupations where employees work with their arms over their heads and their necks extended, like a painter or electrician.

Repeated or prolonged side bending can lead to unilateral facet impingement, nerve root irritation, lateral ligament sprains, or disc problems. This is likely to happen to shot putters or javelin throwers who have their heads bent laterally or to telephone receptionists who have their heads tilted over the

ASSESSMENT   INTERPRETATION

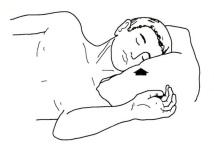

Fig. 2-14 Insidious onset—excessive cervical side bending during sleep (pillow too thick.

phone. Hearing-impaired athletes may rotate or laterally bend their necks when turning their ears closer to sounds.

Occupations requiring constant lifting can aggravate a neck lesion (especially an intervertebral disc herniation) because of the compressive forces.

Prolonged static work positions with a forward head posture, such as keyboard and terminal operators, have a high incidence of neck and shoulder pain and muscle spasm.

Sleeping Position

What is the athlete's head and neck position during sleep? (Fig. 2-14)

Sleeping positions with too thick or too thin a pillow or not enough support can lead to undue stress on the cervical joints. This is important to determine, since it can be the cause of, or add to, the athlete's injury. Sleeping in the prone position subjects the cervical region to hyperextension and rotation for long periods of time.

Tension and Stress

Is the athlete under a lot of tension or stress?

Excess stress from sport, work, or life-style, can lead to neck problems. Tension in the suboccipitals, erector spinae, and trapezius muscles can subject the cervical spine to compressive forces. Fatigue from stress can affect the athlete's posture, which can add to problems.

Chronic Problems

Has this injury occurred before?

If so, fully describe the previous episode.

Athletes such as football players can have reoccurring brachial plexus overstretch or nerve root impingement problems.

Athletes with cervical hypermobility can have reoccurring neck sprain problems.

Reoccurring problems are common with poor cervical posture.

Athletes with poor posture can have ongoing degenerative changes especially in the facet joints and the intervertebral disc.

Reenacting the Mechanism

Can the athlete demonstrate the mechanism of injury (if it is not too painful) or the position that causes the most discomfort?

Have the athlete demonstrate the cervical positions and movements that occurred at the time of injury. This helps clarify their description of what happened and helps determine which structures were stressed. If the athlete can remember the posi-

ASSESSMENT

INTERPRETATION

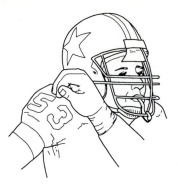

Fig. 2-15 Sport mechanics. Football has a high incidence of neck injuries.

tion of the head or neck during the injury it will help determine if rotation only or rotation with forward bending was involved.

Positions that increase the cervical discomfort may help determine the structure at fault and also what positions the athlete should avoid.

Sport Mechanics

Ask relevant information about the amount of force involved in the sport.

Ask about protective equipment.

Ask where the force was concentrated at the head, neck, trunk, or legs.

The amount of force involved often helps determine the degree of injury.

Contact sports, especially football and hockey, have a high incidence of neck and neck-related injuries.

Diving, horseback riding, gymnastics, wrestling, rugby, and soccer have sport-related cervical injuries.

Protective equipment such as helmets dissipate and deflect cervical compression injuries (Fig. 2-15).

A cervical roll or high shoulder pad limit cervical backward bending and side bending.

A force concentrated at the skull can cause significant direct damage to the cervical spine, but also a concussion component to the brain must be considered and evaluated. Forces to the trunk or legs can cause whiplash mechanisms that can cause severe cervical spine injuries because of the inertia of the head and the relatively weak neck structures and musculature.

Pain

Location

Where is the location of the pain?

Determining whether the pain is local or referred depends on the depth of the involved structure. Injured superficial structures cause pain that is easy for the athlete to localize because the pain is perceived at the location of the lesion (i.e., skin, fascia, superficial ligament, periosteum, superficial muscle, or tendon). Deeply injured structures, viscera, and neural tissue injuries are more difficult to localize and pain is usually referred or radiates away from the lesion site. Deep muscle pain can be referred along the related myotome. Deep ligmentous or boney injuries can have pain referred along the involved sclerotome. Deep nerve root injuries have pain that is usually referred to the dermatome and myotome served by the nerve.

ASSESSMENT

INTERPRETATION

Local

Can the athlete locate the pain with one finger?

A specific facet joint problem, muscle strain, or ligament sprain may cause more local pain but muscle spasm often obscures the exact location. If the athlete can pinpoint the pain, he or she will often indicate a trigger point rather than the lesion site.

Referred from the cervical spine (Fig. 2-16)

Pain from the cervical spine can be referred to the head, face, temporomandibular joint, thoracic spine, scapula, shoulder joint, upper arm, elbow joint, forearm, and hand (Fig. 2-16). As a rule, pain is normally referred distally from the structure causing the pain and is rarely referred proximally. Head, jaw, and face pain does not follow this rule because pain can be referred to other structures supplied or derived (embryologically) from the same spinal level.

Cervical referred pain can be classified in two basic forms:
1. Somatic pain syndromes
2. Radicular pain syndromes

Somatic pain syndromes have referred pain from a musculoskeletal element of the cervical spine (no nerve root compression signs) and may include:
- cervical and shoulder myofascial trigger points (Travell and Simons)
- trapezius, sternocleidomastoid, semispinalis cervicis and capitis, splenius capitis and cervicis, multifidus, and suboccipital muscles
- ligament, capsule, fascia, and periosteum (Kellgren)
- facet joints (Mooney and Robertson)
- dural tube (Cyriax, Upledger)
- intervertebral discs (Cyriax)

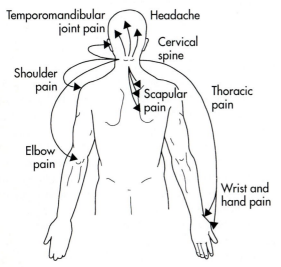

Fig. 2-16 Pain referred from the cervical spine.

ASSESSMENT

INTERPRETATION

Radicular pain syndromes involve a compression or irritation of spinal nerves or nerve roots. There are always neurological signs such as dermatome and/or myotome and/or reflex changes. These nerve or nerve root irritations can be caused by:
- osteophytes of the uncus joints or facet joints
- intervertebral disc herniation (i.e., posterolateral protrusion)
- facet joint effusion
- fibrotic thickening of dural sleeve

Athletes with cervical pain may have combinations of these pain syndromes.

Headache Pain (Fig. 2-17)

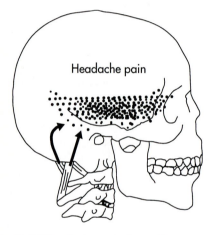

Fig. 2-17 Headache pain from the upper cervical spine.

Patients with headaches and neck pain predominantly have involvement of the upper cervical facet joints, according to Maitland's work. The incidence of C0-C1 (atlanto-occipital [O-A] joint) and C2-C3 facet involvement was slightly higher than C1-C2 (atlanto-axial [A-A] joint); from C3-C4 on, the incidence declined rapidly.

Headaches of a cervical origin usually cause occipital or suboccipital headache pain, although frontal, temporal, supraorbital, or parietal headache pain has been reported. Unilateral occipitofrontal headache pain is often caused by atlanto-occipital (C0-C1) joint problems.

According to Bogduk, any structure innervated by any of the upper three cervical nerves can refer pain to the head and face. If head pain spreads below the occiput it is usually from the atlanto-axial joint (C1-C2) or C2-C3 facet joint. If the pain is only occipital it is likely to come from the atlanto-occipital joint (C0-C1).

The head is formed embryologically from the first and second cervical segments. Therefore headaches can arise from the atlanto-occipital or atlanto-axial joints (including their ligaments, capsule, and local suboccipital muscles).

There are usually spasm and tenderness in the suboccipital muscles on one or both sides while the athlete's pain is mainly in the occipital area.

Some athletes may complain of fatigue, light-headedness, dizziness, nausea, tinnitus, and blurry or dull vision. Cervical headache sufferers usually describe the pain as a deep ache or, less commonly, as a throbbing sensation.

Although most headache pain comes from the upper facet joints and the suboccipital muscles, sometimes it comes from cervical spondylosis and acute intervertebral disc syndrome.

Headaches from a disc protrusion can radiate pain from the midcervical spine area, down to the scapular region, up to the temple, to the forehead, and behind one or both eyes. With an intervertebral disc herniation, the valsalva maneuver and/or coughing will accentuate the pain.

ASSESSMENT   INTERPRETATION

The first cervical level tends to refer pain to the top of the head; the second cervical level tends to refer pain behind one eye in the temporal area. The lower cervical area can refer pain to the occiput.

Headaches are frequent in the older athlete with osteoarthritic changes in the facet joints or degenerative disc disease.

Cervical headaches are usually precipitated or aggravated by cervical motions or sustained cervical postures, such as prolonged forward bending while working at a desk or back bending during dental work. Cervical headaches are usually of moderate severity and occur daily or two to three times per week. These headaches usually build up as the day progresses and are aggravated by activity.

Patients who wake up in the morning with a headache often have an upper cervical articulation dysfunction causing the pain. They often sleep with inadequate neck support or with the cervical spine in poor alignment.

Sudden headaches or shooting pains do not usually indicate cervical origin.

Facial Pain

The face is formed from the second cervical segment embryologically so pain in the facial region may come from the neck. Pressure from an intervertebral disc herniation or an articular facet irritation can refer pain to the face. Discomfort can include vertigo and tinnitus. Auditory and temporomandibular joint problems can also cause these problems and should be ruled out through an assessment (see Chapter 1).

Eye Pain

Eye pain and symptoms can occur with cervical dysfunction. Blurring of vision, tearing, retro-orbital pain in one or both eyes can occur. This may occur from an irritation of the cervical sympathetic nerve supply.

Temporomandibular Pain

Movement of the upper cervical spine is coupled with jaw movements, especially during chewing. The short posterior cervical musculature (rectus capitis, cervicis, and obliques) is active during jaw movement. Excessive or abnormal movements of the temporomandibular joint can cause trigger points in the cervical musculature and lead to neck pain. Instability or trigger points in the cervical joints and musculature, especially suboccipital muscles, can cause temporomandibular dysfunction and temporomandibular joint pain.

Throat Discomfort

Complaints of a sore, tight throat and abnormal swallowing patterns can be attributed to a loss of the normal cervical curva-

ASSESSMENT

INTERPRETATION

ture. The head assumes the forward head posture with tightness in the suprahyoid muscles and stretch weakness in the infrahyoid muscle. This muscle imbalance around the hyoid bone leads to difficulty in swallowing and can cause a sensation of throat soreness or tightness.

A sensation of a "lump in the throat" may be caused by irritation of the anterior root branches from C2 and C3 (descendens cervicalis nerve) that joins the hypoglossal nerve to form the ansa hypoglossi nerve. The ansa hypoglossi nerve serves the hyoid muscles and therefore causes an alteration in hyoid movement.

Thoracic, Clavicular, and Scapular Pain

The pain may be from an underlying thoracic injury or referred from a lower cervical problem (Fig. 2-18). According to Cloward, cervical disc protrusions can refer pain down the thoracic spine.

- A protrusion at C3-C4 refers pain adjacent to the C7-T1 interspinous area.
- Pain along the periosteum of the clavicle can be sclerotomal pain referred from C4.
- A protrusion at C7-T1 refers deep pain adjacent to T6-T7.

Cervical disc pain can center into localized areas around the scapula.

- Pain at the spine of the scapula can be the C7 dermatome.
- Pain at the supraspinatus fossa can be the C5-C6 dermatome.
- Pain at the anterior superior area of the shoulder girdle can be from the C4 dermatome.
- Pain along the periosteum of the vertebral border of the scapular and coracoid process can be referred from the C5 sclerotome.

Myofascial trigger points in the cervical spine musculature can also cause scapular (levator scapulae, scalenes) and thoracic pain (Travell and Simons). Scapular pain can be caused by an intervertebral disc protrusion, a nerve root impingement, or a facet joint impingement.

C8, T1, T2 nerve root compression or facet dysfunction can cause lower scapular pain.

Recent research has shown that the cervical facet joints can refer pain in predictable patterns of nonsegmental origin (Fig. 2-19). The pain patterns for the following facet joints are:

- C2-C3 pain extends into the posterior neck upper cervical area and up to the occiput.
- C3-C4 pain extends over the posterolateral cervical region into the suboccipital area (following the course of the levator scapulae).
- C4-C5 pain extends over a triangular area from the midline to the posterolateral border of the neck parallel to the spine of the scapula.

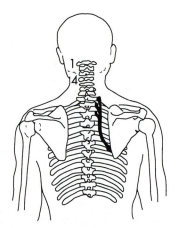

Fig. 2-18 Pain referred to the thoracic spine from the lower cervical spine.

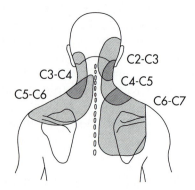

Fig. 2-19 Cervical facet joint pain patterns.

ASSESSMENT

INTERPRETATION

- C5-C6 pain extends in a triangular pattern over the posterior yolk of the neck over the front, top, and back of the shoulder girdle.
- C6-C7 pain extends below the spine of the scapula over the posterior aspect of the neck and scapular region.

Chest Wall Pain

Stimulation of the lower cervical levels of the cervical interspinous ligaments can produce pain in the chest wall (Kellgren).

Studies show that electrical and mechanical stimulation of the cervical intervertebral discs produces posterior chest wall and scapular pain.

Pressure on the cervical posterior longitudinal ligament can cause anterior chest pain.

A lesion at the level of C6-C7 may cause neural or muscular pain in the chest, raising the concern of angina pectoris. This pain may be increased by exertion, referred down the arm, and compression felt on the chest wall. Heart disease must be ruled out in this case.

Shoulder Pain (Fig. 2-20).
- *radicular pain syndromes*
- *somatic pain syndromes*

Shoulder pain is often a radicular syndrome from the cervical spine with sharp, shooting pain. Paresthesia or numbness is often experienced in the involved dermatome; sometimes muscles weaken and reflexes are affected.

The shoulder joint is supplied by C5 and a spinal nerve or nerve root irritation can refer pain to the joint. Sclerotomal pain from C5 can be referred into the acromioclavicular joint, sternoclavicular or glenohumeral joint, as well as along the humerus itself. The abductors and adductors are supplied by the cervical nerve roots C5 and C6 respectively and can be weak or painful if these roots are injured.

A problem with the neural supply may cause shoulder joint discomfort. Cervical spondylosis and intervertebral disc protrusion often refer pain to the shoulder region. The referred pain is sharp and well localized with paresthesia and numbness in the sensory distribution of the nerve root.

Somatic pain syndromes in the cervical spine and cervical region can refer pain to the shoulder from:
- injury to the cervical interspinous ligaments (Kellgren)
- myofascial trigger points in paraspinal and scapular musculature, scalenes, trapezius (Travell and Simons)
- facet joints, C4-C7

With a frozen shoulder there is often midcervical joint dysfunction.

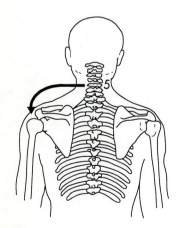

Fig. 2-20 Shoulder pain referred from the midcervical spine.

Elbow Pain (Fig. 2-21)

Pain radiating down the arm usually arises from the lower cervical spine (C5-C7). This is usually caused by a cervical nerve

ASSESSMENT   INTERPRETATION

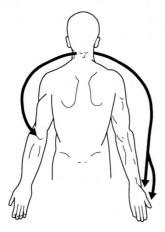

Fig. 2-21 Elbow, wrist, and hand pain referred from the mid and lower cervical spine.

root irritation from a disc herniation or cervical spondylosis (radicular pain syndrome). The tender area or trigger point pain is often over the lateral epicondyle.

According to Kellgren, elbow pain can occur from stimulation of the cervical interspinous ligament (C6, C7, C8, T1).

Myofascial trigger points in the scalenes can refer pain into the posterior aspect of the elbow (Travell and Simons).

Sclerotomal pain from C5-C7 can refer pain into the elbow joint and along the ulna and radius.

Wrist and Hand Pain (see Fig. 2-21)

Wrist and hand pain rarely occurs from the cervical region. When it does occur it is a dull, boring type ache that radiates along a broad surface of the wrist and hand.

The area of pain depends on the cervical level of the problem.
- Pain spread mainly on the radial surface can be referred from C6 cervical level. The C6 sclerotome can refer pain along the radius and into the first metacarpal bone.
- Pain more on the ulnar surface can be radiated more from the C7-C8 cervical level.
- Sclerotomal pain from C7 projects into the third and fourth metacarpal along with portions of the ulna and radius.
- Sclerotomal pain from C8 affects the ulna and fourth and fifth fingers.

Myofascial trigger points in the scalenes can also refer pain into the radial aspect of the forearm, wrist, and hand (Travell and Simons). Kellgren found forearm, wrist, and hand referred pain from the cervical interspinous ligaments (C7, C8).

Cervical Spine Pain

Neck pain arising from structures outside the cervical spine include:
- tumors, trauma, or disease of the spinal cord
- brain lesions (recent trauma or tumor)
- heart (coronary artery disease)

ASSESSMENT   INTERPRETATION

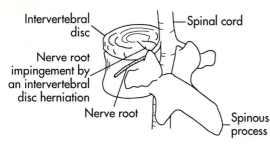

Fig. 2-22 Intervertebral disc herniation and nerve root impingement.

- apex of lung (Pancoast tumor)
- diaphragm (spasm, trauma)
- gallbladder (cholecystitis, biliary calculi)
- aorta (aneurysm)
- other somatic or visceral structures having same cervical nerve root innervation

All of these conditions will have other signs and symptoms that will help determine the structure at fault.

Onset
How quickly did the pain begin?

Immediate

Immediate pain indicates a more acute lesion such as:
- intra-articular facet displacement
- acute torticollis
- cervical ligament sprain or tear (interspinous, anterior longitudinal, capsular, supraspinous)
- cervical muscle strain
- acute disc herniation (Fig. 2-22)
- acute cervical nerve root impingement (see Fig. 2-22)
- acute brachial plexus stretch

Gradual

A gradual onset of pain or discomfort usually indicates a gradual swelling or a chronic degenerative process and occurs with:
- degenerative disc disease
- a whiplash injury that may develop pain 24 hours after trauma
- chronic muscle strain or ligamentous sprain (including postural or occupational etiologic factors)

Type of Pain
Can the athlete describe the pain?

Different musculoskeletal structures give rise to different types of pain.

Sharp Pain

- skin, fascia (i.e., laceration)
- superficial muscle (i.e., trapezius)
- superficial ligament (i.e., supraspinous)
- periosteum (i.e., spinous process)

ASSESSMENT

INTERPRETATION

Sharp, Shooting Pain

- facet or disc impingement of a nerve root
- local cutaneous nerve impingement

Dull, Aching Pain

- bone, subchondral (i.e., neoplasm, degenerative cervical disease)
- deep muscle (i.e., rectus capitis, splenius cervicis)
- deep ligament (i.e., posterior longitudinal)
- deep fibrous capsule (i.e., degenerative cervical facet disease)

Twinges with Movement (when structure is stretched)

- superficial ligament (i.e., around facet joints)
- superficial muscle (i.e., sternocleidomastoid)

Sharp, Burning Pain (burner or stinger)

- neural plexus, (i.e., brachial plexus when stretched)
- nerve root, neural sheath, dural sheath, or nerve trunk when stretched

Tingling, Numbness

- peripheral nerve (facial nerve)
- nerve root irritation from herniated intervertebral disc, facet joint, cervical spondylolysis, or spondylolisthesis
- circulation problem, (i.e., cervical rib, thoracic outlet problem)

Stiffness

- muscle spasm
- facet joint capsular swelling (effusion)
- osteoarthritic or degenerative changes in the facet joints
- ankylosing spondylitis

Sharp Pain with Coughing, Swallowing, Sneezing, or Straining

This pain is normally caused by increased intrathecal pressure (pressure within the spinal cord) caused by a space occupying lesion.
- intervertebral disc herniation
- acute facet or muscle lesion
- tumor
- osteophyte

Pain with coughing that is felt on the anterior or anterolateral aspect of the throat may suggest an anterior intervertebral disc herniation.

Throbbing Pain

- vascular congestion accompanying inflammatory processes in the vertebral joints (i.e., capsule, ligaments, etc.)

ASSESSMENT

INTERPRETATION

Timing of Pain
On Waking

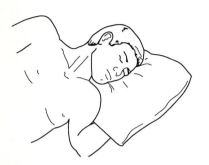

Fig. 2-23 Head and neck position during sleep.

Determine the athlete's sleeping position and pillow usage (Fig. 2-23). Sponge rubber pillows may not allow the head to rest fully because the head bounces and the muscles of the cervical spine and shoulders remain under tension. The pillow may not support the spine adequately or keep the cervical spine in good alignment.

If the athlete sleeps in the prone position, the neck is extended and rotated, which can lead to pain and dysfunction.

If the athlete sleeps supine, this prolonged flexed position can lead to increased intervertebral disc pressure and problems.

If the athlete sleeps in side lying, without the spine in good alignment (pillow too thick or too thin), neck pain may result.

If there is pain on waking, rest may not help the condition, or the cervical spine position was not supportive.

At the End of the Day

Does the athlete's daily activities allow free body movements rather than maintaining one position? Holding the head or upper body rigidly can produce tension, stiffness, and pain.

The anatomical structures that support the head and allow movement become fatigued as the day progresses. Underlying pathologic conditions can become painful, especially if the daily posture allows a forward head posture or repeated mechanical irritation.

All Day

All day discomfort suggests that the injured site is still acute, very irritable, or of a chronic arthritic nature.

If the pain worsens as the day progresses and decreases with rest, this pain is often associated with poor postural habits.

With Certain Movements

Feeling pain with certain movements indicates that an articular or muscular component of the cervical spine is injured. Symptoms that are produced with a certain movement are usually of a mechanical nature and require systematic testing to determine what aggravates and relieves the symptoms.

Night Pain

Symptoms of a mechanical nature are usually relieved by rest and the pain is decreased on waking (provided the appropriate cervical support is given during the night). Symptoms caused by an active inflammatory response or metastatic tumor will not be relieved by rest and may be even more uncomfortable or stiff in the morning.

These include:

ASSESSMENT

INTERPRETATION

- degenerative facet joint disease
- staphylococcal or tuberculous infection
- inflammatory arthritis or osteitis
- neoplastic disease of the cervical spine (primary or secondary, malignant or benign)

Sensations

What sensations does the athlete feel?

Vertigo, Tinnitus

Vertigo and tinnitus can originate from the upper cervical region (C1, C2 dysfunction) or from an obstruction of the vertebral arteries (secondary to a dens defect or cervical osteophytes). It develops from prolonged cervical back bending (i.e., painting a ceiling), a postural forward head carriage, repeated cervical rotation, or rising from a supine to a sitting position or vice versa. This sensation can also be referred from inner ear (vestibular apparatus in semicircular canals) or temporomandibular joint problems.

Since these symptoms can also be caused from vertebral artery or basilar insufficiency, vertebral artery tests should be done before functional testing if this symptom occurs.

Paresthesia, Hyperesthesia, Dysesthesia (or Hypesthesia), Anesthesia

- paresthesia causes abnormalities of sensation that include pins and needles, tingling, hot or cold feelings, heaviness, fullness, puffiness
- hyperesthesia causes increased skin sensitivity
- dysesthesia causes diminished skin sensitivity
- anesthesia causes a sensation loss that can be objectively confirmed

A complaint of pins and needles, numbness, or increased sensitivity in areas supplied by one peripheral nerve indicates pressure or damage to the cervical nerve root or local cutaneous nerve.

Determine the dermatome and corresponding cervical nerve supply if the nerve root is suspected. The nerve supply from the nerve root to the extremity can be impinged anywhere along its length (i.e., cervical rib, thoracic outlet problem, or brachial plexus injury) (Fig. 2-24). The tingling or numbness can radiate to the dermatomes of the head, cervical spine, shoulder, arm, and/or hand.

Determine if the sensation changes are not dermatomal but are from a local cutaneous nerve.

Tingling can also be caused by a circulatory problem. The subclavian artery can be affected as it passes through the thoracic outlet and anywhere along its distribution.

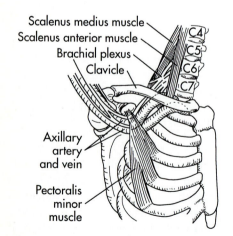

Fig. 2-24 Thoracic outlet syndrome. Impingement of the neurovascular structures.

Scalenus medius muscle
Scalenus anterior muscle
Brachial plexus
Clavicle
C4
C5
C6
C7
Axillary artery and vein
Pectoralis minor muscle

ASSESSMENT

INTERPRETATION

Catching

If a sensation of catching occurs during a particular part of the range of motion, it signifies an articular lesion or synovial fringe impingement in the facet joint, an instability of a cervical segment, or both.

Snapping

An audible and palpable click or snap of the neck during cervical rotation can be from:
- irregularity at the joint articulations
- a tendon over a boney prominence
- hypermobility of the cervical vertebrae

Locking

A subluxation of one of the facet joints can cause the cervical spine to become locked in side bending and rotation.

Function

What daily activities are difficult or painful?
What alleviates the discomfort?
What aggravates the area?

Daily Function

Daily activities that prove painful help determine the lesion and the severity of the problem.

The athlete may find that certain actions alleviate the pain. For example he or she may express that lying down or a hot tub relieves the pain. Incorporate these suggestions into a rehabilitation program. If the athlete is better when moving or worse when still, static positioning may cause pain because there is a postural component to the problem.

Determine what aggravates the injury. This may tell you what the condition is and what movements the athlete should avoid.

Athletes with an acute facet joint or torticollis with associated muscle spasm may feel less pain with no movement and may physically hold the neck to support it.

Particulars

Has the athlete seen a physician, orthopedic surgeon, physical therapist, physiotherapist, osteopath, chiropractor, athletic trainer, athletic therapist, or other medical personnel?
What was the diagnosis?
Were there x-rays?
What recommendations and/or prescriptions were given?
At the time of injury what was the method of transportation (car, ambulance) and the most comfortable position for the cervical spine?

Record medical personnel's name, address, and diagnosis.
Record the x-ray results and where they were done.
Record the physician's recommendations and prescriptions.
The method of transportation indicates the severity at the time of injury. The cervical position of comfort during transportation helps determine the structures that are injured.
The ability of the athlete to return to sport and daily activities helps determine the degree of the injury and their willingness to return.
The treatment at the time of injury is important in determining whether the inflammation process was controlled or increased. Ice and immobilization can help limit the secondary edema but heat will increase swelling.

ASSESSMENT

INTERPRETATION

Was the athlete able to return to sport immediately?

What treatment was carried out (ice, heat, immobilization) at the time of injury and now?

Has the injury occurred previously? If yes, get full details such as when it happened, how it was treated, and was the treatment successful.

Does the athlete currently participate in sport, daily functions, and occupation?

Has the athlete had a previous upper quadrant injury (i.e., frozen shoulder) for which the cervical spine may be compensating?

If the athlete is able to work or return to sport, make sure that he or she is ready and will not aggravate the injury or predispose it to reoccurrence.

If this is a reoccurrence, record all the details of the previous injury, including:
- date of injury
- mechanism of injury
- diagnosis
- length of disability
- treatment and rehabilitation

Any mechanical dysfunction of the upper quadrant can result in altered cervical mechanics and dysfunction. The following are common upper quadrant dysfunctions that can lead to cervical problems.
- Temporomandibular joint problems lead to upper cervical compensatory movements.
- Glenohumeral pathology (i.e., frozen shoulder) alters the shoulder girdle and its musculature, causing dysfunction in the cervical spine.
- Brachial plexus injuries can cause limitations in cervical motions and eventual dysfunction.
- Thoracic spine hypomobility problems can lead to cervical hypermobility and related problems.

OBSERVATIONS

The upper body must be exposed as much as possible.

Head Carriage

Observe the athlete's head carriage during his or her walk to the examining table and during coat, shirt, or sweater removal.

Notice the athlete's ability and willingness to move the head and cervical spine throughout the assessment routine.

Notice the temporomandibular joint and mandible position and movement during the athlete's response to questions.

Any muscle spasm or cervical pain will cause the athlete to hold the head and neck stiffly during gait and during the remainder of the assessment. Temporomandibular joint, C1, and C2 function often influence one another because of their proximity. Dysfunction may be noted during static posture and while answering questions during the assessment.

Standing or Sitting

Anterior View

Look at the following:

ASSESSMENT   INTERPRETATION

Cranial position (cervical side bending and rotation)

If the cervical spine is side bent toward and rotated away from the side of pain, the athlete may have torticollis or wry neck (Fig. 2-25).

According to McNair (see Grieve G, Manual Therapy, Chapter 34), the categories and causes of wry neck are:

1. muscular
   - adult
     post-trauma
     post-viral infection (i.e. tonsillitis)
   - adolescent
     post-viral
   - child
     congenital torticollis
     contracture SCM
2. acquired wry neck from hearing loss or visual defects
3. atlanto-axial fixation
4. spasmodic and hysterical torticollis
5. acute cervical locking (facet or intervertebral disc dysfunction)
   - traumatic onset
   - sudden onset
   - spontaneous onset

The history-taking should determine which type of torticollis problem exists. Chronic or acquired torticollis will have contracture changes in the sternocleidomastoid.

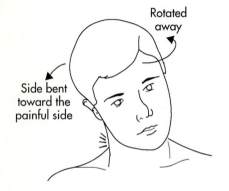

Rotated away

Side bent toward the painful side

Fig. 2-25 Acute torticollis—wry neck.

Sternocleidomastoid or Upper Trapezius Muscles

Normally the sternocleidomastoid muscle is barely visible, but if the muscle is visible and prominent at its clavicular insertion the muscle is in spasm. This muscle spasm may be protective for underlying pathology or from poor postural habits. Muscle spasm of the upper trapezius muscles can also be protective or a product of poor postural habits.

Pectoralis Major and Minor Muscles

Muscle imbalance changes from faulty posture cause tightness in pectoralis major and minor muscles. Tightness in these muscles tends to pull the entire upper quadrant, including the cervical spine, to imbalance.

Deep Neck Flexor Muscles

The deep neck flexor muscles tend to weaken and atrophy quickly. Atrophy of these muscles, with tightness of the sternocleidomastoid, causes a forward head posture and its related problems (see Forward Head Observation, Lateral View).

Digastric Muscle

Straightening of the throat line is usually a sign of increased tonus in the digastric muscle. This tightness can lead to difficult swallowing.

ASSESSMENT

INTERPRETATION

Scars

Scars at the front of the neck can be from a previous tracheotomy or thyroid surgery.

Temporomandibular Joint

Temporomandibular joint asymmetry can indicate dysfunction that causes referred problems into the cervical spine. If this is suspected, a full temporomandibular assessment is necessary (see Chapter 1).

Ischemia into the Upper Extremity

Look for ischemia caused by circulatory problems. Some cervical or upper thoracic pathologic conditions can affect the autonomic nervous system and alter blood flow.

Irritation of the cervicothoracic sympathetic chain, reflex dystrophy, or the thoracic outlet can cause circulatory changes such as coldness, hand swelling, sweating, and piloerection.

Muscle Wasting in Upper Limbs

Muscle atrophy may be noticeable at the shoulder or into the forearm and hand, especially in the deltoid, biceps, and forearm muscles. Atrophy indicates either a nerve root problem that affects a specific myotome or weakness following surgery or a chronic lesion.
- C5 nerve root irritation (atrophy of deltoid, supraspinatus, and infraspinatus)
- C6 nerve root irritation (atrophy of biceps, brachioradialis, brachialis, and wrist extensors)
- C7 nerve root irritation (atrophy of triceps and wrist flexors)
- C8 nerve root irritation (atrophy of thumb extensors and wrist ulnar deviators)
- T1 nerve root irritation (atrophy of thumb abductors and dorsal interossei of the fingers)

If there is muscle atrophy, the nerve root irritation has been present for 2 weeks or longer.

Symmetry of the Upper Extremity

The level of the clavicles, acromioclavicular joints, and sternoclavicular joints should be equal bilaterally. The entire shoulder girdle is the platform for the muscles that control the cervical spine and upper quadrant. If it is not level, compensatory structural changes and muscle imbalances will occur throughout the kinetic chain. If the asymmetry is caused by dysfunction in the shoulder girdle or the limb, an assessment of the area is necessary because the cervical dysfunction that it causes may be secondary to the actual problem.

Lateral View

Look for the following:

ASSESSMENT

INTERPRETATION

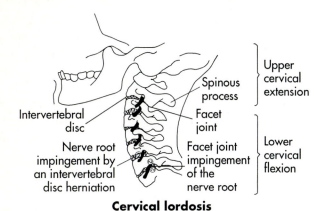

Upper cervical extension

Spinous process

Intervertebral disc

Facet joint

Nerve root impingement by an intervertebral disc herniation

Facet joint impingement of the nerve root

Lower cervical flexion

Cervical lordosis

Fig. 2-26 Lateral view of the cervical spine. Locations for impingement.

Forward Head (Fig. 2-26)

A forward head is associated with upper cervical extension, lower cervical flexion, upper thoracic extension, and midthoracic flexion. The abnormal positioning of the head on the upper cervical spine will affect the entire quadrant and possibly the entire body posture. The upper vertebral cervical joints contain receptor systems in the connective tissue and muscles that regulate static and dynamic postures and produce reflex changes in the motor unit activity of all four limb muscles.

The normal cervical spine posture is maintained by the contraction of the posterior cervical musculature, especially the suboccipital muscles, to overcome gravity and to balance the anterior cervical muscles.

However, in the forward head position, there is shortening of the suboccipital muscles. This pulls the occiput posteriorly and inferiorly, resulting in upward and backward displacement of the mandible in its fossa. This causes shortening of the suprahyoid muscles, lengthening of the infrahyoid muscles, and elevation of the hyoid bone and can lead to painful myofascial trigger points in the involved muscles and referred headaches.

This position also forces the masseter and temporalis to contract antagonistically against the shortened suprahyoid muscles, which tends to pull the mouth open. This can lead to temporomandibular joint dysfunction or myofascial trigger points in the masseter and temporalis muscles.

Because of the tight suboccipital muscles, the upper trapezius muscle shortens, resulting in scapular elevation. The levator scapulae can then shorten or develop myofascial trigger points that refer pain laterally to the cervical spine and on the vertebral border of the scapula. The forward head position and the increased cervical lordosis will then lead to thoracic kyphosis.

With the forward head posture, the dorsal scapular nerve can be compressed by the scalene muscle or a cervical rib, resulting in scapular pain and pain along C5-C6 dermatome. The suprascapular nerve can also be stretched by the forward head pos-

ASSESSMENT   INTERPRETATION

ture (increased distance between C5-C6 segment and the nerve's insertion into the acromioclavicular joint and infraspinatus muscle). This can lead to pain or dysfunction in the supraspinatus and infraspinatus muscles and in the acromioclavicular and glenohumeral joints. The dorsal scapular nerve entrapment causes weakness in the rhomboids and levator scapulae muscles, which augments or maintains the forward head and rounded shoulder posture.

Carrying the head in front of the center of gravity requires continuous cervical and cranial extensor muscle work that leads to fatigue, spasm, and pain.

Increased cervical lordosis causes cervical spondylolysis and premature wear and tear in the intervertebral discs. The spinous processes and facet joints are approximated with excessive lordosis that leads to ligament sprain, muscle fatigue, and articular joint degeneration in the lower cervical vertebrae (see Fig. 2-26).

A forward head can therefore lead to dysfunction and pain throughout the upper quadrant resulting from direct mechanical dysfunction or secondary compensatory actions.

Muscle Wasting (deltoid, triceps, forearm musculature)

Muscle wasting from a nerve root impingement or injury (intervertebral disc or facet, brachial or cervical plexus, thoracic outlet) should be suspected.

Anterior Glenohumeral Position

An anterior glenohumeral position can reduce the thoracic outlet and cause circulatory or neural problems to the upper extremity. If this is suspected, the thoracic outlet tests should be carried out during the functional tests.

Excessive Thoracic Kyphosis

Excessive thoracic kyphosis can cause excessive cervical lordosis and related problems.

Posterior View (Fig. 2-27)

Look for the following:

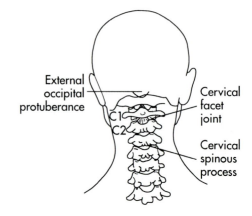

Fig. 2-27 Posterior aspect of the cervical spine. Boney alignment.

External occipital protuberance

Cervical facet joint

Cervical spinous process

C1
C2

ASSESSMENT   INTERPRETATION

Cranial Position

Check the cranial position and resulting compensatory mechanics. If the head is side bent toward and rotated away form the direction of pain, a torticollis can exist.

If the athlete has a short neck and low posterior hairline, with gross limitation in ranges, he or she may have Klippel-Feil Syndrome (congenital fusion of the cervical spine). Associated facial asymmetry, torticollis, webbing of the neck, Sprengel deformity, and scoliosis may also be present.

Spinous Process Alignment

The cervical and thoracic spinous processes should line up vertically in a straight line without any concave or convex curves. If there are curves, it suggests cervical joint dysfunction, unilateral muscle spasm, or compensatory spinal alterations.

Muscle Spasm (suboccipitals, erector spinae, trapezius, levator scapulae)

Muscle spasm of these muscles occurs with nearly all the cervical conditions; it protects the underlying cervical dysfunction. According to Yanda, the upper trapezius, levator scapulae, and suboccipital muscles will develop tightness. Poor posture (forward head) or trauma can accelerate the tightness and lead to muscle imbalances, which can lead to cervical dysfunction.

Scapular Position and Interscapular Space

Weakness of the scapular retractors (rhomboids, serratus anterior) will cause the scapula to rotate and wing, resulting in increased interscapular space. Tightness of the upper trapezius and levator scapulae accompany this weakness. This pattern of weakness accompanies the forward head position and leads to excess stress in the cervicocranial and cervicothoracic junctions.

A very small and elevated scapula may be present on one side. This is called Sprengel deformity (embryological, undescended scapula) and it is sometimes attached to the cervical spine by the omohyoid muscle.

Downward and lateral displacement of the scapulae occurs with middle and lower trapezius muscle weakness. Prominence of the vertebral border of one scapula (winging) suggests long thoracic nerve neuritis with weakness or paralysis of the serratus anterior on that side.

Prominence of both scapular vertebral borders suggests problems with serratus anterior (myopathic lesion) or its nerve root.

Shoulder Joint

One shoulder lower than the other, without scoliosis, suggests a leg-length discrepancy.

ASSESSMENT   INTERPRETATION

Lesion Site

Look for the following:

Deformities or Changes in Boney Contour

Any significant spinal deformity may indicate a severe injury. Further assessment may not be possible. If the athlete has not had an x-ray, immobilize and transport immediately.

Muscle Spasm

Protective muscle spasm around the involved spinal segment is common. Muscle atrophy at the lesion site usually indicates a recurring cervical condition, degenerative joint changes, or chronic pathology.

Muscle Hypertrophy or Atrophy

Muscle hypertrophy can develop if muscle actions are repeated with resistance in one direction (i.e., football players usually develop hypertrophy of the trapezius muscles).

Redness, Swelling, or Bruising

Redness, swelling, or bruising can indicate local inflammation, infection, or contusion.

SUMMARY OF TESTS

FUNCTIONAL TESTS

Rule out
    Temporomandibular joint
    Thoracic outlet or inlet syndrome
    Upper and midthoracic spine dysfunction
    Fixed first rib or first rib syndrome
    Cervical rib syndrome
    Fracture
Tests in Sitting
    Active cervical forward bending
    Resisted cervical forward bending
    Active cervical back bending
    Resisted cervical back bending
    Active head flexion
    Resisted head flexion
    Active head extension
    Resisted head extension
    Active cervical rotation
    Resisted cervical rotation
    Active cervical side bending
    Resisted cervical side bending

ASSESSMENT

INTERPRETATION

Tests in Supine Position
Passive head flexion and cervical forward bending
Passive cervical rotation
Passive cervical side bending

SPECIAL TESTS

Vertebral artery test
Quadrant test
Traction test
Compression test
Valsalva test
Swallowing test
Upper limb or brachial tension test
Slump test
Myotome testing
Dermatome testing
Cutaneous nerve testing
Reflex testing

Rule Out

If the joints of the upper limb cannot be ruled out, arthrology scans of the shoulder, elbow, wrist, and hand may be done (see Introduction, Arthrology Scans).

Temporomandibular Joint

Rule out the TMJ throughout the history-taking and observations. Conduct active tests of jaw opening, closing, protrusion, and retrusion.

Pain, clicking, or locking during these movements indicate temporomandibular dysfunction. If the temporomandibular joint cannot be ruled out, a complete TMJ assessment is necessary (see Chapter 1).

It is important to rule out temporomandibular joint because:

- TMJ, cervical spine, and cranium share some of the same muscles (i.e., suprahyoid, suboccipitals, sternocleidomastoid); therefore any muscle spasm or dysfunction in one can alter all three areas.
- upper cervical spine and TMJ often have the same symptomology when dysfunction is present (i.e., facial pain, tinnitus, auditory and visual disturbances, vertigo).
- TMJ and cervical spine must work together during jaw movements; therefore abnormality in either part will affect the other (i.e., during jaw opening there is upper cervical joint extension).
- myofascial trigger points (Travell and Simons) from the cervical spine can refer pain into the TMJ (i.e., suboccipital muscles, sternocleidomastoid); therefore it is difficult to determine the primary location of the problem.

ASSESSMENT

INTERPRETATION

Thoracic Outlet (or Inlet) Syndrome

Rule out a thoracic outlet syndrome throughout the history-taking and observations.

These tests can be done to rule out circulatory or neural involvement from the thoracic outlet.

This is a term used to describe compression on the neurovascular bundle in the thoracic outlet that can cause pain, tingling, or decreased circulation in the arm or hand. Some of the notable vascular symptoms include:

- swelling or puffiness in the limb or hand
- bluish discoloration of the hand
- feeling of heaviness in the limb or hand
- a pulsating lump above the clavicle

Some of the frequently reported neural symptoms include:

- paresthesia in C8 or T1 nerve roots
- muscle weakness, muscle wasting in T1 nerve root
- difficulty with fine motor tasks of the hand
- finger flexor cramps
- pain in the hand, forearm, and arm

The neurovascular bundle contains the brachial plexus, the subclavian artery, and vein. This is not to be confused with a cervical root impingement.

The compression can occur when the size or shape of the thoracic outlet is altered. The outlet can be altered by exercise, trauma, pregnancy, a congenital anomaly, an exostosis, or postural changes.

The compression can be caused by:

- reduction of the outlet because of a cervical rib or ligamentous cord from the seventh cervical transverse process
- a reduced interscalene triangle between scalene anterior and medius or an extra head on the scalene muscle called scalene minimus
- reduced space between the scalenes and first rib
- reduced costoclavicular space between the clavicle and first rib
- reduced costocoracoid space between the coracoid process and the clavipectoral fascia or pectoralis minor tendon
- reduced space caused by a droop shoulder on an athlete who overdevelops one side of the upper body or the dropping of the entire shoulder girdle in a middle-aged athlete
- reduced space caused by a large clavicular callus formation following a clavicular fracture

Adson Maneuver (Figs. 2-28 and 2-29)

Palpate the radial pulse on the affected side.

Ask the athlete to take a deep breath and hold it while extending the neck and turning the head toward the affected side. Apply downward traction on the extended shoulder and arm while palpating the radial pulse.

The pulse may diminish or become absent.

This test determines if a cervical rib or a reduced interscalene triangle is compressing the subclavian artery. The compression of the artery is determined by the decrease or absence of the radial pulse. The difficulty with this maneuver is that it may be positive in an asymptomatic patient.

ASSESSMENT

INTERPRETATION

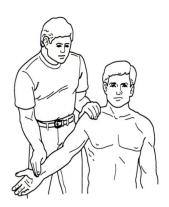

Fig. 2-28 Adson maneuver 1.

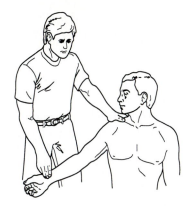

Fig. 2-29 Adson maneuver 2.

In some athletes a greater effect on the subclavian artery is exerted by turning the head to the opposite side, so both can be tried.

Costoclavicular Syndrome Test

Ask the athlete to stand in an exaggerated military stance with the shoulders thrust backward and downward. Take the radial pulse before and while the shoulders are held back.

This test causes compression of the subclavian artery and vein by reducing the space between the clavicle and first rib. A modification or obliteration of the radial pulse indicates that a compression exists. Pain or tingling into the arm can also occur. If this test causes the symptoms that are the athlete's major complaint, a compression problem is at fault.

A damping of the pulse may occur even in a healthy athlete who does not have this syndrome because this position can close a normal thoracic outlet.

Hyperabduction Test (Fig. 2-30)

The athlete can fully abduct the shoulder or repeatedly abduct the shoulder. Take the radial pulse before the test and after prolonged or repeated abduction.

Repeated or prolonged positions of hyperabduction can close down the outlet.

This position is often assumed during sleep, in certain occupations (painters, electricians), and in certain sports (volleyball, tennis).

The subclavian vessels are compressed in two locations: (1) between the pectoralis minor tendon and the coracoid process and (2) between the clavicle and first rib. Pain, a diminishing of the pulse, or reproduction of the athlete's symptoms indicates that a compression exists.

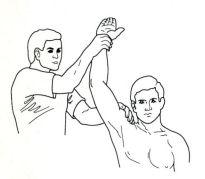

Fig. 2-30 Hyperabduction test.

ASSESSMENT

INTERPRETATION

Upper and Midthoracic Spine Dysfunction

Rule out the upper and midthoracic spine throughout the history-taking and observations.

A history of thoracic or chest wall pain suggests thoracic involvement.

Problems with excessive thoracic kyphosis, excessive scapular protraction, or tightness of the anterior chest musculature indicates thoracic restrictions or pathologic conditions.

The upper thoracic spine (T1-T4) is examined, along with the normal cervical functional tests, while palpating between the spinous processes to localize the movement. If the range is full and pain free, perform an overpressure in each position. If the pain during testing is felt in the upper thoracic area, the injury is probably to the upper thoracic spine rather than the lower cervical spine. Overpressures can be directed lower to involve the upper thoracic spine if the upper cervical area is symptom free.

Test the midthoracic spine (T4-T8) with the athlete seated and the lumbar spine pushed against the back of the chair.

Have the athlete clasp the hands behind the cervical spine from cranium to the cervical thoracic junction with the flexed elbows together in front to prevent cervical spine movement (Fig. 2-31, A).

Have the athlete forward bend and move the shoulders toward the groin area (if full and pain free, do an overpressure) (Fig. 2-31, B).

The athlete backward bends (Fig. 2-32, A) without extending the lumbar spine or allowing cervical movement (Fig. 2-32, B). Again, an overpressure can be done by gently localizing the movement to each intervertebral area.

For thoracic side bending (Fig. 2-33, A), the athlete maintains the cervical thoracic grasp but moves the elbows out to the side into the frontal plane, then side bends only through the tho-

If there is upper thoracic spine pathology, the pain or symptoms will be reproduced during the cervical functional testing. A thoracic problem is indicated by the location of the pain and by the range where the pain is reproduced.

Generally, the end of range or overpressures in forward bending, side bending, and rotation will reproduce the upper thoracic symptoms. If there is a midthoracic spine dysfunction, the midthoracic tests will reproduce the symptoms and pain in the involved segment. Thoracic spine dysfunction tends to refer pain into the chest area, local thoracic spine, or ribs.

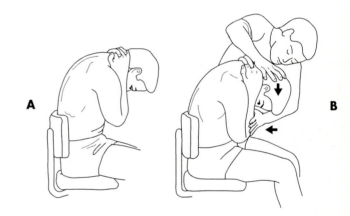

Fig. 2-31 A, Active thoracic forward bending. **B,** Active thoracic forward bending with overpressure.

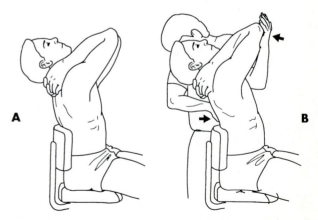

Fig. 2-32 A, Active thoracic back bending. **B,** Active thoracic back bending with overpressure.

ASSESSMENT

INTERPRETATION

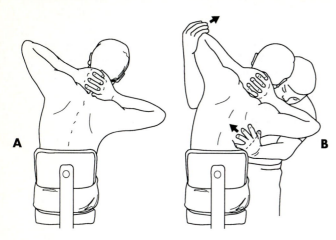

Fig. 2-33 A, Active thoracic side bending. **B,** Active thoracic side bending with overpressure.

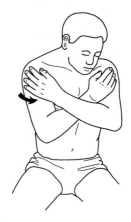

Fig. 2-34 Active thoracic rotation (with slight forward bending).

racic spine (Fig. 2-33, *B*) (overpressures can be done with pressure, with one hand on the patient's elbow and the other at the angle of the ribs). During side bending the pelvis and buttocks should not move or lift off the plinth.

For thoracic rotation (Fig. 2-34), the athlete's arms are crossed in front of the body. Ask the athlete to rotate while in slight flexion because this isolates the midthoracic spine.

Fixed First Rib or First Rib Syndrome

Rule out first rib syndrome throughout the history-taking and palpations.

This syndrome is characterized by:

- local pain or tenderness in the supraspinatus fossa
- burning feeling over the upper trapezius on the side of the pain
- paresthesia or aching in the C8 or T1 dermatome (arm, forearm, or hand)
- heaviness of the affected upper limb
- sympathetic nervous system changes in the limb through the cervicothoracic ganglion (sweating, swelling, piloerection)

Palpate the first rib, the transverse process of T1 and the costotransverse joint of T1, checking for pain or any of the above symptoms.

Cervical rotation to the painful side is restricted and back bending may be painful.

The condition is aggravated by pulling activities such as hoeing and raking.

There are very strong fascial connections with the first rib and the thoracic spine and clavicle. Any rib dysfunction can lead to thoracic and cervical dysfunction and can even affect the sympathetic nervous system.

The first rib should move upward and laterally to the upper limb on deep inspiration. If the rib is fixed in an elevated position, through injury or costal cartilage calcification, the first ribs move bilaterally and the sternum's manubrium must move as a single unit about a transverse axis through the costotransverse joints (*Gray's Anatomy*). This can cause costotransverse joint dysfunction, which can lead to thoracic and cervical spine compensations.

ASSESSMENT

INTERPRETATION

Cervical Rib Syndrome

Rule out the presence of a cervical rib throughout the history-taking, observations, thoracic outlet tests, and palpation.

History responses that include subclavian artery compression and pressure on the eighth cervical and first thoracic spinal nerves (motor or sensory involvement) can indicate the presence of cervical rib syndrome.

The cervical rib may be observable. Palpate for a costal element to the seventh cervical vertebra. If it is present, it is palpable at the level of the clavicle between the anterior and middle scalene muscle.

The cervical rib may have a rib head, neck, and tubercle with or without the rib shaft.

The presence of the cervical rib can affect the thoracic outlet and cervical function. According to Travell and Simons, the cervical rib patient is prone to developing myofascial trigger points and referred pain in the scalene muscles. If the thoracic outlet is compromised, there can be circulatory changes and pins and needles of the median and ulnar nerve (blanching and cyanosis of the hands).

Fracture

If a fracture is suspected from the history-taking or observations, do not carry out any functional tests of the cervical spine. Block the head and neck to prevent movement. Test the extremity myotomes and dermatomes to determine if there is nerve root or spinal cord involvement (C4-T1). Call for an ambulance while monitoring the athlete's vital signs. Immobilize and assist in transport if necessary. Do not allow head or neck movement during transport. Record and forward the history, observations, and your findings to the involved medical personnel.

Tests in Sitting

Active Cervical Forward Bending (with overpressure) (80°) (Fig. 2-35)

Ask the athlete to nod the head forward and attempt to put the chin to the chest. Instruct the athlete to keep the teeth closed during this movement. If there is no pain but the range of motion is limited, apply an overpressure with gentle pressure forward on the back of the skull. Palpate between the cervical

Full range allows the athlete's chin to touch his or her chest with the teeth clenched.

Pain, weakness, or limitation of range of motion can be caused by an injury to the muscle or its nerve supply. The prime movers are:
- Sternocleidomastoid (both sides contracting together)
- Cranial nerve 11 and ventral primary division of C2-C3 (spinal accessory nerve)

ASSESSMENT

spinous process for the amount of gapping or joint opening.

Robin McKenzie advocates repeating this test 5 to 15 times ensuring that the head always returns to the upright position.

The patient is seated with the back supported. Active forward bending is repeated to determine if the cervical problem is caused by dysfunction (defined by McKenzie as pain resulting from the stretching of adaptively shortened or contracted soft tissue) or derangement (intervertebral disc protrusion). The patient is asked if the pain decreases or centralizes during the repetitions or if the pain increases or spreads.

INTERPRETATION

The accessory movers are:
- Longus capitis
- Longus colli
- Scalenes anterior, medius, and posterior
- Rectus capitis anterior
- Infrahyoid group
- Rectus lateralis

Most of the range of flexion occurs in the central cervical region. The atlanto-occipital joint range during flexion and extension is approximately 18° and the atlanto-axial joint range of flexion and extension is about 13°. The midcervical joints can get 30° to 40° of range.

During flexion the upper vertebral body tilts and slides forward and the intervertebral foramen is 20% to 30% larger than in extension. During forward bending in the normal spine with all cervical segments contributing, the occipital condyles roll forward on the atlas while the atlas glides backward (relative to the occiput) and tilts upward. This allows the posterior arch of the atlas and occiput to approximate.

The cervical vertebrae joint surfaces tend to gap during forward bending with the most movement between C4, C5, and C6. This mobility also causes the most stress in these joints. The C6-C7 and C7-T1 cervical segments have less gapping and mobility. If the range is limited but pain free, apply a gentle overpressure. This overpressure is limited by injury to the:
- posterior longitudinal ligament
- capsular ligaments between the articular processes
- ligamentum flavum
- interspinous ligaments
- ligamentum nuchae
- posterior muscles of the neck
- intervertebral disc (posterior fibers)

Neck flexion stretches both the cervical and thoracic musculature and dura mater during the overpressure.

If pain occurs centrally or unilaterally in the neck or scapular region, the cause may be a cervical or thoracic herniated disc. With a thoracic herniation, pain with scapular approximation also occurs. A stress fracture of the C7 or T1 spinous process (clay shoveler's fracture) from unaccustomed exertion in a unfit athlete (digging or lifting weights) causes pain during active flexion.

McKenzie's interpretation of the repeated test results include:
- pain that does not change is a dysfunction or postural problem
- pain that becomes more centralized or decreases indicates an intervertebral disc derangement that will improve if this exercise is done during rehabilitation
- pain that becomes greater or moves down the arm indicates an intervertebral disc derangement that will *not* improve if this exercise or action is done

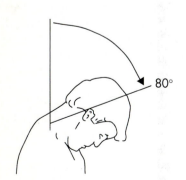

80°

Fig. 2-35 Active cervical forward bending.

ASSESSMENT

INTERPRETATION

Resisted Cervical Forward Bending

The athlete attempts to forward bend the cervical spine. Resist the movement while instructing the athlete to attempt to move only the head and neck and not lean with the entire body.

The isometric movements are done in the neutral position with one hand on the athlete's forehead and the other hand on the back of the head.

Pain and/or weakness can occur from an injury to the muscle or its nerve supply (see Active Forward Bending).

Active Cervical Back Bending (70°) (Fig. 2-36)

Ask the athlete to look as far back overhead as possible. Have the athlete move only the head and not lean with the entire body or extend through the lumbar or thoracic spine.

Full range allows the plane of the athlete's nose and forehead to be horizontal to the floor. Do not attempt an overpressure in cervical back bending. Facet joint surfaces and spinous processes in the cervical spine (C2-C6) approximate during back bending.

Pain, weakness, or limitation of range of motion can be caused by an injury to the muscle or its nerve supply.

The prime movers are:

- Trapezius—spinal accessory nerve CN 11 and ventral divisions
- Semispinalis capitis—dorsal primary divisions of the cervical nerves
- Splenius capitis—dorsal primary divisions C4-C8
- Splenius cervicis—dorsal primary divisions C4-C8
- Semispinalis cervicis—dorsal primary divisions of spinal nerves
- Sacrospinalis (erector spinae group)—dorsal primary divisions of adjacent spinal nerves

The following muscles are also prime movers:

- Iliocostalis cervicis
- Longissimus capitis
- Longissimus cervicis
- Spinalis capitis
- Spinalis cervicis

The capsular pattern of the cervical facet joints has limitations of an equal degree in side flexion and rotation in the same direction and some (or great) limitation in back bending.

This capsular pattern can indicate any of the following conditions:

- osteoarthrosis of the facet joint
- spondylitic arthritis
- rheumatoid arthritis
- recent fracture
- bone disease

Back bending is limited by an injury to the:

- anterior longitudinal ligament
- posterior cervical arches

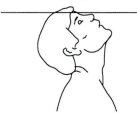

Athlete's forehead and nose should be horizontal to the floor

Fig. 2-36 Active cervical back bending.

ASSESSMENT

INTERPRETATION

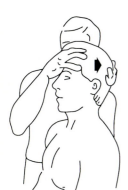

Fig. 2-37 Resisted cervical back bending.

- cervical forward bending muscles that are on stretch
- spinous processes

The atlanto-occipital joint can be injured if it is forced into back bending (when the cervical spine is back bent the atlas tilts upward, resulting in compression between the atlas and occiput).

A recent fracture of a vertebral body leads to marked limitation of movement in each direction, especially of back bending.

A clay shoveler's fracture (stress fracture) of C7 or T1 causes pain during active and passive extension. The fracture occurs from repeated lifting or shoveling action in an unfit athlete.

If the forced cervical back bending has caused a severe ligament sprain or subluxation, the sternocleidomastoids can go into muscle spasm, pulling the head forward. The athlete will then have great difficulty in accomplishing active cervical back bending. For this reason, do not demand cervical back bending if the athlete is reluctant to do the movement.

Resisted Cervical Back Bending (Fig. 2-37)

Have the athlete attempt to extend the head and cervical spine without leaning backward.

Resist the head in the neutral position with one hand on the back of the athlete's head and one hand on the front of the head.

Pain and/or weakness can occur from an injury to muscle or its nerve supply (see Active Back Bending). These muscles are usually stronger than the cervical forward bending muscles. The posterior spinal muscles are sometimes strained when the head is forced into flexion while the athlete is extending the neck against a resistance (i.e., wrestling, weight lifting, gymnastics).

Active Head Flexion (nodding, with overpressure) (Fig. 2-38)

Ask the athlete to tuck the chin in without forward bending the cervical region. The teeth should be gently clenched. You should demonstrate this position. If there is no pain, a gentle overpressure can be applied. Gently push the mandible inward with one hand while resting the other hand on the back of the athlete's head. Tip the head forward.

McKenzie advocates repetition of this action 5 to 15 times, ensuring that the motion be actively taken to the full end of range of flexion (retraction).

As described with Active Forward Bending, the McKenzie repeats help determine if the pain is caused by a postural problem, dysfunction, or derangement. The athlete is asked if the pain is increased or decreased by the repetitions.

The athlete is asked to perform this movement because nodding occurs primarily at the atlanto-occipital (O-C1) and atlanto-axial (C1-C2) joints. According to Grieve, during controlled artificial head nodding motion at the atlanto-occipital joints, the occipital condyles glide backward on the atlas; the atlas moves forward and cranially in relation to the occiput. Pain, weakness, or limitation of range can be caused by an injury to the muscles or their nerve supply.

The prime movers are:
- Rectus capitis anterior—ventral rami of C1 and C2 spinal nerves
- Suprahyoid—facial nerve, inferior alveolar nerve, hypoglossal nerve
- Infrahyoid—ansa cervicalis, hypoglossal nerve

The accessory movers are:
- Longus capitis
- Rectus capitis anterior and lateralis (bilaterally)

When the infrahyoid muscles contract, the mandible is lowered. However, if the mandible is fixed by a contraction of the masticator muscles (masseter and temporalis), the infrahyoid and suprahyoid muscles produce head flexion or nodding.

ASSESSMENT

INTERPRETATION

Head flexion (retraction) and then cervical extension combination motion is also advocated by McKenzie to determine if repetition of the action 5 to 15 times, increases, decreases, centralizes, or peripheralizes (spreads) the pain.

All of the prime movers flatten the cervical vertebrae and are therefore very important in reducing cervical lordosis and supporting the cervical column at rest.

Limitation of head flexion of the occiput on the atlas (atlanto-occipital joint) is caused by an injury to the:

- articular capsules of the atlanto-occipital joint
- posterior atlanto-occipital ligament (membrane)
- posterior longitudinal ligament

Limitation or pain with flexion in the atlanto-axial joint is caused by an injury to the articular capsule of the atlanto-axial joint and the ligamentum flavum.

The membrane tectoria, the alar ligaments, and the ligamentum nuchae, which connect the axis with the occipital bone, become taut with head flexion and help to limit movement.

The head extensors, if strained, also cause pain when they are placed on stretch at the end of range. The overpressure helps determine the injured structure.

McKenzie's interpretation of the repeated test results include:

- pain that does not change is a dysfunction or postural problem
- pain that becomes more centralized or decreased is a derangement (IVD: intervertebral disc herniation) and this exercise will help correct the problem
- pain that becomes greater or moves down the upper limb indicates a derangement (IVD) and this motion should be avoided during the healing process

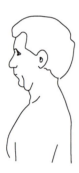

Fig. 2-38 Active head flexion.

Resisted Head Flexion

Apply pressure under the chin while the athlete tries to pull the chin toward the throat. Cup your hand under the athlete's mandible while standing behind him or her. Place the other hand on the back of the athlete's head to prevent the rebound effect. The athlete's teeth must be closed. This test may *not* be possible if the athlete has temporomandibular dysfunction.

Pain and/or weakness can occur from an injury to the muscle or its nerve supply (see Active Head Flexion).

The short neck flexor muscles often need strengthening if the athlete has poor postural habits and a constant excessive cervical lordosis position.

This also acts as a myotome test for the integrity of the C1 cervical spinal segment and its nerve roots.

Active Head Extension (Fig. 2-39)

Have the athlete tilt the head backward without neck movement (thrust the chin out).

Demonstrate this to the athlete.

Apply an overpressure if there is no pain and the range is not full.

As with forward bending and head flexion, the patient is seated and

This movement concentrates on the atlanto-occipital and the atlanto-axial joints, and is limited by the impact of the occipital condyles on the atlas.

The posterior arches of the atlas and axis are approximated.

During forced head extension, the posterior arch of the atlas can be compressed and fractured. Pain, weakness, or limitation of range of motion can be caused by the muscles or their nerve supply.

ASSESSMENT	INTERPRETATION

McKenzie repeats active head extension (protrusion) 5 to 15 times to determine what happens to the patient's pain and to determine the structure at fault. The patient is asked if there is more or less pain after the repetitions.

The prime movers of the atlanto-axial joint are:
- Rectus capitis posterior major—dorsal ramus of the first spinal nerve
- Obliquus capitis inferior—dorsal ramus of the first spinal nerve.

The prime movers of the atlanto-occipital joint are:
- Rectus capitis posterior major and minor—dorsal ramus of the first spinal nerve
- Obliquus capitis superior—dorsal ramus of the first spinal nerve
- Semispinalis capitis—dorsal rami of the cervical spinal nerves
- Splenius capitis—lateral branches of the dorsal rami of the middle cervical spinal nerves
- Trapezius (upper part)—spinal accessory nerve

Pain, weakness, or limitation of range of motion of the atlanto-occipital joint is caused by an injury to the anterior longitudinal ligament or the atlanto-occipital joint capsule.

Pain, weakness, or limitation of range of motion of the atlanto-axial joint is caused by an injury to the atlanto-axial capsule or the anterior longitudinal ligament. If the head flexor muscles are strained or contused this movement will cause pain also.

The interpretation of McKenzie repeat testing again determines if the problem is a derangement or dysfunction and if this repeated action will help or hinder the healing process.

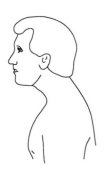

Fig. 2-39 Active head extension.

Resisted Head Extension

As the athlete attempts to poke the chin forward, cup the chin and resist this movement. Place the other hand on the back of the athlete's head. The athlete's teeth must be clenched.

Pain and/or weakness can occur from an injury to the muscle or its nerve supply (see Active Head Extension).

Active Cervical Rotation (70° to 90°) (Fig. 2-40)

Have the athlete turn the head as far as possible to the right and left with the chin slightly tucked.

Demonstrate this before conducting the test.

Compare the movement bilaterally.

McKenzie testing has the patient flex the head (retract the chin) then rotate toward the side of pain. The effect on the patient's symptoms are recorded. This same action is then repeated 5 to 15 times and the effects on the symptoms are recorded.

Normally, during rotation, the chin does not quite reach the frontal plane of the shoulder. Usually the first 45° of axial rotation takes place at the atlanto-axial joint and the remainder occurs in the lower cervical spine. If there is an injury to the atlanto-axial joint the initial segment of rotation will cause pain. The rotation at the atlanto-occipital joint is negligible.

According to Grieve, during rotation to the left, the left inferior cervical articular facet glides backward and downward on the adjacent superior articular facets on the same side. The inferior facets of the opposite side glide forward and upward. Therefore there is approximation of the joints on the left with gapping on the right. There is side flexion to the left with left rotation.

ASSESSMENT

INTERPRETATION

If repetition has no effect, it may be necessary to have the patient add a manual overpressure to the motion and repeat it 5 to 15 times to determine what happens to the pain. This is then repeated in the opposite direction.

Rotation always occurs with some side bending because the cranium has to side bend to the opposite side to stay vertical during rotation.

Pain, weakness, or limitation of range can come from the prime movers or their nerve supply.

The prime movers for right cervical rotation are:

- Left sternocleidomastoid—spinal accessory (C2, C3)
- Left trapezius (upper fibers)—spinal accessory (C2, C3)
- Right splenius capitis—lateral branches of the dorsal rami of middle cervical nerves
- Right splenius cervicis—lateral branches of the dorsal rami of lower cervical nerves

The accessory movers are:

- Left scalenes
- Left transversospinalis
- Right obliquus capitis inferior
- Right rectus capitis posterior major
- Left obliquus capitis superior

For rotation of the atlanto-occipital to the right, the prime movers are:

- Left obliquus capitis superior
- Right obliquus capitis inferior
- Rectus posterior minor (returns the head to neutral)

For the atlanto-axial joint rotation to the right, the prime movers are the right capitis obliquus inferior, and the left rectus major will return the head to neutral.

Pain and/or limitation is caused by:

- opposite alar ligaments (connecting the occiput and axis)
- atlanto-occipital ligaments
- atlanto-axial articular capsule and ligaments
- injury to one of the rotator muscles on stretch

A cervical rotation overstretch injury that subluxes the facet joint will have a marked restriction of rotation to the affected side. The head will be rotated away and flexed to the opposite side. It is difficult to tell if a subluxation or dislocation has occurred and this must be referred for further consultation.

A dislocation will have severe discomfort. Nerve root tingling or shooting pain with active rotation can be the result of irritation of a spinal nerve or nerve root caused by:

- hypermobility of a cervical facet joint
- adhesions about the nerve
- subluxation of a facet joint

An audible and palpable click or snap during neck rotation can be caused by:

- a tendon over a boney prominence
- irregularity at the facet joint
- creation of negative pressure release in a facet joint

Because of the amount of axial rotation at C1-C2 the vertebral artery can cause some symptoms of vertigo, nausea, visual prob-

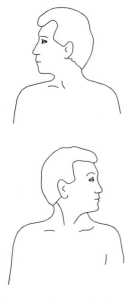

Fig. 2-40 Active cervical rotation.

ASSESSMENT

INTERPRETATION

lems, or tinnitus. This does not usually appear in the younger athlete, but can appear in the master athlete, with osteophytes from the facet joint projecting laterally or from their intervertebral joint.

Acute torticollis can cause a marked limitation in active cervical side bending toward the painful side and rotation away.

A cervical facet joint capsular pattern has equally limited side flexion and rotation, some or a great deal of limited back bending, and full forward bending.

Disc lesions can cause limitations in active rotation and side flexion to the same side while the other cervical movements may be full. A painful arc during rotation or side flexion can also occur with a disc lesion.

The interpretation for McKenzie retraction and rotation repeats are used to determine which actions decrease or centralize the pain from an intervertebral disc protrusion. The action that achieves this is used to help rehabilitate the patient. If the repeats do not change the pain at all, then McKenzie believes the cervical problem is a dysfunction (adaptively shortened or contracted soft tissue) or a postural problem.

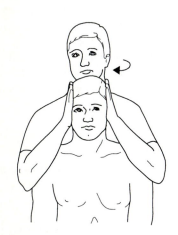

Fig. 2-41 Resisted cervical rotation.

Resisted Cervical Rotation (Fig. 2-41)

The athlete attempts to rotate the head. Apply resistance with one hand on each side of the athlete's head with your forearms and elbows over the athlete's trapezius muscles for stabilization. Be careful not to apply pressure on the mandible because this can aggravate the temporomandibular joint.

Do not allow any head movement—it must be a purely isometric contraction.

Pain and/or weakness is caused by an injury to the muscles or their nerve supply (see Active Cervical Rotation).

Cervical rotation is also a test for the C2 myotome.

Active Cervical Side Bending (lateral flexion, with overpressure, 20° to 45°) (Fig. 2-42)

The athlete tilts the head in an attempt to place the ear on one shoulder.

Repeat to the opposite side.

Rotation should not occur and the athlete should not lift the shoulder toward the ear.

Compare bilaterally.

If there is no pain or restriction an overpressure can be done.

McKenzie testing has the patient flex the head (retraction) first, then side bend as far as possible. The patient's symptoms are recorded. This same

About 8% of side bending occurs at the atlanto-occipital joint and a negligible amount occurs at the atlanto-axial joint. The remainder of the range occurs mainly in C2-C5, with a small amount in the lower cervical region. Side bending of C2-C6 is accompanied by rotation to the same side with backward gliding of the concave side facets.

Pain or limited side bending and rotation occurs if there is an injury to the:

- facet joint
- intervertebral disc
- sternocleidomastoid
- brachial plexus or cervical nerve roots
- fixed first rib
- upper costotransverse joints

ASSESSMENT

INTERPRETATION

motion is repeated 5 to 15 times, always returning to neutral. The effects on pain are recorded.

If the repetitions have no effect, the patient may be instructed to do a manual overpressure and repeat the motion 5 to 15 times. Side bending is then tested to the opposite side.

This movement is painful or limited along with cervical rotation and back bending if there is a capsular pattern (see conditions causing capsular pattern in Active Cervical Rotation).

Damage to the brachial plexus or cervical nerve roots may not cause limitation of range and pain but will cause transitory paresthesia, anesthesia, or decreased motor function (i.e., paralysis).

The facet joint injury causes pain when the neck is side bent to the injured side and rotated to that side.

Pain, weakness, or limitation of range can come from the muscles or their nerve supply.

The prime movers are:
- Sternocleidomastoid—CN 11 and ventral primary divisions of C2, C3, and the spinal accessory nerve
- Longissimus cervicis—dorsal rami of lower cervical spinal nerves
- Rectus capitis anterior—ventral rami of C1 and C2 spinal nerves
- Rectus capitis lateralis—ventral rami of C1 and C2 spinal nerves
- Scalenes (anterior, medius, posterior)—branches from the ventral rami of C3 to C8 cervical spinal nerves
- Trapezius—spinal accessory nerve and ventral rami of C3 and C4 cervical spinal nerves (multifidus, intertransversarii)

The accessory movers that cause extension, side bending, and ipsilateral rotation are:
- Levator scapulae
- Splenius cervicis
- Semispinalis capitis
- Semispinalis cervicis
- Erector spinae—the longissimus and iliocostocervicalis components

The interpretation of McKenzie repeats determine which motion helps improve an intervertebral disc derangement problem and which action will aggravate it. The motion that centralizes or decreases the pain is the motion to be added to the rehabilitation program. If the pain remains unchanged by the action, McKenzie believes the patient has a postural or dysfunctional problem, not an intervertebral disc protrusion.

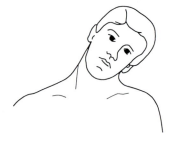

Fig. 2-42 Active cervical side bending.

Resisted Cervical Side Bending

Face the athlete and place your hands on each side of the athlete's head.

The athlete attempts side bending to each side.

Your forearms and elbows rest on the athlete's shoulder area.

Pain and/or weakness can occur from an injury to the muscle or to its nerve supply (see Active Cervical Side Bending).

This is a test for the C3 myotome.

Dysfunction of the costotransverse joint or the first rib on the involved side will cause pain on side bending to that side. The rib is pulled upward when the scalenes contract. Active and passive scapular elevation and shoulder flexion can also cause pain at the rib or costotransverse joint at the base of the neck.

ASSESSMENT

INTERPRETATION

Tests in Supine Position

Passive Head Flexion and Cervical Forward Bending (Fig. 2-43)

Cradle the athlete's head securely with both hands.

Move one hand down to palpate the spinous process of the second cervical vertebra while nodding the head forward.

The head is then brought into flexion as the other hand palpates for spinous process gapping.

The cervical region is forward bent slowly until pain or an end feel is reached.

Ensure that the cervical muscles are relaxed during the passive test.

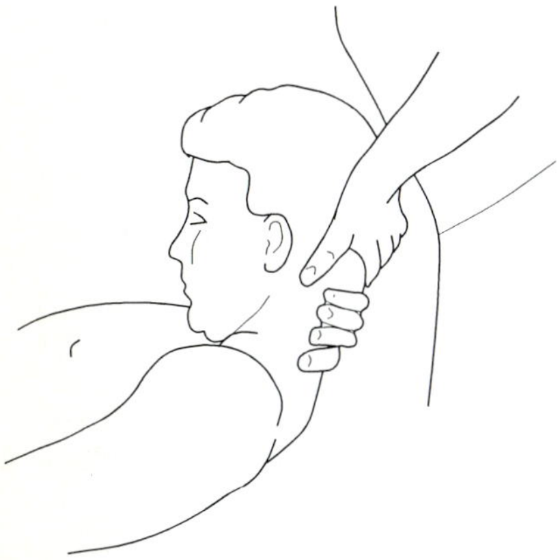

The passive head flexion tests movement initially between the occiput and the atlas and then the atlas and axis. Restriction is difficult to palpate for but if the athlete experiences pain with head flexion an injury here can be expected.

Any local muscle spasm or tenderness between the occiput and the axis can be palpated.

Pain or limitation of range at the atlanto-occipital joint is caused by an injury to the:
- atlanto-occipital capsule
- posterior atlanto-occipital ligament (membrane)
- posterior longitudinal ligament

Pain or limitation of range at the atlanto-axial joint is caused by an injury to the:
- atlanto-axial joint capsule
- alar ligaments
- ligamentum flavum (restricts head flexion between the axis and the occiput)

This area may be tense and point tender from poor postural head carriage, stress, or after prolonged bed rest for a concussion injury.

The majority of forward bending occurs in the middle cervical interspaces, especially between C5 and C6.

There will be point tenderness of the ligaments at the cervical segment with dysfunction.

Pain or limitation of range in the inferior cervical segment can be caused by an injury to the:
- posterior longitudinal ligament
- articular capsule of the involved cervical facet joint
- interspinous or supraspinous ligaments
- ligamentum flavum
- posterior neck muscles
- posterior fibers of the intervertebral disc of the cervical or thoracic vertebrae
- the posterior dural sleeve or dura mater of the cervical and thoracic levels
- meningeal irritation (i.e. meningitis)
- nerve root or spinal cord irritation

Painless limitation can be caused by osteoarthritis in the older patient.

Fig. 2-43 Passive head flexion and cervical forward bending.

Passive Cervical Rotation (Fig. 2-44)

Place hands on each side of the athlete's head. The athlete's head is rotated until pain or an end feel is reached. Palpate behind the mastoid process with the index fingers during the head

When the neck ligaments are sprained by a rotational force the neck musculature spasms to flex and turn the head away from the injured site. Reenacting the over-rotation with a passive stretch will cause pain.

Gross limitation of passive movements in the athlete with an

ASSESSMENT

rotation. The left transverse process moves toward the left mastoid process with right rotation and vice versa.

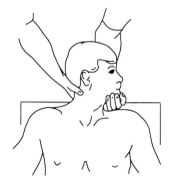

Fig. 2-44 Passive cervical rotation.

Passive Cervical Side Bending (Fig. 2-45)

Place one hand under the athlete's head while the other hand palpates the transverse processes on each side. Rock the head from side to side while palpating for gapping of the transverse processes on one side and closing of the transverse process on the compressed side. Take the head into full side bending until an end feel is reached.

INTERPRETATION

early bone-on-bone end feel in rotation and side flexion can be caused by ankylosing spondylitis.

Limitation in the elderly patient is often due to osteoarthritic changes.

The amount of passive rotation is also determined by the torsional deformity of the intervertebral disc.

Although there is only a small amount of torsional deformity between two cervical vertebrae, there is quite a bit along the entire length of the cervical column. An equal limitation of rotation and side bending and some (or a great deal of) limitation of back bending indicates a capsular pattern, as previously mentioned.

The most limitation of rotation is caused by an osteoarthrosis of C1 and C2.

A cervical facet joint problem will cause discomfort at the passive end of range with rotation (and side bending) to the involved side.

As with active cervical rotation, overpressure limitation or pain can come from an injury to the:
- opposite alar ligament (connecting the occiput and axis)
- atlanto-occipital ligaments
- atlanto-axial capsule and ligaments
- rotator muscles on stretch
- facet joint on the restricted side
- nerve root
- vertebral artery
- intervertebral disc

As with active side bending with overpressure, the movement will be painful, weak, or limited in range of motion with an injury to the:
- facet joint (on the involved side)
- intervertebral disc
- side bending muscles on stretch
- brachial or cervical plexus on stretch

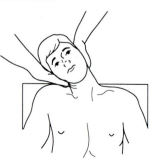

Fig. 2-45 Passive cervical side bending.

ASSESSMENT   INTERPRETATION

SPECIAL TESTS

Vertebral Artery Test

An athlete with vertigo, giddiness, syncope, disequilibrium, nausea, tinnitus, drop attacks, vision problems, or blackouts in his or her history may have a problem with the vertebral artery, and this test can help determine if it is an inner ear or vertebrobasilar arterial insufficiency.

These tests will help detect any deficiency in the circulation through the vertebral artery in the atlanto-axial region (Fig. 2-46). The artery can be damaged or occluded here because of the stretch placed on it from the amount of rotation of the axis on the atlas (Fig. 2-47). This also tests the vertebral artery as it courses between the 6th and 7th cervical vertebrae. Rotation may impair blood flow in the ipsilateral side. This special test should be done first, since several other tests can not be done if this is positive.

If the history and observations of the athlete indicate a vertebral artery occlusion, this test should be done before the functional test.

Because of the dangerous implications of vertebral artery occlusion, if the results are positive, the athlete should be sent for further medical evaluation with a qualified physician or specialist in this area of expertise. *No further testing should be done.*

This test may be positive in the elderly athlete with arteriosclerosis, cervical spondylosis, arthrosis, atheroma of vertebral arteries, or significant osteoarthritic changes in the cervical spine.

It may also be positive in the young athlete with a history of rheumatoid arthritis because of the possibility of the subluxation of the atlas.

The vertebral artery can be occluded in other ways. In some individuals the vertebral artery is abnormal and originates from the posterior aspect of the subclavian artery. As a result it gets kinked and occludes during cervical rotation.

Deep bands of cervical fascia can also occlude the artery during rotation.

External projecting osteophytes from the uncovertebral joints, usually at the C5-C6, can also occlude the vertebral artery during rotation.

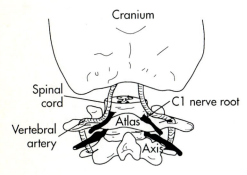

Fig. 2-46 Posterior aspect of the cervical spine. Vertebral artery through the foramen of the atlas.

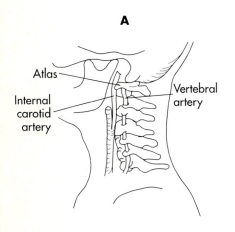

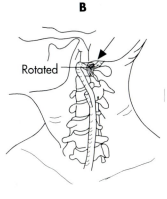

Fig. 2-47 A, Lateral view of cervical spine and of the vertebral artery. **B,** Cervical rotation and vertebral artery relationship.

ASSESSMENT

INTERPRETATION

If the test produces tingling into the arm, nerve root occlusion is suggested.

Test 1

The athlete stands with eyes closed, shoulders flexed to 90°, and the arms extended.

Ask the athlete to rotate the head to one side and hold it for a minute. The outstretched arms are observed for any movement. The head is turned in the opposite direction and held for a minute also.

Swaying of the arms away from the parallel, or if one arm drops lower than the other, suggests cerebellar ischemia.

Test 2

Part 1

With the athlete in supine lying, the therapist takes the athlete's head in both hands and brings the neck into full back bending and right rotation. This is held for 30 seconds.

The eyes are observed for nystagmus (jittering of the pupils), and the sensations felt by the athlete are recorded (i.e., vertigo, nausea). Repeat with back bending and left rotation.

If a positive response is noted, smoothly and quickly return the head to neutral.

Any nystagmus or shaking of the eyes suggests a vertebral artery problem or an inner ear problem (semicircular canals). Repeating the test with the head held allows you to rule out an inner ear problem. If dizziness or nystagmus continues when the head is held, the vertebral artery is at fault because no fluid is moving in the semicircular canals when the head is held. No traction or manipulations should be done on any athlete with vertebral artery deficiencies.

Part 2

With the athlete in the sitting position, hold the athlete's head to keep it from moving. The athlete is then instructed to turn the body to one side and then the other side. Watch the eyes and have the athlete comment on his or her feelings during the test.

Quadrant Test

This test is done when there is no pain with the active and passive cervical movements, yet you suspect a facet injury. These tests should not be done if the vertebral artery test has proven positive.

A localized facet or joint restriction will cause pain on the involved side during this test. If the test causes a reproduction of the arm or shoulder referred pain, this confirms a nerve root irritation. The upper quadrant procedure tests the upper cervical joints, and the lower quadrant procedure tests the lower cervical facets. The atlanto-occipital and atlanto-axial joints do not have facet joints, therefore the upper quadrant test determines if these joints have restrictive patterns.

ASSESSMENT

INTERPRETATION

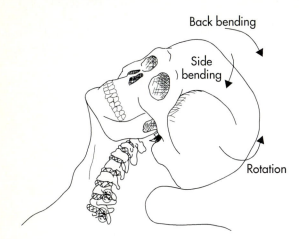

Fig. 2-48 Lower quadrant test.

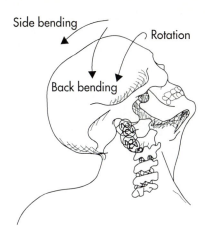

Fig. 2-49 Upper quadrant test.

Lower Quadrant (Fig. 2-48)

With the athlete in the supine position, passively back bend, then side bend and rotate the head in the same direction. Test one side and then the other side.

Upper Quadrant (Fig. 2-49)

Passively back bend, then side bend the head as above, but rotate to the opposite side. Test one side and then the other side.

Traction Test

With athlete in the supine position, apply traction with one hand under the occiput and the other hand under the mandible. If there is a temporomandibular joint problem the hand must be positioned on either side of the head rather than under the mandible.

This traction test should be done only after the vertebral artery test has proved negative.

The athlete must close the teeth.

The traction is applied gently and the athlete is told to raise the hand if any pain occurs during the traction.

This test will open the joint space and the neural foramen, which may relieve pain in the joint capsule of the facet joints.

It may alleviate the pressure of the intervertebral disc protrusion, which may reduce the nerve root pain.

It helps to reduce the muscle spasm in the area and promote muscle relaxation.

The test may cause pain in the athlete with joint hypermobility or after a cervical ligament sprain.

If traction relieves the pain, this may be an important component for cervical rehabilitation.

ASSESSMENT   INTERPRETATION

This test is done in neutral to assess the upper cervical spine, then repeated with gradual cervical forward bending of 20° to 30°.

The midcervical, lower cervical, and upper thoracic spine can all be evaluated in the forward bent position. Approximately 20° forward bending tests the midcervical spine. Approximately 20° to 35° forward bending tests the lower cervical and upper thoracic spine.

Compression Test

This compression test should be done only if the vertebral artery test was negative.

Method 1

With the athlete in a supine position, gently press the head down caudally. Ask the athlete if there is any local referred pain and, if so, to describe it.

If the compression causes pain in the cervical spine the pain may come from a facet joint or between the transverse or spinous processes. This compression narrows the neural foramen.

If the compression causes referred pain into the shoulder or down the arm, a nerve root problem and specific dermatomes can be determined.

Nerve root problems can come from an intervertebral disc herniation, facet joint dysfunction, or uncovertebral joint osteophyte impingement.

Method 2 (Foramen Compression Test)

The athlete side bends toward the pain-free side while the therapist presses down on the head.

When the head is compressed in a bent position, pain that radiates into the arm indicates pressure on the nerve root on that side.

Valsalva Test

The athlete is asked to hold his breath and bear down as though having a bowel movement.

The athlete is asked if there is any local or referred pain and if so to describe it.

This test increases the cerebral spinal fluid pressure and venous pressure (intrathecal pressure).

The pressure problem is caused by a space occupying lesion. This can be:
- intervertebral disc lesion
- tumor
- an osteophyte

This test can cause pain that may radiate along a specific dermatome.

ASSESSMENT   INTERPRETATION

Swallowing Test

Ask the athlete to swallow several times.

Difficulty or pain during swallowing can be caused by:
- central anterior intervertebral disc herniation
- a boney osteophyte
- tumor or infection to the soft tissue
- hematoma following a direct blow

Upper Limb or Brachial Tension Test (Elvey) (Fig. 2-50)

This is a progressive test and the order is very important. The athlete's pain should be assessed in each position before the next joint movement is added. If the athlete's symptoms are reproduced in any position, determine the damaged structures. There is no need to progress.

This test is important to determine if nerve tension is causing the cervical, shoulder, or upper limb symptoms. When the history indicates shoulder pain, it may be difficult to determine whether the origin of pain is from the cervical spine, shoulder joint, or myofascial trigger points. This test tells the therapist that it is from a neural origin (especially C5-C7 nerve roots).

This is a progressive test and is done to place tension on the cervical nerve roots, nerve root sheaths, and the brachial plexus.

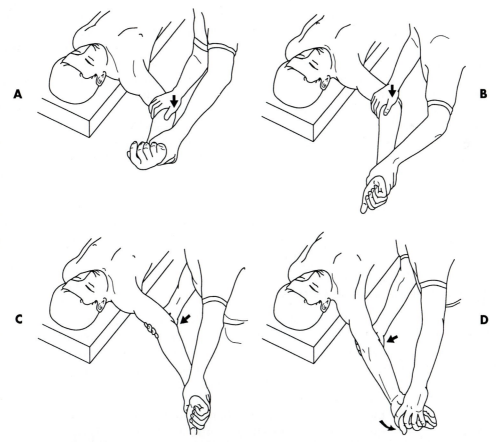

Fig. 2-50 Upper limb or brachial tension test (ULTT) (Elvey). **A,** Shoulder component. **B,** Forearm component. **C,** Elbow component. **D,** Wrist and hand component.

ASSESSMENT

INTERPRETATION

The athlete is in a supine position with the head in a neutral position. With the shoulder extended about 10°, abduct the arm in the frontal plane (usually 110° to 130°) to the point of full stretch. Then adduct the arm slightly until the shoulder is pain free. Then externally rotate the glenohumeral joint (approximately 60°) to the point of pain (the elbow is flexed) (Fig. 2-50, *A*). Next, internally rotate the glenohumeral joint slightly until the shoulder is pain free.

If there is no reproduction of symptoms, supinate the forearm (do not allow shoulder elevation) (Fig. 2-50, *B*) and then extend the elbow slowly (Fig. 2-50, *C*). Stabilize the shoulder to prevent shoulder girdle elevation. If there is no reproduction of symptoms, the wrist and fingers are extended while maintaining supination and elbow extension (Fig. 2-50, *D*). The athlete extends the joints actively. Then you can apply a gentle overpressure if the active movement was pain free. With the wrist and finger extension maintained, release the elbow and allow it to flex. Note any changes in the symptoms as the neural tension is released.

If there is any brachial plexus or nerve root injury, this test will be painful.

When the test is begun at the shoulder, tension or pain can initially come from the thoracic outlet, especially with a first rib syndrome or cervical rib. When the lower brachial nerve roots are affected, ulnar arm and hand symptoms are reproduced.

Shoulder instability from a previous dislocation can cause apprehension or pain in the externally rotated position; therefore take the tension off the glenohumeral joint by allowing a slight degree of internal rotation. The athlete should feel only an anterior shoulder joint stretch. If the athlete feels shoulder pain, it is likely from the cervical spine or brachial plexus, not the shoulder joint, since the joint is no longer stressed.

If the athlete is pain free, the forearm is supinated and the elbow is gently extended. Determine if there are any shoulder or arm symptoms. The athlete should feel an anterior elbow joint stretch and still some anterior shoulder stretch. If the athlete feels shoulder pain or is unable to fully extend the elbow, cervical or brachial nerve root pathology may be causing the discomfort and inhibiting elbow range. When you conduct an elbow assessment, the elbow range will be full.

The elbow will only show this restriction in the upper limb tension test position.

If the athlete is symptom free, the wrist and finger extension is added next. Determine if there is any shoulder or upper limb referred pain during the joint extension. The athlete should feel a deep ache or stretch in the elbow, forearm, and hand. There can also be some tingling in the thumb or fingers. This is normal—but this test sequence should not cause any shoulder pain, just a mild stretch sensation in the anterior shoulder region. The athlete is able to determine if this test reproduces his or her shoulder or brachial plexus pain. If it does, this pain is coming from the cervical nerve roots or the brachial plexus.

The pain should abate as the elbow is flexed, since the neural tension has been released.

Slump Test (Neuromeningeal Tension Test) (Fig. 2-51)

The athlete is high sitting with the arms behind the back. The athlete flexes the thoracic spine (slump) and the therapist holds this position with their forearm (Fig. 2-51, *A*). The athlete is then asked to forward bend the cervical region as far as possible and the therapist maintains this position with their hand (Fig. 2-51, *B*). You can apply an overpressure if the movement is pain free. Then ask the athlete to extend the knee as far as possible while the cervical

This test determines the mobility of the pain-sensitive neuromeningeal structures in the vertebral canal and/or intervertebral foramen down the entire length of the spinal canal. The athlete will indicate where pain or symptoms are felt. This test becomes important when cervical neural impingement is suspected (intervertebral disc herniation, dural sleeve adhesions, meningeal inflammation). If pain disappears when the neck is extended, it confirms that the pain stems from a neuromeningeal structure.

ASSESSMENT

INTERPRETATION

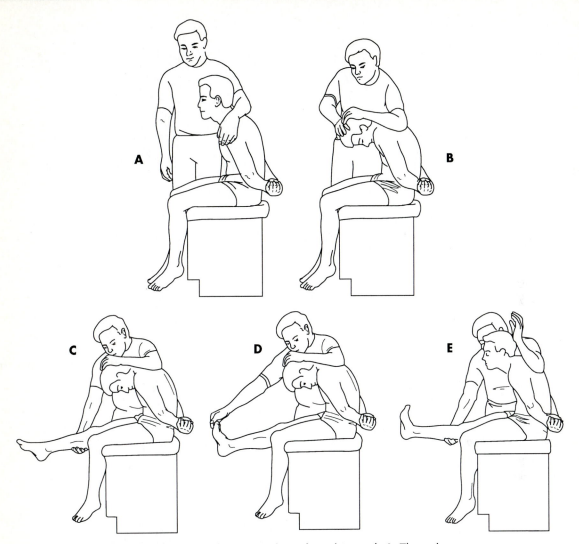

Fig. 2-51 Slump test (neuromeningeal tension test). **A,** Thoracic spine component. **B,** Cervical spine component. **C,** Knee component. **D,** Ankle component. **E,** Release of cervical forward bending.

and thoracic forward bent position is maintained (Fig. 2-51, *C*). Next, ask the athlete to dorsiflex the ankle joint as far as possible (Fig. 2-51, *D*). Apply an overpressure if this is pain free. Release the cervical spine flexion and record if the symptoms change (Fig. 2-51, *E*).

Myotome Testing (Fig. 2-52)

The muscles of the neck and upper limb are innervated by one or more seg-

Any muscle or muscle group weakness during the testing suggests trauma to the spinal cord or its nerve roots.

ASSESSMENT   INTERPRETATION

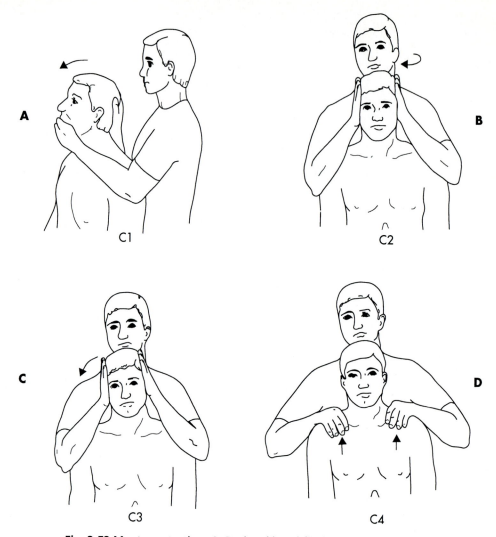

Fig. 2-52 Myotome testing. **A,** Resisted head flexion. **B,** Resisted cervical rotation. **C,** Resisted cervical side bending. **D,** Resisted shoulder elevation.

ments of the spinal cord. By testing muscular movements, you can determine which cervical segment or motor nerve root supplying the muscles is damaged.

There are several differences of opinion on certain muscle innervation, and several muscles are innervated by more than one cervical segment.

The myotomes are tested by resisting the muscle or muscle group that is served by each cervical spinal level. The athlete contracts the muscles being test-

The spinal cord injuries may affect several spinal levels with gross movement limitations. All the nerve segments below the lesion site will be affected.

Damage to the individual cervical roots can be caused by a facet impingement, a boney spur, direct trauma, an overstretch, or irritation from a herniated intervertebral disc.

The first cervical root emerges between the occiput and the atlas, and the eighth root emerges between the seventh cervical and first thoracic vertebrae. If an intervertebral disc herniates, it will usually affect the nerve root below (i.e., C6 herniation affects C7 nerve root). Herniated discs are usually unilateral and only affect one side of the athlete, but the protrusion on occasion can be central and affect both sides. There are usually sensory

ASSESSMENT

INTERPRETATION

ed isometrically while you resist the movement, where possible. The test is done bilaterally and is compared for equal strength.

changes from a herniation but there can be motor function changes only, or both sensory and motor changes.

C1 Spinal Segment Test—Resisted Head Flexion (Fig. 2-52, A)

The athlete attempts head flexion against the therapist's resistance under the chin (see Resisted Head Flexion).

This maneuver resists the short flexors of the neck:
- Rectus capitis lateralis—ventral rami C1, C2 spinal nerves
- Rectus capitis anterior—ventral rami C1, C2 spinal nerves
- Longus capitis—ventral rami C1, C2, C3 spinal nerves
- Infrahyoid—C1, C2, C3

C2 Spinal Segment Test—Resisted Cervical Rotation (Fig. 2-52, B)

Resist the athlete's rotation (see Resisted Cervical Rotation). Test both right and left rotation.

This tests the cervical rotators supplied mainly by C2:
- Longus capitis—ventral rami C1, C2, C3
- Sternocleidomastoid—spinal accessory C2, C3

Cervical nerve root pressure at C1 and C2 is caused by osteoarthrosis at the atlanto-axial joint with an osteophyte against the C2 root.

C3 Spinal Segment Test— Resisted Cervical Side Bending (Fig. 2-52, C)

See Resisted Cervical Side Bending in functional testing section.
Test bilaterally.

This tests the cervical side benders supplied mainly by C3:
- Trapezius—accessory nerve and ventral rami C3, C4
- Longus capitis—ventral rami C1, C2, C3
- Longus cervicis— dorsal rami C2-C6

The third cervical root pressure is rarely affected.

C4 Spinal Segment Test—Resisted Shoulder Elevation (Fig. 2-52, D)

Attempt to depress the shoulders while positioning yourself over the athlete. The athlete elevates the shoulders and attempts to hold them up.

Put pressure over the diaphragm to determine its tonus as an alternative test while the athlete attempts to depress the diaphragm.

This tests the shoulder elevators supplied mainly by C4:
- Trapezius—accessory and ventral rami C3, C4
- levator scapulae—C3, C4

The fourth cervical root pressure is rare.
This tests the diaphragm muscle as well (C3, C4, C5)

C5 Spinal Segment Test—Resisted Shoulder Abduction

Resist the athlete's shoulder abduction. The athlete abducts and holds the arms up while the therapist attempts to push them down.

This tests the shoulder abductors supplied mainly by C5:
- Deltoid—axillary nerve C5, C6
- Supraspinatus—suprascapular nerve C4, C5, C6
- Infraspinatus, teres minor, rhomboids, biceps

The fifth cervical root pressure comes from:
- intervertebral disc herniation
- traction palsy of this root—brachial plexus stretch
- facet impingement

C6 Spinal Segment Test—Resisted Elbow Flexion (see Fig. 4-26)

Resist elbow flexion in midrange and/or wrist extension.

This tests the elbow flexors supplied mainly by C6:
- Biceps brachii—musculocutaneous nerve C5, C6

ASSESSMENT

INTERPRETATION

This is done and compared bilaterally.

- Brachialis—musculocutaneous nerve C5, C6, and radial nerve C7
- Brachioradialis—radial nerve C5, C6, C7

The wrist extensors supplied mainly by C6:
- Extensor carpi radialis longus and brevis
- Extensor digitorum
- Extensor digiti minimi
- Extensor carpi ulnaris
- Extensor pollicis brevis and longus
- Extensor indicis

The sixth cervical root pressure comes from:
- intervertebral disc herniation
- a cervical rib
- a brachial plexus stretch
- a facet impingement

C7 Spinal Segment Test—Resisted Elbow Extension (see Fig. 4-28)

Resist elbow extension in midrange bilaterally and/or wrist flexion if a C7 problem is suspected. If one group is weak, test the other to confirm nerve root involvement.

This tests the elbow extensors supplied mainly by C7:
- Triceps—radial nerve C6, C7, C8
- Anconeus—radial nerve C7, C8, T1

Wrist flexors supplied mainly by C7:
- Pronator teres
- Flexor carpi radialis longus and brevis
- Palmaris longus
- Flexor digitorum superficialis
- Flexor pollicis brevis

The seventh cervical root pressure is the most common root affected by a herniated disc or a facet impingement. The triceps will definitely be weak and if there is prolonged pressure, atrophy of pectoralis major may be visible.

C8 Spinal Segment—Resisted Thumb Extension

Resist thumb extension and/or the wrist ulnar deviators bilaterally. If weakness is found in one muscle group, confirm nerve root involvement with testing the other muscle group.

This tests the thumb extensors supplied mainly by C8:
- Extensor pollicis longus—posterior interosseous C7, C8
- Extensor pollicis brevis—posterior interosseous C7, C8

This tests the ulnar deviators supplied mainly by C8:
- Extensor carpi ulnaris—posterior interosseous C7, C8
- Flexor carpi ulnaris—ulnar nerve C7, C8

The eighth cervical root compression can come from:
- a cervical rib
- traction palsy of the lower brachial plexus
- an intervertebral disc lesion
- a fractured clavicle
- aneurysm of the arch of the aorta
- disease of the pulmonary apex

T1 Spinal Segment Test—Resisted Finger Abduction

Resist finger abduction by having the athlete splay the fingers while you

This tests the muscles mainly supplied by T1:
- Abductor pollicis brevis—median nerve C8 and T1

ASSESSMENT

INTERPRETATION

resist them two at a time bilaterally.

You can also resist finger adduction because most of the hand intrinsics are supplied by T1.

- Abductor digiti minimi—ulnar nerve C8 and T1
- Dorsal interossei—ulnar nerve C8 and T1

The first thoracic root compression comes from:
- disc herniation (rare)
- a cervical rib
- a fractured clavicle
- brachial plexus stretch

Dermatome Testing (Fig. 2-53)

The dermatome is an area of skin supplied by one spinal segment. There is considerable overlap between these segments, and researchers vary slightly in their sensory field mapping.

Use a safety pin and touch the skin surface while the athlete looks away or closes the eyes. The athlete reports where the pin prick is felt and if it is sharp or dull. Use the point or broad side of the pin and touch the dermatomes. Several points in each dermatome should be tested (approximately eight). The tests should be done bilaterally, testing and comparing dermatomes on each side (i.e., touch deltoid area C5 on right side, then on the left side, while the athlete reports and compares sensations). The dermatome, if affected, can be further tested with hot and cold test tubes or a cotton ball along the involved dermatome(s).

An area of numbness that follows a dermatome pattern supplied by one spinal nerve indicates a spinal nerve irritation. Because the dermatomes overlap and because of individual dermatome variations, the area of anesthesia, paresthesia, or hyperesthesia can vary. Altered sensation in a dermatome area can be affected by:
- herniated intervertebral disc (affects level below)
- nerve root irritation or neuritis
- traction or contusion to the nerve trunk, root, or brachial plexus
- a thoracic outlet problem
- cervical spondylosis or osteoarthritis

If the area of numbness follows a peripheral nerve, it indicates that there is a peripheral nerve entrapment or injury. If the area of decreased sensation goes around the circumference of the limb, this indicates a sensory nerve deficit resulting from a vascular insufficiency.

Pain that follows a dermatome, myotome, or sclerotome pattern does not always indicate a nerve root or peripheral nerve problem. It can be referred from muscles, joints, ligaments, or other structures supplied by the same spinal nerve level.

True nerve root pain (radicular pain) is of a sharper nature and there will be changes in muscle strength (myotome) and/or reflexes at the involved spinal segmental level or levels.

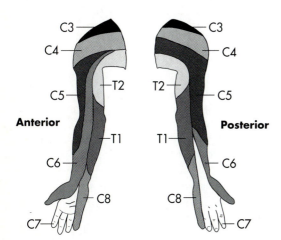

Fig. 2-53 Dermatomes of the upper limb.

ASSESSMENT

INTERPRETATION

Alterations in sensations and pain from somatic structures other than the nerve root will have dull, achy pain, and there will be no alterations in myotomes or reflexes.

If you can determine the cervical spine level of the nerve root problem through dermatome testing, this is very valuable for determining the condition and for determining the best rehabilitation.

Cutaneous Nerve Testing

Test the skin areas with a pin as described previously, but prick the skin in the cutaneous skin supply regions (see Fig. 3-50).

- test C1—no cutaneous branches
- test C2—vertex temple, forehead, occiput, lower mandible, chin, lateral side of head and ear
- test C3—back of the neck and scalp, side of the neck, and down to the first rib
- test C4—back of neck, side of the neck, clavicle and over the acromion, first intercostal space
- test C5—lower shoulder, radial arm, and forearm
- test C6—central portion of the anterior upper arm and forearm, radial side of forearm and thumb
- test C7—central portion of the dorsal forearm, palm, and middle three fingers
- test C8—ulnar border of lower forearm, wrist, and hand (fifth finger)
- test T1—ulnar side of the forearm and a bit of the upper arm
- test T2—inner side of axilla, pectoral, and midscapular areas

Reflex Testing

Reflex testing should be done when there is a sensory (dermatome) or muscle (myotome) deficit and/or if a neurological problem is indicated.

An excessive response (hyperactive) reflex usually indicates an upper motor disorder or lesion (cardiovascular attack, stroke).

A sluggish or hypoactive reflex indicates there is an impingement, entrapment, or injury of a lower motor nerve (spinal or peripheral nerve).

Normal reflexes vary in each individual so they must be compared bilaterally to determine the individual's norm.

ASSESSMENT

INTERPRETATION

Biceps Reflex (C5) (Fig. 2-54)

The athlete's forearm is placed over your forearm so that the biceps is relaxed. Your thumb is placed over the biceps tendon in the cubital fossa (flex elbow with resistance to ensure you are over the tendon). Tap the thumb with a reflex hammer. The biceps should jerk slightly. Repeat six successive times.

An equal reflex bilaterally indicates that the C5 neurological level is normal.

A hypoactive reflex could indicate:
- fifth cervical root impingement or traction palsy
- herniated intervertebral disc C4
- musculocutaneous nerve injury

Brachioradialis Reflex (C6) (Fig. 2-55, A)

Support the athlete's forearm in a neutral position. Using the flat edge of the reflex hammer, tap the brachioradialis tendon at the distal end of the radius. Repeat six successive times.

The muscle should contract and the wrist jerks.

A hypoactive reflex can indicate:
- sixth cervical nerve root impingement or traction palsy
- radial nerve injury
- cervical rib or other thoracic outlet neurological problem

Triceps Reflex (C7) (Fig. 2-55, B)

With the athlete's forearm in a pronated position, tap the triceps tendon where it crosses the olecranon fossa with the reflex hammer. You should see or feel a slight jerk. Repeat six successive times.

C7 nerve root is the most common root impinged, yet the triceps jerk is rarely affected even though the triceps muscle is weakened.

The triceps reflex can be hypoactive from a:
- C7 nerve root problem
- radial nerve injury
- thoracic outlet neurological problem

PALPATIONS

Palpate boney and soft tissue for point tenderness, temperature differences, swelling, adhesions, calcium

According to Janet Travell, myofascial trigger points in muscle are activated directly by overuse, overload, trauma, or chilling and are activated indirectly by visceral disease, other trigger points, arthritic joints, or emotional distress.

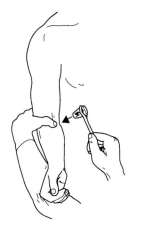

Fig. 2-54 Biceps reflex (C5).

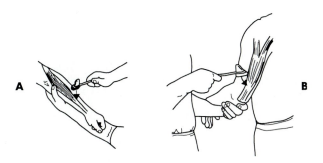

Fig. 2-55 A, Brachioradialis reflex (C6). **B,** Triceps reflex (C7).

ASSESSMENT

INTERPRETATION

deposits, muscle spasms, and muscle tears.

Palpate for muscle tenderness, lesions, and trigger points.

Palpate the cervical region with the athlete in a supine position with the head supported on a pillow.

The athlete must be relaxed.

Myofascial pain is referred from trigger points that have patterns and locations for each muscle. Trigger points are hyperactive taut bands in a skeletal muscle or the muscle's fascia that are acutely tender on palpation and evoke a muscle twitch. These points can evoke autonomic responses (i.e., sweating, pilomotor activity, local vasoconstriction).

The cervical musculature is very important in orienting the head and body in space. These muscles are highly innervated and receptive to changes in proprioception of the head in relation to the body.

Anterior Aspect (Fig. 2-56)

Boney
Thyroid Cartilage, Hyoid Bone, Trachea, and C6 Carotid Tubercle

The thyroid cartilage, hyoid bone, or trachea can be fractured, although this is uncommon in athletics. Because of the possibility of respiratory problems, significant trauma with point tenderness or problems in breathing or swallowing should be referred to a trained laryngologist as soon as possible.

The hyoid bone is a horseshoe-shaped bone at the level of approximately C3. Palpate the bone gently with the thumb and finger. With swallowing, the hyoid moves.

The hyoid cartilage is below the hyoid bone, level with approximately C4-C5. This cartilage, called the "Adam's Apple," moves with swallowing also.

The first tracheal ring is below the thyroid cartilage at the level of C6. This ring is an important part of the trachea and must be palpated gently to avoid a gag response.

Lateral to the tracheal ring is the carotid tubercle of C6 transverse process. The carotid pulse can be felt in this area.

Cervical Rib

A cervical rib that can lead to thoracic outlet problems may be palpable in the fossa above the clavicle at the base of the neck.

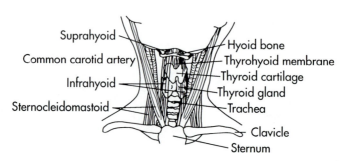

Suprahyoid — Hyoid bone
Common carotid artery — Thyrohyoid membrane
— Thyroid cartilage
Infrahyoid — Thyroid gland
Sternocleidomastoid — Trachea
— Clavicle
— Sternum

Fig. 2-56 Anterior aspect of the neck.

ASSESSMENT

INTERPRETATION

Soft Tissue
Sternocleidomastoid

The sternocleidomastoid can spasm on one side, causing a torticollis deformity. Palpate the full length of the muscle for swelling or defects. Both sides go into reflex spasm following a whiplash or a significant hyperextension or side flexion mechanism.

There are myofascial trigger points in the sternal and clavicular portions of the sternocleidomastoid muscle. Active trigger points are found along the length of the sternal portion of the muscle and refer pain around the eye and into the occipital region of the head, auditory canal, and even the throat (during swallowing). Active trigger points in the deeper clavicular portion refer pain to the frontal area, ear, cheek, and molar teeth.

Platysma Muscle

The myofascial trigger points for the platysma muscle are usually in front of the sternocleidomastoid muscle and refer a prickling pain to the skin below the mandible.

Anterior Vertebral Muscles

The anterior vertebral muscles, the suprahyoid and infrahyoid, can be palpated for point tenderness.

Suprahyoid and Infrahyoid Muscles

The suprahyoid muscles, according to Yanda, tend toward shortening when a forward head posture is assumed or just gradually with time. Palpate the suprahyoid muscles (digastric, stylohyoid, geniohyoid, and mylohyoid muscles) for tightness and trigger points.

Lengthening of the antagonists, the infrahyoid muscles, also occurs with time. They consist of the sternohyoid, sternothyroid, thyrohyoid, and omohyoid muscles. Palpate the infrahyoids for lack of tonus and trigger points.

This muscle imbalance will result in an elevated hyoid bone.

Parotid Gland

The parotid gland is about 5 cm in length. It runs under the upper border of the mandibular condyle in line with the masseter muscle and extends backward toward the ear. With infection or mumps the gland enlarges and becomes point tender.

Submandibular Gland

The submandibular gland is irregular in form and about the size of a walnut. It is located under the mandible at the angle of the jaw. With infection this gland can be enlarged, particularly with throat and upper respiratory infections.

ASSESSMENT   INTERPRETATION

Submandibular and Cervical Lymph Nodes

Infection can also cause enlargement of the submandibular and cervical lymph nodes under the mandible and anterior to the sternocleidomastoid. Because of its location the sternocleidomastoid can go into spasm unilaterally or bilaterally if there is an infection.

Carotid Pulse and Peripheral Pulses

The carotid pulse can be palpated between the trachea and sternocleidomastoid and compared bilaterally.

The peripheral pulses (ulnar and radial) can have altered blood flow on one side if the subclavian artery is compressed in the thoracic outlet. Compare the pulses bilaterally.

Posterior Aspect

The posterior structures can be palpated in prone lying, if the athlete supports the forehead with his or her hands and the muscles are relaxed in that position.

Alternatively, the athlete's posterior neck structures can be palpated in supine lying while you compress the pillow supporting the athlete's head.

Boney
External Occipital Protuberance, or Inion

The external occipital protuberance, or inion, is a bump in the midline of the occipital region on the center of the nuchal line. It acts as a reference for the center of the skull.

Superior Cervical Segment

Palpate the axis spinous and transverse processes to determine their depth and prominence and to determine if there is rotation of the axis on the atlas. Palpate the facet joints for point tenderness suggesting dysfunction.

Inferior Cervical Segment

A prominent C3 spinous process frequently is associated with headaches. A prominent C4 spinous process is often associated with midcervical dysfunction. The C5, C6, C7 spinous processes or facet joints may be point tender, since these segmental levels have the most mobility and dysfunction.

ASSESSMENT

INTERPRETATION

Spinous Processes

The spinous processes from C2 to C7 are palpable (C1 is not palpable). The spinous processes should all be in good alignment with one another. Any deviation or rotation of a process should be recorded.

Deviations in alignment can be caused by:
- unilateral facet joint dislocation
- cervical joint dislocation or rotation
- a fractured spinous process
- muscle spasm
- developmental anomaly

Gentle posterior anterior oscillatory pressure (PAs) on each spinous process helps to determine the mobility at each level and whether pain is elicited with palpation. Pain is often experienced at the cervical segment that has dysfunction.

Gentle transverse oscillatory pressures against the lateral aspect of the spinous process can also be performed to determine pain and level of dysfunction. These pressures may reproduce the athlete's symptoms when they are applied to the cervical level of dysfunction.

Transverse Processes

Gentle posterior anterior oscillatory pressures (PAs) and transverse oscillatory pressures can be applied to the tip of the transverse processes as well. These are done to reproduce the athlete's symptoms or pain and determine the cervical level that is in dysfunction. The amount of mobility of each segment should also be determined.

Facet Joints

These joints can be palpated more individually by side bending the neck to each side gently while palpating.

The facet joints are about 1 inch lateral from the spinous process on each side. Palpate these joints for point tenderness. Point tenderness can be caused by:
- facet sprain
- facet unilateral dislocation or subluxation
- osteoarthritic changes in the facet joint
- a facet joint impingement problem

Soft Tissue (Fig. 2-57)
Trapezius

The trapezius muscle runs from the external occipital protuberance down to T12 and is divided into upper, middle, and lower fibers. Palpate the muscle for spasm or point tenderness.

Overstretch in forward bending can injure the muscle.

Significant neck trauma will cause the muscle to spasm to protect and splint the cervical spine.

The upper fibers of the trapezius muscle tend to develop tightness with cervical injury and poor posture. The middle and lower trapezius muscle fibers tend to develop weakness and

ASSESSMENT   INTERPRETATION

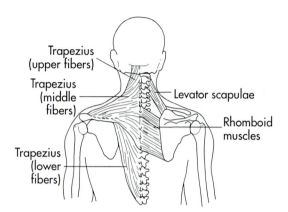

Fig. 2-57 Posterior cervical musculature.

inhibition. Because of this muscle imbalance, the body posture moves toward a forward head position and protracted scapula. This altered posture puts stress on the cervicocranial and cervicothoracic junctions. Deviations in alignment can also be caused by unilateral muscle spasm. There are several trigger points especially in the upper fibers.

The upper fibers of trapezius myofascial trigger points refer pain unilaterally along the posterolateral neck and head. The middle fibers of trapezius have a trigger point on the midscapular border of the muscle, which refers pain toward the spinous process of C7 and T1.

A trigger point can sometimes be found distal to the acromion, causing pain to the acromion process or top of the shoulder. The lower fibers of trapezius have a trigger point mid-belly and it can refer pain to the cervical paraspinal area, mastoid process, and acromion. A trigger point over the scapula below the scapular spine can refer a burning pain along the scapula's vertebral border.

These myofascial trigger point locations and pain patterns are taken from Travell and Simons work.

Ligamentum Nuchae

The ligamentum nuchae is a fibroelastic membrane or intermuscular septum from the external occipital protuberance to the spine of the seventh vertebra. It is not directly palpable but point tenderness in that area can be caused by a ligamentous sprain in a forward bending overstretch.

Levator Scapulae

Levator scapulae attach to and control both the scapula and the cervical spine. Often with cervical dysfunction, the muscle spasm of the levator causes scapular and eventually glenohumeral dysfunction. According to Yanda's work, the levator scapula is a muscle that has a tendency to develop tightness.

ASSESSMENT   # INTERPRETATION

There are often myofascial trigger points in this muscle when cervical or shoulder girdle dysfunction exists. The trigger points are located at the angle of the neck and the pain stays locally there as well as projecting down the vertebral border of the scapula (Travell and Simons).

Rectus Capitis (Major and Minor) and Obliquus Capitis (Superior and Inferior)

Rectus capitis muscles are often in spasm if upper cervical dysfunction exists, especially problems with the atlanto-occipital joint and atlanto-axial joint. These suboccipital muscles elicit local pain deep in the upper neck region. Looking upward for a prolonged period of time or a forward head position leads to overuse and discomfort of these muscles. The recti and oblique muscles have myofascial trigger points that refer pain deeply into the head.

Semispinalis Capitis and Semispinalis Cervicis and Multifidus

Semispinalis capitis and semispinalis cervicis, or multifidus, can be strained with injuries involving forced forward bending and rotation. These muscles overwork with reading or doing paper work at a desk with the head in sustained flexion. The semispinalis cervicis has a trigger point just below the occiput and pain is referred into the back of the head.

The semispinalis capitis has a trigger point right over the occipital bone and causes frontal headaches.

The multifidus muscle has a trigger point lateral to approximately the fifth cervical spinous process with referred pain into the neck and down to the vertebral edge of the scapula.

Splenius Capitis and Splenius Cervicis

These muscles develop overuse discomfort when the head and neck is held in extension or rotation for a prolonged period of time. Muscle spasm results with the athlete's complaint of a stiff neck.

Splenius capitis has a myofascial trigger point midbelly that refers pain to the top of the head. Splenius cervicis trigger points can refer pain to behind the eye and into the base of the neck.

Rhomboids (Major and Minor)

According to Yanda's work, the rhomboids tend to develop weakness and inhibition with time. This will lead to scapular protraction and eventual shoulder girdle dysfunction. Trigger points can develop in the rhomboid muscles when there are cervical pathologic conditions.

Upper or Proximal Cross Syndrome (Yanda)

Typical muscle imbalance problems tend to follow a predictable trend in the upper quadrant. There are muscle groups that develop tightness while others develop weakness and inhi-

ASSESSMENT   INTERPRETATION

bition. These palpations along with your observations will confirm the following upper or proximal cross syndrome.

The muscles that are tight are:

- Suboccipital
- Pectoralis major and minor
- Upper trapezius
- Levator scapulae
- Sternocleidomastoid

The muscles that are weak are:

- Serratus anterior
- Deep cervical flexors
- Rhomboids (major and minor)
- Middle and lower trapezius

Topographically, when the weakened and shortened muscles are connected they form a cross pattern. This pattern is important to be aware of because of the resulting forward head, thoracic kyphosis, rounded shoulders, and protracted scapula that will lead to altered upper quadrant mechanics. The body naturally follows this pattern but injury or poor posture can accelerate this process. These altered mechanics lead to dysfunction and eventual breakdown at the weakest link, which is often the cervical spine.

Lateral Aspect

Boney
Transverse Processes

The transverse process of the atlas is felt through the overlying tissue between the mastoid process and the mandibular angle. The transverse processes may be palpated with passive cervical rotation or side bending to help locate them.

C4-C5 is in line with the thyroid cartilage and C6 is in line with the top of the trachea.

A cervical rib on C7 may be palpable just above the clavicle at the base of the neck.

Soft Tissue (Fig. 2-58)
Sternocleidomastoid (see Anterior Aspect of Palpation)
Scalenes

The scalenes medius and anterior, levator scapulae, and splenius capitis can all be palpated, and are especially tender if the athlete has experienced an overstretch in side bend or rotation. Note any point tenderness, trigger points, or muscle spasm. Muscle spasm of the scalenes muscles can typically occur with thoracic outlet problems. Trigger points located in the anterior, medius, or posterior scalenes muscles can refer pain anteriorly to the chest wall, laterally to the upper extremity, and posteriorly to the vertebral scapular border. Pain can also be referred into the pectoral region, the biceps and triceps muscles, the radial

ASSESSMENT   INTERPRETATION

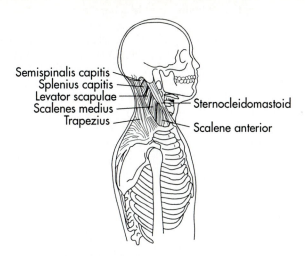

Semispinalis capitis
Splenius capitis
Levator scapulae
Scalenes medius
Trapezius

Sternocleidomastoid

Scalene anterior

Fig. 2-58 Lateral view of the muscles of
the cervical spine.

forearm, thumb, and index finger. Because of all these referred
patterns, the scalenes muscles must be palpated for trigger
points that refer to these areas.

When the anterior and medius scalenes are tight or shortened
they can entrap the brachial plexus in the thoracic outlet.

BIBLIOGRAPHY

Albright J et al: Head and neck injuries in college football: an 8-year analysis, Am J Sports Med 13(3):147,
1985

Anderson JE: Grant's Atlas of anatomy, Baltimore 1983,
Williams & Wilkins.

Aprill C, Dwyer A, and Bogduk N: Cervical zygapho-
physeal joint pain patterns. II: A clinical evaluation,
Spine, Vol 15, Number 6:458-461, 1990.

APTA: Review for advanced orthopaedic competencies.
Personius W: The cervical spine, Chicago, 1989.

Bland JH: Disorders of the Cervical Spine, Toronto, 1987,
WB Saunders Co.

Bogduk N: Cervical causes of headache and dizziness. In
Grieve G: Modern manual therapy of the vertebral
column, Edinborough 1986, Churchill Livingstone.

Booher JM and Thibodeau GA: Athletic injury assessment, Toronto, 1985, Times Mirror/Mosby College
Publishing.

Clinical symposia, CIBA 24:2, 1972, Ciba-Geigy Corp.

Cloward RB: Cervical discography: a contribution to the
etiology and mechanism of neck, shoulder, and arm
pain, Ann Surg 150:1052, 1959.

Cyriax J: Textbook of orthopedic medicine, diagnosis of
soft tissue lesions, vol 1, London 1978, Bailliere
Tindall.

Daniels L and Worthingham C: Muscle testing, techniques of manual examination, Toronto, 1980, WB
Saunders Co.

Donatelli R: Physical therapy of the shoulder, New York,
1987, Churchill Livingstone.

Dwyers A, Aprill C, and Bogduk N: Cervical zygapophy-
seal joint pain Patterns I: A study of normal volun-
teers, Spine, Vol 15, November 6:453:457, 1990.

Dzioba F: Non-sport diving caused spinal fractures, The
Physician and sportsmedicine 11(11):38, 1983.

Elvey RL: Brachial plexus tension tests and the
pathoanatomical origin of arm pain. In Idszack RM
(ed): Aspects of manipulative therapy, Australia, 1981,
Lincoln Institute of Health Sciences.

Evjenth O and Hamberg J: Muscle stretching in manual
therapy: a clinical manual, the spinal column and the
TM joint, Vol II, Alfta, Sweden, 1980, Alfta Rehab
Forlag.

Feldrick J and Albright J: Football survey reveals 'missed'
neck injuries, Physician Sportsmed 11:78, 1976.

Fielding J et al: Athletic injuries to the atlantoaxial articulation, Am J Sports Med 6(5):226, 1978.

Fisk JW: The painful neck and back, Springfield, Illinois, 1077, Charles C. Thomas.

Goodman CC and Snyder TE: Differential diagnosis in physical therapy, Toronto, 1990, WB Saunders Co.

Gould JA and Davis GJ: Orthopaedic and sports physical therapy: Toronto, 1985, The CV Mosby Co.

Grant R: Physical therapy of the cervical and thoracic spine, New York, 1988, Churchill Livingstone.

Grieve G (ed.): Modern manual therapy of the vertebral column, Edinburgh, 1986, Churchill Livingstone.

Grieve G: Common vertebral joint problems, Edinbergh, 1988, Churchill Livingstone.

Gunn CC: Reprints on pain, acupuncture & related subjects, Vancouver, 1979.

Hoppenfeld S: Physical examination of the spine and extremities, New York, 1976, Appleton-Century Crofts.

Kapandji IA: The physiology of the joints, Upper Limb, Vol I, New York, 1983, Churchill Livingstone.

Kellgren JH: On the distribution on pain arising from deep somatic structures in the charts of segmental pain areas, Clin Sci 4:35, 1939.

Kendall FP and McCreary EK: Muscle testing and function, Baltimore, 1983, Williams & Wilkins.

Kessler RM and Hertling D: Management of common musculo-skeletal disorders, Philadelphia, 1983, Harper and Row.

Klafs CE and Arnheim DD: Modern principles of athletic training, ed 5, St Louis, 1981, The CV Mosby Co.

Kornberg C and Lew P: The effect of stretching neural structures on grade one hamstring injuries, J Sports Phys Ther 10(12):481, 1989.

Kraus H: Clinical treatment of back and neck pain, New York, 1970 McGraw-Hill.

Kulund D: The injured athlete, Toronto, 1982, JB Lippincott.

Ladd A and Scranton P: Congenital cervical stenosis presenting as transient quadriplegia in athletes, J Bone Joint Surg 68(A):1371, 1986.

Laver R: Hockey's rash of neck injuries puzzles doctors, The Globe and Mail, Toronto, February 11, 1984.

Magee DJ: Orthopaedics conditions, assessments, and treatment, Vol II, Alberta, 1979, University of Alberta Publishing.

Magee DJ: Orthopaedic physical assessment, Toronto, 1987, WB Saunders Co.

Maitland GD: The slump test: examination and treatment, Aust J Phys 31:215, 1985.

Maitland GD: Peripheral manipulation, Toronto, 1977, Butterworth & Co.

Mannheimer JS and Lampe GN: Clinical transcutaneous electrical nerve stimulation, Philadelphia, 1986, FA Davis Co.

McKenzie RA: The cervical and thoracic spine, New Zealand, 1990, Spinal Publications.

Mueller F and Blyth C: An update on football deaths and catastrophic injuries, The Physician and Sportsmedicine 14(10):139, 1986.

Nitz A et al: Nerve injury and grades II and III sprains, Am J sports Med 13(3):177, 1985.

Nuber G and Schafer M: Clay shovelers' injuries, Am J Sports Med 15(2):182, 1987.

O'Donaghue D: Treatment of injuries to athletes, Toronto, 1984, WB Saunders Co.

Orlando K: Testing the cervical spine. Presentation, Sheridan College, March, 1987.

Palmer K and Louis D: Assessing ulnar instability of the metacarpophalangeal joint of the thumb, J Hand Surg 3:545, 1978.

Petersen L and Renstrom P: Sports injuries, their prevention and treatment, Chicago, 1986, Year Book Medical Publishers, Inc.

Reid DC: Functional anatomy and joint mobilization, Alberta, 1970, University of Alberta.

Reid DC: Sports injury assessment and rehabilitation, New York, 1992, Churchill Livingstone.

Rocabado M: Diagnosis and treatment of abnormal craniocervical and craniomandibular mechanics, 1981, Rocabado Institute.

Roy S and Irvin R: Sports medicine, prevention, evaluation, management, and rehabilitation, New Jersey, 1983, Prentice-Hall.

Saunders HD: Classification of musculoskeletal spinal conditions, J Orthop Sports Phys Ther 1(1):3, 1979.

Schneider RC: Head and neck injuries in football, Baltimore, 1973, Williams & Wilkins.

Tator C: Report on major injuries due to sports or recreational activities, Sports Medicine News, Bobby Orr Sports Clinic 3(1):2, 1987.

Tator C and Edmonds V: Sports and recreation are a rising cause of spinal cord injury, The Physician and Sports Medicine 14(5):157, 1986.

Tomberlin JP et al: The use of standardized evaluation forms in physical therapy, J Orthop Sports Phys Ther 1:348, 1984.

Torg JS: Epidemiology, pathomechanics and prevention of athletic injuries to the cervical spine, Med Sci Sports Exercise, 17(3):295.

Torg J et al: Neurapraxia of the cervical spinal cord with transient quadriplegia, J Bone Joint Surg 68(A):1354, 1986.

Torg J et al: The epidemiologic, pathologic, biomechanical, and cinematographic analysis of football-induced cervical spine trauma, Am J of Sports Med 18(1):50-57, January/February 1990.

Travell JG and Simons DG: Myofascial pain and dysfunction: the trigger point manual, Baltimore, 1983, Williams & Wilkins.

Vereschagin K et al: Burners, don't overlook or underestimate them, The Physicial and Sportsmedicine, Vol 19 #9:96-104, Sept 1991.

White AA and Panjabi MM: Clinical biomechanics of the spine, Toronto, 1978, JB Lippincott.

Williams PL and Warwick R: Gray's anatomy, New York, 1980, Churchill Livingstone.

Worthy DR and Selvik G: Movements of the craniovertebral joints. In Grieve G: Modern manual therapy of the vertebral column, Edinborough, 1986, Churchill Livingstone.

Zohn D: Musculoskeletal pain, diagnosis and physical treatment, ed 2, Toronto, 1988, Little Brown & Co, Inc.

CHAPTER 3
Shoulder Assessment

For several reasons the shoulder girdle is a difficult area to examine: it has many movements, many components, many conditions, and there is a good chance of the existence of multiple lesions at this site. Also pain that manifests in the shoulder area is seldom caused by a shoulder joint problem. Pain can be referred to the shoulder from the cervical spine, the thoracic spine, the first costovertebral joint, the first costosternal joint, the temporomandibular joint, the elbow joint, and the viscera. Therefore these joints and structures may need to be ruled out before examining the shoulder joint.

Examination of the shoulder girdle must include:

- acromioclavicular joint
- glenohumeral joint
- sternoclavicular joint
- scapulothoracic articulation
- first costosternal joint
- first costovertebral joint

Related problems that must be ruled out include:

- heart problems: a coronary (myocardial infarction), angina, pericarditis, which may radiate pain to the left shoulder
- lung or diaphragm problems: spontaneous pneumothorax; pulmonary tuberculosis; lung cancer, abscess, and Pancoast tumor, which relay pain along the same nerve roots of C4 and C5
- chest problems: aortic aneurysm, nodes in the axilla or mediastinum, breast disease (benign or malignant), and hiatal hernia, which can refer pain to the local area and shoulder
- cervical problems: intervertebral disc herniation or degeneration, facet joint effusion, nerve root irritation, which may also radiate pain to the shoulder and scapula
- spinal fracture: a cervical or thoracic spinal fracture, which can radiate pain to the shoulder muscles in the area, as well as produce local pain
- elbow problems: humeroulnar, humeroradial, or radioulnar joint dysfunction or pathology can also refer pain into the shoulder and humerus
- temporomandibular joint problems: TMJ degeneration or effusion, which can refer pain through the neck region and into the shoulder
- rib problems: costovertebral joint or costosternal joint dysfunction, according to Cailliet, which can influence shoulder function and first rib restrictions that can influence the clavicle and thoracic spine and in turn affect shoulder function
- thoracic spine problems: thoracic spine dysfunction can also limit shoulder movements and range
- abdominal problems: ruptured spleen, pancreas pathology can refer pain to the left shoulder; liver pathology and gallbladder disease can refer pain to the right shoulder

For these reasons it is very important to find the true cause of the problem because treatment and rehabilitation will then be more successful.

The shoulder girdle is a very mobile, complex structure that gives a good deal of mobility to the upper extremity at the expense of joint stability.

Usually the movements of the humerus and the scapula are smooth and well coordinated. Harmony exists between the muscle contractions of the prime movers, stabilizers, neutralizers, and the antagonists. A disturbance of any of these muscles will alter this pattern and the smooth motion through the shoulder girdle will be lost. Any injuries to other components of this unit, such as the scapula, the acromioclavicular joint, or the sternoclavicular joint, can affect the entire shoulder girdle and even the kinetics of the whole upper quadrant.

Shoulder girdle overuse injuries are very common in swimming and the throwing sports; traumatic shoulder girdle injuries are relatively common in football and hockey.

The close-packed position of the glenohumeral joint is maximal abduction and lateral rotation.

The close-packed position of the acromioclavicular joint is 30° of glenohumeral abduction, although Kaltenborn believes it is 90° of abduction.

The close-packed position for the sternoclavicular joint is glenohumeral extension, although according to Kaltenborn it is maximal arm elevation.

The resting, or loose-packed, position for the glenohumeral joint is 55° of abduction and 30° of cross-flexion (horizontal adduction).

The resting, or loose-packed, position for the acromioclavicular joint and the sternoclavicular joint is the normal physiologic position with the arm resting at the side.

The capsular pattern of the glenohumeral joint is limited lateral rotation, abduction, and medial rotation, in descending order of degree of restriction.

The capsular pattern for the acromioclavicular and sternoclavicular joints is pain at the extremes of range of motion.

ASSESSMENT

INTERPRETATION

HISTORY

Mechanism of Injury

Direct Blow

Was it a direct blow?

Contusion

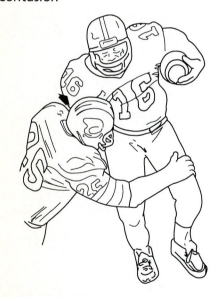

Fig. 3-1 Direct blow to the shoulder. Blocker's exostosis.

Contusions in the shoulder area are significantly reduced by the use of shoulder pads.

Contusions over the acromioclavicular joint are the most frequent, and deltoid contusions on top of the shoulder still occur in sports in which shoulder pads are not used.

Deltoid midbelly contusions occur frequently in hockey and lacrosse—sports in which sticks are used to crosscheck opponents.

Contusions over the front of the shoulder (between the coracoid process and the head of the humerus) may result in axillary nerve damage.

Contusions to the upper arm over the biceps or triceps muscles are also frequent because they occur below the deltoid-cap protection of the shoulder pads.

A *blocker's exostosis* is caused by repeated contusions to the attachment of the deltoid on the lateral aspect of the humerus. A periostitis and, eventually, an exostosis can develop here (Fig. 3-1).

The coracoid process can be contused when a marksman's gun recoils and hits this area.

Fracture (Fig. 3-2)
CLAVICLE

A greenstick fracture of the shaft of the clavicle is a frequent athletic injury, especially in the preadolescent and adolescent.

A fracture of the distal end of the clavicle (distal to the coracoclavicular ligaments) can occur when the acromion is hit downward in relation to the clavicle. It can also be fractured as a result of falling on the shoulder or outstretched arm. This readily occurs in contact sports, skiing, wrestling, and cycling. The

ASSESSMENT   INTERPRETATION

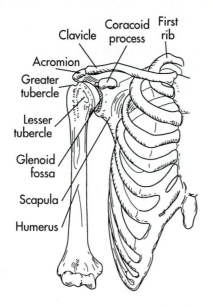

Acromion
Greater
tubercle
Lesser
tubercle
Glenoid
fossa
Scapula
Humerus

Clavicle   Coracoid   First
            process   rib

Fig. 3-2 Anterior boney aspect of right shoulder girdle.

fracture is usually located in the outer third of the clavicle where the bone curves. There is deformity, point tenderness, and pain with any shoulder movement on the involved side.

ACROMION

A fracture of the acromion can also occur with a fracture of the distal end of the clavicle. Such fractures are caused by direct blows in a downward direction over the acromion.

SCAPULA

A fracture of the scapula is very rarely sustained during athletic maneuvers; a violent, direct force is usually the cause of the injury. There are a few reported cases in football, ice hockey, and rugby.

A fracture of the glenoid is usually caused by very violent trauma with a fall on to the flexed elbow.

HUMERUS

Humerus fractures are the result of a fall on the outstretched arm but can be caused by a direct blow.

Fractures of the upper humerus are often through the neck of the humerus.

A fracture of the humeral head is also rare but can be caused by a direct blow or a fall on the shoulder.

A fracture can develop at the proximal epiphysis of the humerus in the young throwing athlete.

Fractures of the shaft of the humerus demonstrate the classical fracture signs: pain, deformity, and point tenderness. However, a significant force up the arm or across the upper arm is needed to fracture the humerus.

ASSESSMENT

INTERPRETATION

Sprain, Subluxation, Dislocation

GLENOHUMERAL JOINT

1. Anterior dislocation (frequent)
2. Posterior dislocation (occasional)
3. Inferior dislocation (rare)
4. Multidirectional instability

1. Anterior dislocation—This type of injury is caused by an indirect force such as a fall on the outstretched arm or elbow. The classical position for an anterior glenohumeral dislocation is shoulder abduction (at an angle of 90°), external rotation (at an angle of 90°), and cross-extension and then a force that increases the cross-extension or rotation (Fig. 3-7). It can be dislocated also by a posterior force to the upper humerus that dislocates the head anteriorly. With the anterior dislocation the head of the humerus will be in front of the glenoid fossa. There will be a hollow area underneath the acromion.

   The resulting damage can be:
   - anterior glenohumeral capsule or ligament sprain or tear
   - coracohumeral ligament sprain
   - a tear or detachment of the labrum of the glenoid cavity

   Other associated injuries that can occur as a result of the anterior dislocation are:
   - Bankart labral lesion, which is an injury to the glenoid rim and anterior capsule ligaments that become detached and no longer function to stabilize the humeral head.
   - Hill-Sachs lesion, which is a compression fracture of the humeral head or a defect in the posterolateral humeral head from repeated humeral head trauma
   - Brachial plexus or axillary nerve damage
   - A humeral neck fracture (more common in the elderly)
   - Avulsion of the greater tuberosity (more common in young athletes)

   Recurrent dislocation of the shoulder is frequently a problem with athletes. Once a shoulder is dislocated, 70% to 90% will redislocate. In the McLaughlin and Rowe study of shoulder dislocations, recurrence in patients under the ages of 20 and 30 is 94% and 90% respectively. According to Henry and Genung the majority of all dislocations occurring before the age of 20 recur without regard to care given. The second dislocation follows within 18 months in 50% of these patients and the other 50% may not experience recurrence for up to 5 years. This recurrence is often a result of inadequate immobilization time, labrum damage or capsular detachment in a normal shoulder, or as a result of congenital problems such as inherent glenohumeral joint laxity, shallow acetabulum, or a small humeral head.

   Dislocations involving labral lesions or capsular detachment have a higher recurrence rate than dislocations that only tear the capsule. Approximately two thirds of the dislocations with just capsular tears can heal in a stable position if strictly immobilized for 3 weeks.

   It is important to realize that the axillary, musculocutaneous,

ASSESSMENT

INTERPRETATION

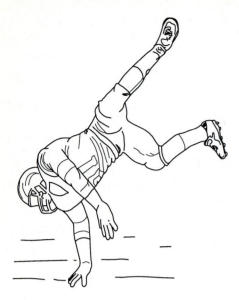

Fig. 3-3 Falling on the outstretched arm.

or ulnar nerve can be damaged from the dislocation, and therefore sensation and muscle function may need to be tested before and after shoulder reduction. Vascular trauma or damage to the axillary artery or vein can occur; therefore pulses and circulation in the upper limb should be monitored before and after reduction.

2. Posterior dislocation—The glenohumeral joint can be sprained or subluxed posteriorly when a direct blow to a flexed elbow forces the humerus backward. Sprains or posterior subluxations can also be caused by a fall on an internally rotated, adducted, outstretched arm. The classical position for a posterior dislocation is shoulder flexion (at an angle of 90°) with the elbow extended and with an axial force experienced through the arm (Fig. 3-3).

   Damage to the posterior capsule and its ligaments, as well as to the posterior rotator cuff muscles, can occur. A full posterior dislocation is not usually incurred by athletes.

3. Inferior dislocation—This rare dislocation occurs when the humerus is dislocated downward. The athlete may have to hold the entire arm above the head because he or she is unable to lower it. The classical injury position is an axial force down the limb when the shoulder is flexed at an angle of 180° (i.e., when diving into shallow water with arms overhead).

4. Multidirectional instability—The shoulder may dislocate in more than one direction or in a combination of directions (anterior, posterior, or inferior). This can be caused by a previous dislocation with lax capsular healing or it may be due to the hypermobility present in loose-jointed athletes. Repeated microtrauma from sporting events can also result in joint laxity (e.g., anterior joint laxity in backstrokers from kick turn forces on the outstretched arm).

STERNOCLAVICULAR JOINT

The sternoclavicular joint is the only articulation joining the shoulder girdle to the body.

The sternoclavicular joint can be sprained with the medial clavicle moving posteriorly, anteriorly, superiorly, or inferiorly. The most common injury causes anterior or superior displacement; posterior or inferior displacement occurs less commonly. The costoclavicular ligaments and/or the sternoclavicular capsular ligaments can be sprained or torn with anterior or superior displacement. The articular disc attaches superiorly to the clavicle and inferiorly to the first costocartilage and rib. If the joint is traumatized this disc can be torn or damaged.

The joint may be forced far enough to cause a subluxation or dislocation of the sternoclavicular joint.

An acute posterior dislocation of the clavicle requires emergency reduction. Because of the location of the trachea, the sub-

ASSESSMENT

INTERPRETATION

clavian artery and vein, aortic arch, and esophagus, the athlete's respiratory status and circulatory system must be monitored and he or she must be transported to a hospital immediately.

ACROMIOCLAVICULAR JOINT

The accepted classification of acromioclavicular joint sprains by Allman includes Types I, II, and III.

Type I consists of intra-articular trauma to the acromioclavicular joint without disruption of the joint capsule or coracoclavicular ligaments.

Type II involves disruption of the acromioclavicular joint, capsule, and ligaments without disruption of the coracoclavicular ligaments.

Type III (Fig. 3-4) consists of acromioclavicular dislocation with disruption of the acromioclavicular capsule, ligaments, and the coracoclavicular ligaments.

The acromioclavicular joint can be sprained by:
- falling on the point of the shoulder with the arm adducted to the side
- falling on the outstretched arm
- falling on the olecranon process of the elbow
- a blow from behind with the ipsilateral arm fixed on the ground, which drives the clavicle forward and away from the acromion
- traction on the humerus that pulls the acromion away from the clavicle
- a direct blow over the acromion so that it is driven inferiorly and depresses the clavicle, which fractures the clavicle or causes a sprain or dislocation of the acromioclavicular joint

According to Fukuda and others, the acromioclavicular and/or coracoclavicular ligaments can be sprained in several ways. With smaller displacement forces, the acromioclavicular ligaments contribute to approximately two thirds of the constraining forces to superior displacement. With larger displacement forces, the conoid ligament contributes the major share. In

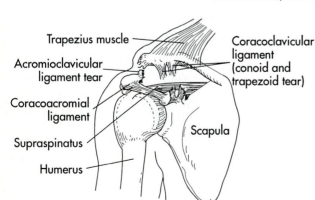

Trapezius muscle

Acromioclavicular ligament tear

Coracoacromial ligament

Supraspinatus

Humerus

Coracoclavicular ligament (conoid and trapezoid tear)

Scapula

Fig. 3-4 Acromioclavicular dislocation (Type III).

ASSESSMENT   INTERPRETATION

the direction of posterior displacement the acromioclavicular ligament contributes approximately 90% of the ligamentous constraint. The trapezoid ligament tends to provide constraint for the axial compressive forces through the acromioclavicular joint.

However, the joint can be subluxed or dislocated if the force is significant. Clinically, the clavicle is often seen displaced superiorly and anteriorly.

If the force continues after the coracoclavicular ligament is torn, the muscle attachments of the deltoid and trapezius to the distal end of the clavicle can be strained or torn.

Repeated trauma causing sprains and joint disruption eventually leaed to the formation of calcium deposits in the ligaments or joint. Because there is a meniscus within the joint, repeated trauma or overuse can lead to osteoarthritic changes.

STERNOCLAVICULAR AND ACROMIOCLAVICULAR JOINT COMBINATIONS (RARE)

A severe acromioclavicular sprain can have an associated minor sternoclavicular sprain and vice versa.

Bursitis
SUBACROMIAL (SUBDELTOID) (FIG. 3-5)

Subacromial bursitis (subdeltoid bursitis) can be exacerbated by a direct blow over the shoulder, which compresses the acromion process into the rotator cuff or into the humeral head. Overuse of the shoulder joint in an abducted and internally rotated position (i.e., in the front crawl stroke in swimming) could inflame the bursa.

Neural Damage
AXILLARY NERVE

Anterior blow to shoulder

A direct blow over the front of the shoulder can damage the axillary nerve or it may be damaged secondarily to an anterior glenohumeral dislocation. The nerve can be damaged during anterior shoulder surgery.

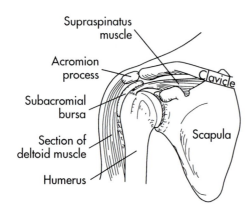

Supraspinatus muscle

Acromion process

Clavicle

Subacromial bursa

Scapula

Section of deltoid muscle

Humerus

Fig. 3-5 Anterior aspect of the right shoulder indicating the location of the subacromial bursa.

ASSESSMENT

INTERPRETATION

SPINAL ACCESSORY NERVE
Anterior blow to the trapezius muscle

A direct blow anteriorly to the undersurface of the trapezius about 1 inch above the clavicle can damage the spinal accessory nerve. A direct blow from a hockey or lacrosse stick or the shoulder of an opposing player can injure this nerve and cause weakness in the trapezius muscle, especially when shoulder shrugging or arm abduction is performed.

MUSCULOCUTANEOUS NERVE
Anterior medial blow to the upper arm

A direct blow to the upper medial aspect of the arm can damage the musculoskeletal nerve or it can be damaged secondary to an anterior glenohumeral dislocation.

SUPRASCAPULAR NERVE
A blow to the base of the neck
Rule out cervical spine, thoracic outlet, and brachial plexus

A direct blow to the base of the neck can injure the suprascapular nerve and cause weakness in the supraspinatus and infraspinatus muscles.

With any muscle weakness or suspected local nerve injury the cervical spine and brachial plexus should be ruled out in the observations and functional testing.

Overstretch
Was it an overstretch?

Shoulder flexion with elbow extension

Shoulder flexion overstretch with elbow extension can cause:
- sprain or tear of the anterior, inferior joint capsule (especially if shoulder flexion is combined with humeral lateral rotation)
- strain or tear of the pectoralis major, teres major, and latissimus dorsi muscles.

Shoulder flexion with elbow flexion

Shoulder flexion overstretch with elbow flexion can cause a strain or tear of the long head of triceps.

Shoulder extension with elbow extension (Fig. 3-6)

Shoulder extension overstretch with elbow extension can cause:
- strain or tear of the biceps tendon, anterior deltoid, and coracobrachialis
- sprain or tear of the anterior coracohumeral ligament, the anterior capsule

Shoulder abduction

Shoulder abduction overstretch can cause:
- strain or tear of the teres major, pectoralis major, or latissimus dorsi muscles
- an inferior glenohumeral sprain or dislocation—when the

ASSESSMENT   # INTERPRETATION

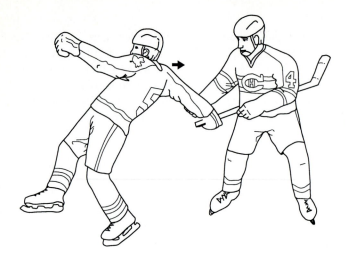

Fig. 3-6 Shoulder extension with elbow extension overstretch.

glenohumeral joint is forced into straight abduction, the inferior capsule and the capsular ligaments can become sprained or torn
- the joint to be subluxed or even dislocated inferiorly (this dislocation is rare and very severe)

Shoulder cross-flexion (horizontal adduction)

Shoulder joint horizontal adduction (cross-flexion) or over-stretch can cause:
- strain or tear of the posterior deltoid, infraspinatus, or teres minor muscles
- sprain or tear of the posterior capsule or posterior gleno-humeral ligaments

Shoulder cross-extension (horizontal abduction)

Shoulder joint cross-extension or horizontal abduction over-stretch can cause:
- strain or tear of the pectoralis major or anterior deltoid muscles
- sprain or tear of the anterior capsule or the anterior gleno-humeral ligaments

Shoulder forced backward or downward while the head is side bent in the opposite direction

A shoulder driven backward or downward with the cervical spine side bent in the opposite direction can cause a brachial plexus injury. The degree of damage can vary from a neuropraxia to an axonotmesis or a neurotmesis.
- A neuropraxia has transient, sharp, burning pain down the shoulder, arm, and hand, followed by numbness, then a return to full functioning in a couple of minutes or, if severe, up to 12 hours.
- An axonotmesis has sharp, burning pain down the limb, followed by muscle limb weakness of the muscles usually

ASSESSMENT   INTERPRETATION

supplied by the upper trunk of the brachial plexus (deltoid, infraspinatus, supraspinatus, and biceps). It can last up to 3 to 4 weeks (must rule out cervical spine).

- A neurotmesis has sharp, burning pain down the limb followed by prolonged muscle weakness of the muscles usually supplied by the upper trunk of the brachial plexus (especially deltoid, supraspinatus, and infraspinatus muscles). There is partial or complete disruption of the neurolemma sheath and full function may never be restored.

Shoulder medial rotation

Medial (internal) rotation overstretch of the shoulder joint can cause a strain or tear of the infraspinatus and teres minor muscles and a sprain or tear of the posterior capsule or the posterior glenohumeral ligaments. This can lead to recurrent posterior glenohumeral instability especially if medial rotation and cross-flexion (horizontal adduction) occurs in the mechanism.

Shoulder lateral rotation

Lateral (external) rotation overstretch of the shoulder joint can cause:
- strain or tear of the subscapularis, pectoralis major, and latissimus dorsi muscles
- sprain or tear of the medial and proximal capsule or the medial glenohumeral ligaments at 60° to 90° of abduction
- sprain or tear of the coracohumeral and medial glenohumeral at 0° to 90° of the shoulder joint (Ferrari)

Shoulder abduction and lateral rotation (Fig. 3-7)

Abduction and lateral rotation overstretch of the shoulder joint can cause:
- sprain or tear of the anterior joint capsule and its ligaments; if the force is excessive the joint can become subluxed or even dislocated anteriorly
- sprain or tear of the glenohumeral ligaments or even a tear of the anterior rotator cuff muscles in the young athlete

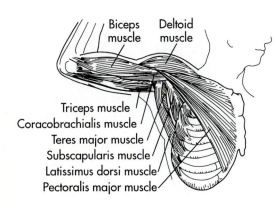

Biceps muscle
Deltoid muscle
Triceps muscle
Coracobrachialis muscle
Teres major muscle
Subscapularis muscle
Latissimus dorsi muscle
Pectoralis major muscle

Fig. 3-7 Shoulder abduction and lateral rotation. Muscles shown.

ASSESSMENT

INTERPRETATION

- partial or full avulsion of the glenoid labrum rim and its attachments (Barker et al.)
- all or part of the greater tuberosity may be avulsed if there is a severe anterior dislocation

Forceful Muscle Contraction

Was it a forceful muscle contraction against resistance that was too great? (Fig. 3-8)

A forceful muscle contraction against resistance that is too great can cause muscle strains around the shoulder joint. Strains can occur to any of the muscles around the shoulder joint or scapula.

The most common strains are to:
- the internal rotators (subscapularis, latissimus dorsi, teres major, and pectoralis major muscles)
- the external rotators (infraspinatus, supraspinatus, and teres minor muscles)
- the long head of the biceps muscle at the superior tip of the labrum; it can even rupture if the force is sufficient. This rupture can occur anywhere along the belly or at its point of origin or insertion

The fascia holding the biceps tendon in its groove can also rupture, allowing the tendon to sublux, usually because of a predisposing shallow groove.

The subscapularis muscle can violently contract in adduction and internal rotation, causing an avulsion of the lesser tuberosity. The athlete will describe a violent external rotation and abduction force (i.e., tackle) that he or she attempts to overcome.

Rotator cuff lesions are more common in the older adult (over 50) because these lesions are associated with degenerative changes in the tendons of the rotator cuff. A rotator cuff muscle tear is usually the result of degenerative thinning, especially in the older throwing athlete who has experienced ongoing impingement syndrome. The supraspinatus tendon can partially or fully tear.

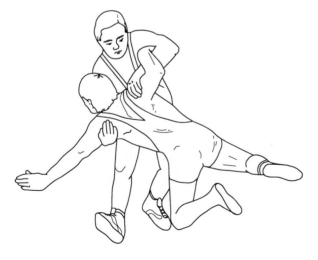

Fig. 3-8 Violent forces at the shoulder joint in wrestling.

ASSESSMENT

INTERPRETATION

Acute ruptures of the rotator cuff muscles of the athlete are often associated with a dislocation or subluxation and usually involve very forceful motion of the shoulder as in wrestling holds or football tackling.

A supraspinatus strain from a forceful abduction can strain the muscle tendon anywhere along its length.

A deltoid strain can be caused by arm-tackling.

Overuse

Was it an overuse, repetitive mechanism?

Overhand Throw (Fig. 3-9)

The mechanical actions involved in the overhand throwing pattern are used in many sports such as volleyball, tennis, baseball, basketball, water polo, and javelin throwing. This repetitive and ballistic action could cause microtrauma to the muscles involved. These muscles are often compressed in the subacromial space, especially the supraspinatus muscle and the long head of the biceps brachii muscle. The position of abduction and external rotation followed by internal rotation could cause an unstable or loose-fitting biceps tendon to sublux or slip out of its groove. With overuse this slipping could lead to tendonitis. Such a position could also cause subluxing of the glenohumeral joint in the athlete who has joint laxity or a previous dislocation. Finally, the overhand throw pattern could lead to eventual glenoid labrum damage.

With electromyographic analysis, it was determined that the supraspinatus, infraspinatus, teres minor, deltoid, trapezius, and biceps brachii have greater electrical activity during the early and late cocking stages, with less activity during acceleration. These muscles probably function primarily to position the shoulder and elbow for the delivery of the pitch. The pectoralis major, serratus anterior, subscapularis, and latissimus dorsi have more activity during the acceleration phases and are primarily responsible for the forward motion of the arm during the pitch.

Wind-up Phase

Each pitcher or thrower has a unique pitching style. The windup is the period between the initiation of motion until the ball is removed from the glove. The cocking phase occurs in approximately 1.5 seconds and accounts for 80% of the entire pitching act.

During windup, the thrower attempts to contract all the antagonist muscles to place the body in a position so that each muscle, joint, and body

Injuries during this phase are rare.

ASSESSMENT   INTERPRETATION

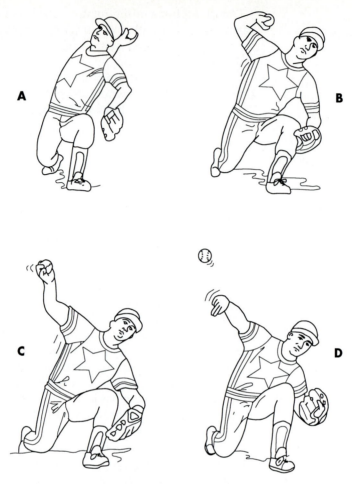

Fig. 3-9 Mechanism of the overhand throw. **A,** Cocking phase. **B,** Acceleration, 1st Phase. **C,** Acceleration, 2nd Phase. **D,** Follow-through phase.

part can contribute its forces synchronously for a powerful release of energy during the pitch.

The right-handed pitcher shifts body weight by flexing the left hip and knee backward and upward while rotating the trunk to the right. The right foot acts as the pivot point.

The pitcher continues to turn to the right until the shoulders and hips are perpendicular to the strike zone (rotated at an angle of 90°).

At the height of the coiling movement and knee lift, the hands separate, and the early cocking phase begins.

Injuries during this phase are rare.

ASSESSMENT

INTERPRETATION

Early Cocking Phase

The hip on the coiled limb begins to extend and abduct as the pelvis and trunk begin to turn toward the plate with the body pivoting over the right leg with the knee slightly flexed. The ball has been lowered in front of the body.

The opposite limb is cross-extended and abducted in front of the body for balance.

The pelvis, hip, and trunk uncoil explosively to the left with the entire right side driving forward with hip and knee extension. The trunk reaches its fastest angular velocity of forward rotation, yet the arm remains behind the shoulder line and there is no forward movement of the ball.

Any lower limb, trunk, or lumbar spine dysfunction can limit or adversely affect this phase, although few upper limb injuries occur during it.

Late Cocking Phase

The late cocking phase begins as the left stride leg comes into contact with the ground.

The shoulder of the throwing arm is at an angle of 90° of abduction and approximately 140° to 160° of external rotation, with about 30° of horizontal abduction (or cross-flexion) (Fig. 3-9, A).

Experienced pitchers develop anterior capsule laxity and the ability to stretch the soft tissue to allow extreme ranges of external rotation.

The posterior deltoid muscle brings the humerus into horizontal abduction while the supraspinatus, infraspinatus, and teres minor muscles must stabilize the head of the humerus. During this time the internal rotators are placed in a stretched position.

The scapular stabilizers contract to maintain a solid base for the glenohumeral movement and the elbow is flexed at an angle of approximately 90°, with the forearm supinated and the wrist in neutral or in a position of slight extension; the body moves forward explosively, leaving the shoulder and arm behind, and the lumbar spine then

Glenohumeral instability may cause pain during the cocking phase of the overhand throw. Pain could be caused by the excessive strain placed on the anterior ligaments. With time, this strain could lead to joint subluxations and tearing of the anterior glenoid capsule and labrum. An anterior-inferior labrum tear leads to more anterior instability.

According to Cain and others, the infraspinatus and teres minor muscles play a critical role in achieving anterior stability in this cocking phase by pulling the humerus posteriorly.

Subacromial impingement problems can also elicit pain here.

An inadequate warm-up routine, a poorly conditioned or fatigued shoulder, a lower limb or lumbar spine injury, and faulty technique can all lead to injury of any segment of the kinetic chain during this phase.

ASSESSMENT

moves into a hyperextended position and force is generated from the trunk, pelvis, and spine into the upper extremity.

Acceleration—First Phase

The acceleration phase begins with the glenohumeral joint in maximum external rotation and terminates with ball release. The time taken for the entire acceleration phase is only 50 milliseconds and accounts for only 2% of the pitching act.

This primary phase of acceleration begins with a powerful internal rotation of the shoulder musculature and the forward motion of the ball (Fig. 3-9, *B*).

According to Perry, the anterior capsule recoils like a spring with the force reversal of internal rotation with incredible torque. The subscapularis, pectoralis major, latissimus dorsi, and teres major muscles contract concentrically while they are in lengthened muscle-stretch positions and the serratus anterior abducts the scapula.

Acceleration—Second Phase

During the second part of the acceleration phase the internal rotation of the shoulder continues while the elbow moves from an angle of 25° to 30° of extension (Fig. 3-9, *C*).

The trunk continues rotating to the left while the humerus horizontally adducts.

There are significant valgus and extension forces through the elbow joint during this period.

The biceps muscles work eccentrically to decelerate elbow extension and the ball is released before full elbow extension while the forearm moves from a supinated to a pronated position.

INTERPRETATION

During the wind-up and acceleration phase of the overhand throw the muscles commonly injured are the internal rotators and the biceps brachii.

The internal rotator muscles, which are the subscapularis, latissimus dorsi, pectoralis major, and teres minor muscles can become injured because of the torque and forces involved but also because these muscles were contracting eccentrically and now have to fire quickly and synchronously and in a concentric manner. As a result, these muscles can develop strains or tendonitis.

The serratus anterior muscle is important here for scapular stabilization and shows intense activity.

The movements of internal rotation and horizontal adduction pull the humeral head anteriorly and can damage the glenoid labrum anteriorly or superiorly, especially if the posterior rotator cuff or posterior deltoid (stabilizing muscles) are weak.

The long head of the biceps muscle can sublux as the glenohumeral joint goes from external rotation to internal rotation. Initially, this may cause biceps tendonitis and can lead to a biceps tendon rupture. Spiral fractures of the humerus resulting from the forces involved have been reported.

Impingement of the structures in the subacromial space can cause pain, especially in the supraspinatus and biceps brachii muscles and the subacromial bursa. Repeated bursitis leads to adhesions that cause further impingement.

During the later acceleration phase, minor tears of the rotator cuff or biceps tendon may occur.

There are considerable forces generated through the medial elbow soft-tissue structures (i.e., medial epicondyle, medial collateral ligament, wrist flexor muscles) that can lead to injury.

The acceleration phases are associated with the greatest forces and have a high incidence of injury during the act of pitching.

There are some case studies that indicate suprascapular neuropathy can also result from the acceleration phase in throwing (Ringel et al.). This may be the result of the stretch placed on the bone.

ASSESSMENT

INTERPRETATION

Follow-through, or Deceleration, Phase

The follow-through phase begins the instant the ball is released. This phase takes approximately 350 milliseconds or 18% of the pitching act (Fig. 3-9, *D*).

Once the left stride foot is planted it starts the deceleration forces of the body.

The trunk bends forward and rotates left with a gradual deceleration and dissipation of torque.

The moment the ball is released, powerful deceleration muscle contractions are necessary to slow the upper limb motion.

The posterior rotator cuff muscles and the posterior deltoid muscles contract eccentrically to prevent the humerus from being pulled out of the fossa.

The scapular stabilizing muscles must contract to control the forward motion of the entire shoulder girdle.

The biceps brachii contracts vigorously to decelerate elbow extension and pronation, and the shoulder girdle forces are gradually dissipated as the glenohumeral joint adducts and the scapula protracts in a cross-body motion.

During the follow-through, the decelerator muscles, the posterior deltoid, triceps, rhomboids, teres minor, and the posterior capsule can be injured.

In some throwers the shoulder may actually sublux anteriorly during the follow-through phase. The athlete develops posterior shoulder pain first as the muscles go into spasm to prevent the humeral head from sliding forward.

Repeated anterior movement pulls the posterior capsule and the triceps and teres minor muscles.

The muscles that are under repeated traction in the follow-through can cause a boney outgrowth at their attachment, especially in the case of the triceps long head or teres minor muscles. Partial tears of the rotator cuff through repeated microtrauma can also occur. Andrews et al. attribute avulsion of the anterior superior labrum and the biceps tendon to excessive forces of the biceps tendon on the labrum with the eccentric biceps contraction during the deceleration phase of throwing.

Backstroke

The repeated flipturns that the backstroker performs can lead to humeral head subluxations anteriorly because of the abducted, externally rotated position of the shoulder.

Drop Shoulder Problems

The continual overhand patterns on one side only can lead to a drop shoulder on that side. This drop shoulder position can reduce the thoracic outlet, leading to compression of its contents (brachial plexus, subclavian artery; see Observation, Anterior View). It also assumes an anterior position that can reduce the subacromial space.

Scapular Pain

Periscapular pain is frequent in shot putters, tennis players, and weight lifters because the scapular muscles become overfatigued in their attempt to anchor the humerus and restrain the scapula during the follow-through phase.

ASSESSMENT

INTERPRETATION

Impingement Syndrome (Fig. 3-10)
Overhand tennis stroke
Front crawl and butterfly swimming strokes
Side arm and overhand throwing act

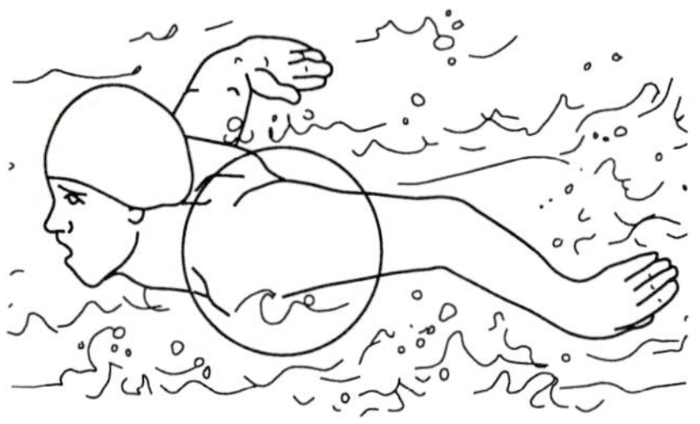

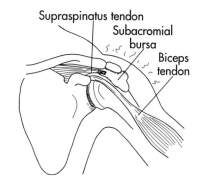

Fig. 3-10 Butterfly swim stroke. Impingement during recovery phase.

Fig. 3-11 Impinged subacromial structures.

The subacromial arch is formed by the acromion, acromioclavicular joint, lateral clavicle, and the coracoacromial ligament.

The strucures in the subacromial space (the supraspinatus tendon, long head of biceps tendon, subscapularis tendon, and the subacromial bursa) can be subject to repeated impingement between the humerus and the acromion (and coracoacromial ligament), as described by Rathburn and McNab, as well as Hawkins and Kennedy.

Repeated abduction (at angles between 70° and 120°), coupled with internal or external rotation and shoulder flexion, can inflame these structures.

This impingement occurs during the tennis serve, the front crawl and butterfly swimming strokes, weight lifting, and overhand and sidearm pitches.

If any of the structures become damaged, inflammation and swelling decreases the subacromial space and impingement discomfort results. This impingement can cause one or all of the following: biceps tendonitis, supraspinatus tendonitis, subacromial bursitis (Rathburn, McNab, Kennedy et al.) (Fig. 3-11).

Because of this impingement an avascular zone can develop in the supraspinatus tendon (1 cm proximal to the insertion) and in the long head of the biceps, where it stretches over the humeral head. This avascular zone can cause necrosis of the tendon cells, calcification, and even tears.

Chronic subacromial bursitis can result if adhesions develop in the bursal wall or if there is a thickening of the muscles in the subacromial space; these adhesions or thickenings will reduce the subacromial space even further.

Neer and Welsh maintain that thickening or a separation of the acromioclavicular joint may cause secondary impingement syndromes. Hawkins and Abrams state that shoulder boney architecture has a role with impingement, from any of the following:

- abnormal shape or thickness of the acromial process
- prominent greater tuberosity
- incompletely fused apophysis

Neer states that an acromion with less slope and a prominent anterior edge may be more susceptible to impingement.

According to Nuber et al., during the front crawl and butterfly strokes the latissimus dorsi and the clavicular head of the pectoralis major muscle were found to be the predominant muscles of propulsion; however, the subscapularis muscle also has a role. The supraspinatus, infraspinatus, and middle fibers of the deltoid were mainly recovery phase muscles. The serratus anterior appeared to have an important role during the recovery phase in the stabilizing of the glenoid cavity. As the inflammation from impingement increases, the rotator cuff muscles may show reflex weakness and may not be able to stabilize the gleno-

ASSESSMENT

INTERPRETATION

humeral head in the glenoid cavity. As a result, the deltoid may overwork to stabilize the head, which in turn leads to greater impingement.

This impingement problem usually develops in the young athlete (swimmer, thrower) but can also occur in the middle-aged athlete who overtrains (squash, tennis). In both cases , the impingement may be aggravated by an imbalance between the internal or external rotator muscle strength. Swimmers and throwers tend to have stronger internal rotators than external rotators.

The anterior glenoid labrum or anterior capsular laxity that may result from a previous dislocation or from repeated subluxation can result in clicking and/or pain during the front crawl or butterfly strokes.

Chronic
Recurring Injuries
   Has the injury occurred before?

Anterior glenohumeral dislocations tend to recur.

Biceps tendonitis recurs especially when overtraining in the throwing act. The biceps tendon is an important stabilizer during throwing and when overworked will inflame. It tends to occur more commonly in the athlete with the anterior or forward glenohumeral joint or impingement syndrome. Biceps tendonitis is common from the serve and overhead strokes in tennis and the front crawl in swimmers. Infraspinatus tendonitis is also common in tennis players and throwing athletes because this muscle is important to shoulder stabilization during the deceleration phase or follow-through in both sports.

Subacromial bursitis tends to recur at 2 to 5 year intervals.

Recurrent subluxations of the long head of biceps are common. This problem often occurs in the throwing athlete during the cocking and early acceleration phases, especially in athletes who have a shallow bicipital groove. The tendon subluxes when the humerus goes from external rotation to internal rotation. A subluxing biceps tendon also occurs more easily if the angle of the bicipital groove is less than 30° or there is a supratubercle ridge that forces the tendon against the transverse ligament, making it easier to sublux.

Reenacting the Mechanism
   Can the athlete reenact the mechanism using the opposite limb?
Note arm position
Note body position
Note shoulder position
   If it is an overuse injury, ask the athlete to demonstrate the painful action with the opposite limb.

Having the athlete demonstrate the mechanism helps clarify the body position and the stress placed on the involved tissue. This helps determine the damaged structure and injury mechanism.

ASSESSMENT   INTERPRETATION

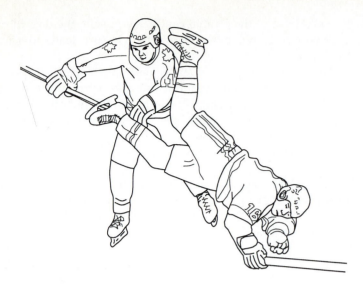

Fig. 3-12 Violent forces in hockey.

Forces in the Sport (Fig. 3-12)

Ask relevant questions concerning the force of the blow or overstretch.

The degree of force that caused the injury helps determine the degree of damage sustained.

Ice hockey subjects the acromioclavicular joint to repeated trauma because of the nature of the sport with body checking, cross-checking with the stick, and contact with the boards.

Gymnastics and wrestling predisposes the shoulder to severe torsional forces, which can cause the rotator cuff muscles to strain or tear. Football and rugby subjects the shoulder and upper arm to significant forces because of the blocking and tackling maneuvres.

Pain

Location (Fig. 3-13)

Where is the pain located?

Pain referred to the shoulder area may come from the:

- Cervical spine
- Shoulder capsule
- Supraspinous fossa
- Ribs
- Thoracic spine (T4 syndrome)
- Elbow, hand, arm
- Myofascial referred pain (trigger points)
- Temporomandibular joint
- Internal organs

The patient can rarely pinpoint the pain's exact location, but he or she can, it is often not the lesion site.

Pain referred to the deltoid insertion is believed to be the referral pattern for the anterior glenohumeral capsule (Travell and Simons). Most common lesions at the glenohumeral joint affect structures derived largely from the C5 segmental level and the pain follows the C5 dermatome.

If the athlete has anterior shoulder pain (C5 dermatome) that the history suggests is referred, all muscles innervated by C5 should be tested (the infraspinatus commonly refers pain there).

If the athlete has local pain in the supraspinous fossa and referred pain into the C8 or T1 dermatomal region, this can be caused by a first rib syndrome, also known as the fixed first rib.

Tendonitis can refer the pain to upper arm (deltoid area) rather than into the muscle from which it originates. In severe conditions, the pain may radiate down the anterolateral aspect of the arm and forearm. The further down the arm the pain spreads, the more severe the lesion.

ASSESSMENT   INTERPRETATION

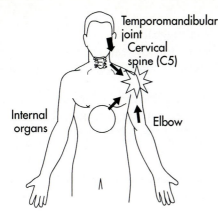

Temporomandibular joint
Cervical spine (C5)
Internal organs
Elbow

Fig. 3-13 Pain referred to the shoulder area.

According to Travell and Simons, each muscle has a tender trigger point and a referral pain pattern that the therapist can map.

Pain can be referred from the following internal organs:

- heart
- aorta
- lungs
- diaphragm
- gallbladder, spleen, and pancreas

Onset

How quickly did the pain begin?
- Quick onset
- Gradual onset

A quick onset of pain suggests more severe trauma than a gradual onset.

Pain that develops gradually and is associated with repetitive actions is often caused by tendonitis or synovitis and suggests an overuse syndrome.

A gradual onset can also suggest a systemic, infectious condition or a metastatic disease.

Type

Can the athlete describe the pain?

Sharp

A sharp pain could suggest:
- injury to a superficial muscle (e.g., deltoid or triceps)
- injury to a tendon (e.g., biceps or supraspinatus)
- acute bursitis (e.g., subacromial)
- injury to the periosteum (e.g., humerus or clavicle)

Dull

A dull pain could suggest an injury to:
- a tendon sheath (e.g., biceps)
- a deep muscle (e.g., subscapularis or serratus anterior)
- bone (e.g., head of humerus or glenoid cavity)

ASSESSMENT

INTERPRETATION

Aching

An ache could suggest:
- injury to deep muscle (e.g., subscapularis or teres minor)
- injury to deep ligament (e.g., glenohumeral or coracoclav-icular)
- injury to tendon sheath (e.g., biceps)
- injury to fibrous capsule (e.g., glenohumeral)
- chronic bursitis (e.g., subacromial)

Pins and Needles

Pins and needles suggest an injury to:
- a peripheral nerve (e.g., lateral cutaneous of the upper arm)
- the dorsal root of a cervical nerve

Tingling (Paresthesia)

Tingling could be caused by injury to a circulatory or neural structure (e.g., thoracic outlet, brachial plexus, subclavian artery, brachial artery, or cervical nerve root compression). Paresthesia from a thoracic outlet compression typically affects the eighth cervical and first thoracic dermatome. Often there is pain and numbness in the same distribution with aching in the supraclav-icular fossa and anterior shoulder. These sensory symptoms can be aggravated by overhead actions or heavy lifting.

Problems with the brachial plexus will cause numbness and weakness along the involved nerves.

Problems with the cervical nerve roots will cause dermatome, myotome, and reflex changes along the involved segment.

Numbness

Numbness can be caused by injury to:
- the cervical nerve root (dorsal compression)
- peripheral cutaneous nerves

Twinges

Twinges of pain during movements could be caused by:
- subluxations
- muscular strain
- ligamentous sprain

Stiffness

Stiffness is often caused by:
- capsular swelling
- arthritic changes
- muscle spasms

Severity of Pain

What is the degree of pain?
- Mild

The degree of pain is not a good indicator of the severity of the problem because the description of pain varies with the ath-

ASSESSMENT	INTERPRETATION

lete's emotional state, cultural background, and previous injury experiences. For example, an acute subacromial bursitis can limit range excessively and be very painful for a couple of days, then completely subside. A biceps tendon rupture may not be very painful at all, while a mild, first-degree acromioclavicular sprain may be more point tender than a complete third-degree tear.

- Moderate
- Severe

Timing of Pain

When is it painful?
- Nightly or morning pain

Only certain movements cause pain
- What makes it feel better?
- What makes it feel worse?

Night pain often suggests an inflamed bursa, vascular disease, metastatic disease, or shoulder-hand syndrome.

Sleeping postures can cause or add to shoulder problems in the following ways: (1) sleeping with an arm under the head maintains the subacromial impingement position that will augment an already irritated subacromial bursitis or tendonitis and (2) sleeping on one side in an anterior glenohumeral position and with the scapula protracted adds to adaptive shortening of the internal rotators and the anterior capsule with lengthening of the retractors.

Pain that occurs only when specific movements are performed suggests:
- a musculoskeletal problem that is probably contractile
- a possible capsular pattern (limitation in lateral rotation, abduction, and medial rotation)
- an impingement problem that is aggravated when the impingement position is repeated

Usually, acute injuries feel better in a position of rest and chronic conditions feel better during movement. The athlete may support the humerus by holding the elbow in a way that takes the forces off the glenohumeral or acromioclavicular joint.

Repeating the mechanism of injury will cause pain. If performing daily activities aggravates the pain, rest is indicated.

Swelling

What type of swelling is present?

- Local
- Diffuse
- Intramuscular

It is very difficult to see or feel swelling in the shoulder joint or bursae.

After direct trauma, intramuscular swelling in the deltoid, biceps, triceps, or other muscles can often be felt as a tight or hard mass in the muscle.

Function

What is the degree of disability?
Could the athlete continue to participate in his or her sport?
Can the athlete sleep on the affected side?
Is the range of motion or function of the shoulder decreasing gradually?

The degree of disability does not indicate the degree of severity of the injury. For example, an acute bursitis may limit range a great deal. A situation can occur in which the athlete does not experience pain at all, but may not be able to abduct the shoulder. This occurs with a long thoracic nerve palsy or a complete supraspinatus tear.

If performing daily functions increases the pain, the shoulder

ASSESSMENT

INTERPRETATION

must be rested. If the athlete participates in his or her sport after injury, it usually indicates that the injury was not severe enough to limit function.

If the athlete is unable to sleep on the affected side, it suggests an active bursitis.

Chronic shoulder joint dysfunction, severe trauma, prolonged glenohumeral immobilization, bursitis, or tendonitis can lead to a "frozen" shoulder (capsular pattern) where the shoulder joint progressively loses range in lateral rotation, abduction, and medial rotation. The losses of range are the greatest in lateral rotation, then abduction, and, lastly, medial rotation, in descending order of loss. The losses of range become progressively worse until glenohumeral movement can become totally restricted unless early mobilization within healing constraints is instituted.

Instability

Does the shoulder joint feel loose or unstable?

Inherent shoulder joint laxity or post-traumatic laxity predispose the glenohumeral joint to recurrent subluxations or dislocations. The most common recurrent dislocations are anterior dislocations, but posterior and inferior dislocations can also occur.

Damage to the labrum of the glenoid as a consequence of anterior dislocations or subluxations can cause functional instability and mechanical dysfunction.

Instability can also be multidirectional in the loose-jointed athlete or the chronic glenohumeral dislocater.

Sensations

Ask the athlete to describe the sensations felt at the time of injury and present sensations.

Clicking

If clicking occurs with both active and passive motions, suspect a glenoid labrum tear.

Clicking could be secondary to glenohumeral subluxations or dislocations.

Snapping

Snapping could be caused by:
- a biceps tendon as it moves out of the bicipital groove
- a catching of a thickened bursa under the acromion during abduction

Grating

Grating could be caused by:
- osteoarthritic changes

ASSESSMENT

INTERPRETATION

- calcium in the joint
- thickening of the bursa or synovium

Tearing

Tearing could be from a rotator cuff strain or tear.

Locking or Catching

Locking or catching could be caused by:
- a calcium buildup in the joint
- by a piece of articular cartilage fractured off the humerus or the glenohumeral labrum.

Recurrent dislocations can chip pieces off the labrum.

Numbness

Numbness could be the result of:
- nerve root impingement
- cervical rib entrapment
- thoracic outlet problem
- injury to the brachial plexus or a cutaneous nerve

Tingling (Paresthesia)

Tingling suggests:
- neural or circulatory problem
- thoracic outlet problem affecting the subclavian artery

Warmth

Warmth indicates an active inflammation or infection. A red-hot burning sensation is caused by acute calcific tendonitis.

Shoulder "Going Out"

The unstable shoulder may be subluxing or dislocating and self-reducing, which causes this sensation.

Particulars

Previous Injury

Was there a previous injury to the shoulder girdle? Has a family physician, orthopedic specialist, physiotherapist, physical therapist, athletic trainer, athletic therapist, chiropractor, osteopath, neurologist, or any other medical personnel assessed or treated this injury this time or previously?

Repeated trauma or repeated dislocations are important and should be noted.

Any previous musculoskeletal injury to the shoulder or shoulder girdle could affect the entire shoulder complex. The acromioclavicular, sternoclavicular, scapulothoracic, and glenohumeral joints are all part of a kinetic chain; an injury to any one component may affect them all.

Common ongoing or repetitive injuries of the shoulder girdle include:
- acromioclavicular sprains or subluxations
- sternoclavicular sprains or subluxations
- glenohumeral sprains, subluxations, or dislocations
- biceps tendonitis (especially long head)
- supraspinatus tendonitis

ASSESSMENT

INTERPRETATION

- infraspinatus tendonitis
- subacromial bursitis

The symptoms of an idiopathic frozen shoulder usually persist for 9 to 12 months regardless of the treatment. The condition remains acute with progressively more pain for the first few months, then stays the same for a few months, and then gradually improves.

A previous cervical, thoracic, temporomandibular, or elbow injury may also affect the shoulder joint.

A history of cardiac problems can suggest heart pathology or angina as a cause of shoulder pain.

Medical History

Has the injury been x-rayed?
If so, what are the results of the x-ray?
Have any medications been prescribed?
Has there been any previous physiotherapy?
What was the diagnosis?
Was the treatment or rehabilitation successful?

The physician's diagnosis, prescriptions, and recommendations for rehabilitation should be recorded at this time. This should include previous x-ray results and treatment methods that have proven helpful.

OBSERVATIONS

The standing view of the whole body should be observed from the anterior, lateral, and posterior aspects.

The cervical spine, thoracic spine, shoulder, elbow, forearm, wrist, and hands should be exposed to view as much as possible.

The posture should be compared bilaterally, noting both the boney and the soft tissue contours.

Gait (Fig. 3-14)

Movements of the upper body and arms should be observed as the athlete enters the clinic.

By observing the athlete's gait, the therapist can determine the severity of the disorder by the ease with which the athlete moves.

Listing of the cervical spine to the affected side of the cervical region or a loss of the rhythmic arm swing are signs of significant shoulder joint problems.

Protecting the shoulder by holding the arm internally rotated with the elbow flexed indicates an acutely irritated shoulder joint.

Asymmetry of motion can lead to additional problems at the lesion site or in the other joints where compensation is being made.

ASSESSMENT   INTERPRETATION

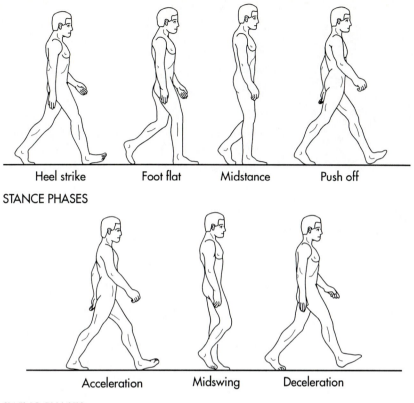

| Heel strike | Foot flat | Midstance | Push off |

STANCE PHASES

| Acceleration | Midswing | Deceleration |

SWING PHASES

Fig. 3-14 Gait—arm swing.

Clothing Removal

If possible, observe as the athlete removes his or her coat, shirt, or sweater.

While the athlete is removing his or her coat, shirt, or sweater, the shoulder, elbow, wrist, and hand should all work together smoothly.

Persons with shoulder-joint problems usually remove the clothing on the uninjured side first and then lift it off the injured side.

Limitations or pain in shoulder abduction and during internal rotation make it particularly difficult to remove clothing.

Standing Position

Anterior View (Fig. 3-15)
Boney
CRANIAL CARRIAGE

The head position could be altered by muscle weakness or spasm in the cervical spine musculature. Often the trapezius or erector spinae muscles will go into spasm to support the structures on the injured side.

ASSESSMENT

INTERPRETATION

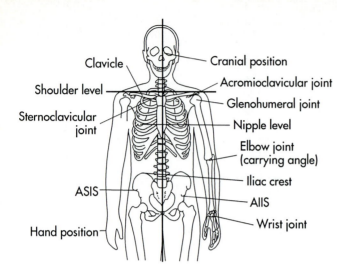

Clavicle — Cranial position
Shoulder level — Acromioclavicular joint
Glenohumeral joint
Sternoclavicular joint — Nipple level
Elbow joint (carrying angle)
ASIS — Iliac crest
AIIS
Hand position — Wrist joint

Fig. 3-15 Anterior view. Boney alignment.

SHOULDER LEVEL

A 'drop' or 'droop' shoulder (according to Priest and Nagel) is a visible depression of the athlete's dominant shoulder as a result of repeated overhand throwing postures and hypertrophy of the dominant arm. It is commonly seen in tennis players because of their serving style and in overhand pitchers. During the overhand motion, the repeated downswing follow-through across the body stretches the shoulder elevators and scapular retractors (the trapezius, levator scapulae, and rhomboids). The shoulder at rest assumes a depressed position because of this and also because of the increased mass of the entire arm and hypertrophy of both muscle and bone. The scapula moves into an abducted position, which reduces the subacromial space and can result in impingement problems.

The depressed shoulder position also reduces the thoracic outlet, leading to potential problems with thoracic outlet compression (subclavian artery and vein, or brachial plexus). The protracted shoulder position can also put tension on the supras-capular nerve, thereby affecting the infraspinatus and supraspinatus muscles.

CLAVICULAR LEVEL

The clavicles should be symmetric. Any swelling or callus formation on the lateral third of the clavicle is a sign of a present or previous clavicular fracture.

ACROMIOCLAVICULAR JOINTS

A "step" deformity where the distal end of the clavicle is above the acromion is a sign of acromioclavicular separation (severe sprain). The degree of the step determines if the ligaments are torn; a complete separation indicates a tear of the

ASSESSMENT   INTERPRETATION

acromioclavicular, coracoacromial, and coracoclavicular ligaments.

Asymmetry can indicate an acute or chronic injury to the acromioclavicular joint.

STERNOCLAVICULAR JOINTS

The sternoclavicular joints should be level. A prominent clavicle on one side of the sternum is a sign of a sternoclavicular joint sprain, subluxation, or complete tear.

GLENOHUMERAL JOINTS

An anterior dislocation of the glenohumeral joint is evident by a prominent acromion laterally, a depressed scapula, and a slightly abducted humerus. There is severe pain and usually the athlete will support the forearm.

The humeral head may be slightly inferior from the normal resting position, with inferior glenohumeral instability. The humeral head may also sit superiorly if there are capsular restrictions secondary to adhesive capuslitis. Many shoulder problems cause deltoid atrophy, so this should be looked for.

ELBOW JOINTS (CARRYING ANGLE)

The carrying angle is the angle created when a line is drawn through the midline of the humerus and another line is drawn through the center of the forearm with the arm in the anatomic position.

The angle of the normal elbow joint is 5° to 10° in males and 10° to 15° in females. If the angle is greater than 15° it is a sign of cubital valgus; if the angle is less than 5° to 10° it is a sign of cubital varus.

The carrying angle of the elbow can develop a cubital varus or valgus when the end of the humerus is subject to malunion or growth retardation at the epiphyseal plate.

A cubital varus can indicate a previous supracondylar fracture of the humerus.

Any changes in the carrying angle or elbow structure can affect the movements of the entire kinetic chain, including the shoulder, forearm, wrist, and hand.

WRIST JOINTS AND HAND POSITION

A wrist and hand that is lower on one side than on the other can indicate a drop shoulder on that side also.

Soft Tissue

Look for muscle hypertrophy or atrophy, especially in the trapezius, biceps, deltoid, pectoralis major, wrist flexors and extensors, and hand musculature.

Unilateral muscle hypertrophy can indicate that the athlete overuses one arm or shoulder to meet the demands of his or her occupation or sport.

If muscle atrophy occurs it is readily observable in the pectoralis major, deltoid, or biceps brachii muscles.

ASSESSMENT

INTERPRETATION

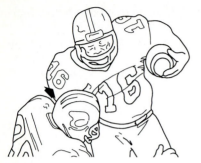

Fig. 3-16 Ruptured biceps tendon (long head).

Atrophy in the deltoid (and teres minor) can be from an axillary nerve injury, which can occur after anterior glenohumeral dislocation.

Atrophy of the coracobrachialis, biceps brachii, and brachialis indicates an injury to the musculocutaneous nerve.

Loss of proper muscle contour may also be the result of a muscle tear or rupture such as the "Popeye" biceps, which develops following a complete rupture of the biceps tendon (Fig. 3-16).

Overdevelopment of the wrist flexors and extensors often occurs in athletes who participate in racquet sports.

Muscle atrophy from a nerve root problem can cause observable atrophy in the hand musculature (C6, C7, or C8).

Muscle atrophy of the elbow, and wrist and hand extensors can result from a radial nerve injury (i.e., following the fracture of a humerus).

Lateral View (Fig. 3-17)
Boney
CRANIAL CARRIAGE (FORWARD HEAD POSTURE)

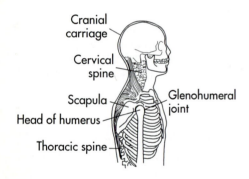

Fig. 3-17 Lateral view. Boney alignment.

A forward head position results in a tight extended suboccipital cervical spine, a flexed mid to lower cervical spine, an extended upper thoracic spine, and elevated scapulae. This position results in uneven forces through the cervical spine facet joints and the intervertebral disc. Stress is also placed on the cervical nerve roots, ligaments, and muscles. This forward head position causes elevated scapulae and anteriorly rotated clavicles, which in turn leads to sternum depression and decreased glenohumeral flexion.

Pain referred from the cervical dysfunction can extend into the scapula, shoulder, arm, and/or hand, as well as the head and cervical region.

The suprascapular nerve can be stretched by this forward head posture, resulting in lateral and posterior shoulder pain, acromioclavicular pain, and infraspinatus and supraspinatus dysfunction.

The dorsal scapular nerve can also be placed on stretch with this posture causing scapular pain.

CERVICOTHORACIC JUNCTION

An abrupt change in the flexed lower cervical spine and extended mid to upper thoracic spine indicates a postural alignment problem that can lead to referred pain in the shoulder.

WINGING SCAPULA(E)

A distracted or winged scapula (or scapulae) can result from an injury to the long thoracic nerve or from a general weakness of the serratus anterior muscle. Poor muscle control of the scapula will result in a poorly positioned glenoid cavity and resulting dysfunction of the glenohumeral joint.

ASSESSMENT

INTERPRETATION

The abducted scapulae may result in compression of the acromioclavicular joint, which in turn can affect the clavicle and its movements during glenohumeral flexion and abduction. Scapular movement, especially rotation, will also be diminished. The subacromial space can be reduced, making impingement of the supraspinatus, biceps, and the subacromial bursa possible.

THORACIC KYPHOSIS

Excessive thoracic kyphosis can be inherited or acquired. The acquired form can be caused by tight medial rotators and adductors. This muscle imbalance commonly occurs in athletes who repeatedly assume a kyphotic position and overuse these muscle groups in their sport (basketball, volleyball, swimming, etc.).

This forward shoulder position adds to shoulder impingement conditions and a reduced thoracic outlet.

ANTERIOR GLENOHUMERAL JOINT

Increased glenohumeral internal rotation stretches the posterior musculature and allows shortening of the anterior musculature and capsule.

According to Rathburn and McNab, the vascular blood supply to the supraspinatus muscle is reduced in the adducted position; therefore the tendon may degenerate more readily in this position.

The accessory movements of humeral head glide and roll are inhibited in the anterior head position so that normal physiological movements may be lost.

The anterior position of the humerus in the glenoid labrum is more likely to develop impingement problems.

A traumatized shoulder will often assume this internally rotated position post injury, especially in patients who have suffered previous shoulder dislocations.

A tight biceps tendon can also pull the humerus forward and capsular adhesions can result.

Soft Tissue

Muscle hypertrophy or atrophy is readily seen in the shoulder region (deltoid, triceps), forearm (extensors, flexors), and the hand (thenar muscles).

Atrophy or hypertrophy of the shoulder, arm, hand, or scapular musculature, as indicated in the anterior view, indicates previous injury or overdevelopment.

Atrophy will be present in groups of muscles that are supplied by the same spinal segment if a nerve root irritation exists. Local neural injuries will cause atrophy in the muscles that they supply.

Posterior View (Fig. 3-18)
Boney
CRANIAL CARRIAGE

See anterior and lateral view.

ASSESSMENT   INTERPRETATION

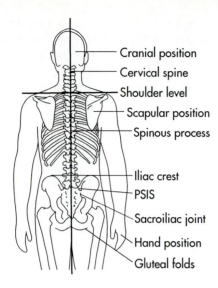

- Cranial position
- Cervical spine
- Shoulder level
- Scapular position
- Spinous process
- Iliac crest
- PSIS
- Sacroiliac joint
- Hand position
- Gluteal folds

Fig. 3-18 Posterior view. Boney alignment.

CERVICAL AND THORACIC SPINOUS PROCESS ALIGNMENT

The spinous processes and the outline of the scapula can be marked with a skin marker.

The spinous processes of the cervical and thoracic vertebrae should line up in a straight line.

A scoliosis or curve in the alignment (structural or functional) should be noted because this can alter the shoulder girdle mechanics.

Overdevelopment of one shoulder and arm can cause a thoracic scoliosis and related back problems.

SCAPULA

Level or winging scapula(e)
Protracted or retracted scapula(e)
Measure the distance from the spinous processes to the vertebral border of the scapula can be measured bilaterally

When one scapula is higher than the other the condition is called Sprengel deformity. Often the scapula is smaller and internally rotated. The range of abduction may be limited on the involved side—this can be bilateral.

Winging of the scapula(e) can be due to a long thoracic nerve injury or a weakness of the serratus anterior muscle.

A protracted scapula can be due to muscle tightness of the pectoralis major and minor muscles and weakness of the rhomboid muscles.

The scapula's vertebral border should be 2 inches from the spinous processes in the resting position.

Weakness of the scapular stabilizers (rhomboids, middle and lower trapezius) or tightness of the levator scapulae and upper trapezius can result in asynchronous scapular movements. When the scapula is not stable the glenoid cavity is not secure and glenohumeral joint dysfunction develops.

HAND POSITION

If the palms of the hands are facing backward, it is a sign of tight medial rotators and adductors.

ASSESSMENT

INTERPRETATION

Soft Tissue

Hypertrophy or atrophy of the musculature, especially the rhomboids, latissimus dorsi, erector spinae, and trapezius

Muscle spasm in trapezius or levator scapulae

Signs of hypertrophy, atrophy, or muscle imbalances should be observed bilaterally.

Often muscle spasms of the upper fibers of the trapezius and levator scapulae occur to help support a painful shoulder injury.

Atrophy of the infraspinatus and supraspinatus can be caused by an injury to the suprascapular nerve as it passes through the suprascapular notch (i.e., may be caused by a backpack with straps over this area) or a rotator cuff tear.

Atrophy of the triceps and wrist extensors can indicate a radial nerve problem.

Lesion Site

Scars or Surgical Repairs

A surgical procedure for recurring dislocations will usually leave a scar at the deltopectoral groove. This repair may restrict lateral rotation.

Swelling

Swelling occurs over an injured acromioclavicular or sternoclavicular joint or muscle lesion.

Swelling or stiffness that extends down the arm can suggest a venous return problem or a reflex sympathetic dystrophy.

Swelling from a severe trauma can cause swelling locally and, because of gravity, can track down the arm.

Redness

Redness or pallor in the upper limb may indicate an arterial problem (i.e., thoracic outlet, reflex sympathetic dystrophy).

Ecchymosis

Because of the pull of gravity, ecchymosis tracks down from the shoulder area into the upper arm, forearm, or hand.

Boney Callus Formation (Fig. 3-19)

Boney callus formation occurs over a fracture site. This occurs commonly with a clavicular fracture, which, in the shoulder girdle can reduce the size of the thoracic outlet, resulting in thoracic outlet compression problems.

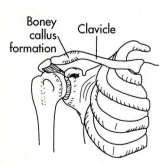

Fig. 3-19 Boney clavicular callus formation.

ASSESSMENT   INTERPRETATION

SUMMARY OF TESTS

FUNCTIONAL TESTS

Rule Out
   Internal organ problems
   Cervical spine
   Temporomandibular joint
   Thoracic spine
   Costovertebral, costotransverse, costochondral joints and rib motion
   Elbow joint
   Thoracic outlet problems
   Systemic conditions
Tests in Sitting
   Active glenohumeral forward flexion
   Passive glenohumeral forward flexion
   Resisted glenohumeral forward flexion
   Active glenohumeral extension
   Passive glenohumeral extension
   Resisted glenohumeral extension
   Active shoulder girdle abduction
   Passive shoulder girdle abduction
   Resisted shoulder girdle abduction
   Active glenohumeral adduction
   Passive glenohumeral adduction
   Resisted glenohumeral adduction
   Active glenohumeral lateral rotation
   Passive glenohumeral lateral rotation
   Resisted glenohumeral lateral rotation
   Active glenohumeral medial rotation
   Passive glenohumeral medial rotation
   Resisted glenohumeral medial rotation
   Resisted elbow flexion with supination
   Resisted elbow extension
   Active shoulder lateral rotation, abduction and flexion (Apley's Scratch Test)
   Active shoulder medial rotation, adduction, and extension

SPECIAL TESTS

Shoulder girdle movements
   Active shoulder girdle elevation
   Resisted shoulder girdle elevation
   Active shoulder girdle depression
   Active shoulder girdle retraction
   Active shoulder girdle protraction
Biceps Tests
   Yergason's test
   Booth and Marvel's test
   Lippman's test

ASSESSMENT   INTERPRETATION

Ludington's test
Hawkins and Kennedy's test or Speed's sign
Drop arm test
Apprehension sign
Anterior-posterior glenohumeral instability
Posterior glenohumeral dislocation test
Impingement signs
Hawkins and Kennedy's test
Neer and Welsh test
Empty can test
Infraspinatus test
Active glenohumeral cross-flexion
Passive glenohumeral cross-flexion
Resisted glenohumeral cross-flexion
Active glenohumeral cross-extension
Passive glenohumeral cross-extension
Resisted glenohumeral cross-extension
Acromioclavicular joint stability
Glide of acromion
Superior-inferior and anterior-posterior glide of the lateral clavicle
Traction
Cranial glide
Compression
Sternoclavicular joint stability
Superior-inferior and anterior-posterior glide of the medial clavicle
Neurological testing
Upper limb or brachial tension test
Reflex testing
Biceps reflex
Brachioradialis reflex
Triceps reflex
Dermatomes – cutaneous nerve supply
Maitland quadrant test
Maitland locking test

ACCESSORY MOVEMENT TESTS

Inferior glide
Posterior glide
Anterior glide
Lateral distraction
Scapular movements

Rule Out

Internal Organ Problems

Ask questions in the history taking regarding cardiac problems, diaphragm or respiratory dysfunction, chest or upper abdominal problems (liver, gall-

These joint clearing tests should be done if symptoms or observations reveal their possible involvement.

Coronary problems (i.e., angina, myocardial infarction) can radiate pain to the left shoulder, sternum, and jaw.

ASSESSMENT

INTERPRETATION

bladder, pancreas, spleen).

Observe for normal respiratory movements and function.

Observe for chest or abdominal scars from a laparotomy, cholecystectomy, or previous heart surgery.

Diaphragm, lung, or respiratory problems can refer pain along the C4 and C5 nerve roots.

A spontaneous pneumothorax can refer pain to the top of the shoulder on the involved side. Chest and upper abdomen problems can refer pain to the shoulder area (spleen, gallbladder, stomach, esophagus, pancreas).

Cervical Spine

Rule out cervical spine through the history-taking, observations, and active functional tests of cervical forward bending, back bending, side bending, and rotation.

Gentle overpressures can be done in forward bending, side bending, and rotation if the range is limited but pain free.

To further clear the cervical spine and brachial plexus, the upper limb or brachial tension test can be done (see Cervical Spine Assessment, special tests).

Often, cervical nerve root impingements will cause pain in the shoulder region, upper arm, or even down the forearm.

Loss of cervical range with individual cervical segment hypomobility or hypermobility can lead to referred pain in the shoulder area. Listen for evidence of dermatome patches of numbness, tingling, or pain during the history-taking.

Limited cervical or elbow ranges suggest more than just shoulder pathology.

Myotome weakness in the history suggests neural pathology.

Trapezius and levator scapulae muscle involvement in particular should be ruled out because these muscles move the scapula and the cervical spine. A problem with either of these muscles will therefore directly influence the shoulder girdle.

Cervical facet joints, ligaments, narrow intervertebral foramen, and osteophytes can all cause cervical radiculitis to the shoulder and therefore involvement of the cervical spine must be ruled out.

Temporomandibular Joint

Rule out TMJ by having the athlete open and close the mouth.

Normal dimensions of the mouth opening should be three fingers width or two knuckles width.

Any decrease in range or signs of pain or clicking during the opening or closing of the mouth can demonstrate temporomandibular pathologic conditions. Any lateral deviation of the mandible during opening indicates temporomandibular joint dysfunction or muscle imbalance. If TMJ dysfunction exists, the resulting forward head posture and myofascial syndromes can cause adaptive shoulder problems.

Thoracic Spine

Rule out thoracic spine dysfunction throughout history-taking and observations. In observations, look for excessive thoracic kyphosis, gibbous deformity (sharp localized posterior angulation of the thoracic curve), or dowager's hump (osteoporosis causing excessive kyphosis). Look for scoliosis (C- or S-shaped curve in the thoracic and/or lumbar spine).

If an upper thoracic dysfunction is

Restrictions of the thoracic spine can refer pain into the shoulder joint.

According to Kellgren, the midcervical and thoracic spine ligaments can refer pain into the glenohumeral joint and can cause irritation of the interspinous ligament of C4-C5, C7-T1, and T1-T2 segments specifically.

Excessive thoracic kyphosis and the rounded shoulder position that accompanies this prevents the glenohumeral, clavicular joints (AC and SC), and scapular joints from functioning normally. The rhomboids and the lower trapezius muscles lengthen while the internal rotators and serratus anterior muscles short-

ASSESSMENT

suspected, have the athlete forward bend, back bend, side bend, and rotate the lower cervical spine while you observe the thoracic function and determine if local pain or dysfunction is present.

If a midthoracic spine dysfunction is suspected, test the athlete with the following motions. With the athlete seated in a low-back chair and the lumbar spine supported, have the athlete clasp hands together with fingers interlaced behind the head. The fingers should run from the occiput to the cervical thoracic junction and are in position to prevent motion of the cervical spine. The flexed elbows are together in front of the athlete's chest (see Fig. 2-31, *A*). Have the athlete forward bend, moving the elbows toward the groin. There should be no lumbar flexion. The athlete then backbends as far as possible over the back of the chair without extending the lumbar spine (see Fig. 2-32, *A*). For thoracic side bending the athlete moves the flexed elbows out laterally in the frontal plane and side bends as far as possible without lifting the pelvis or side bending the lumbar spine (see Fig. 2-33, *A*). For thoracic rotation, the athlete's arms are crossed in front of the body with elbows flexed. The athlete forward bends slightly, then rotates as far as possible (see Fig. 2-34). If the range is restricted in any of these motions, without pain, then overpressures can be done (see Figs. 2-31, *B*; 2-32, *B*; and 2-33, *B*).

Costovertebral, Costotransverse, Costochondral Joints, and Rib Motion

Palpate rib function, especially of the first rib, and of costovertebral movement during inspiration and expiration.

To palpate the rib function, the athlete sits while you palpate anterior posterior movement of the ribs on each side of the chest during normal breathing.

The lateral rib movements can also be palpated.

INTERPRETATION

en. The humerus internally rotates, which can lead to anterior capsule and glenohumeral adaptive shortening or even adhesions. With the adaptive muscle shortening and lengthening, normal muscle function on the shoulder girdle is lost and joint dysfunction can result.

Problems at C7-T1 and T1-T2 spinal segments can refer pain into the armpit and the inner upper arm.

Problems of the midthoracic region can refer pain to the scapula and its surrounding soft tissue.

Dysfunction of the costovertebral or costotransverse joints may cause pain mainly in the posterior triangle of the cervical spine.

Dysfunction in the first and second ribs can affect these joints and, in turn, can affect shoulder movements. During respiration, the costovertebral, costotransverse, and costochondral joints allow a superior-inferior movement (pump handle), which increases the anterior-posterior diameter of the ribs and thorax. The upper ribs move in a "pump handle" fashion while the middle and lower ribs move in a "bucket handle" fashion.

ASSESSMENT   INTERPRETATION

The radiate and intra-articular ligaments of the costovertebral joints and the strong ligaments of the costotransverse joints allow only a slight gliding motion.

Dysfunction of the costovertebral, costotransverse or costochondral joints or rib motion will lead to contraction of pectoralis minor and the scalenes muscles to assist respiratory function. In turn, these muscles will fatigue and can upset the kinetic movements of the cervical spine and shoulder girdles.

Costochondral or costosternal joint pain (often termed costochondritis) can cause point tenderness in the joints involved. In the athletic community, this anterior chest discomfort is primarily caused by direct trauma to the area.

The clavicle and first rib have strong ligamentous and muscular attachments (subclavius); therefore they influence one another.

The serratus anterior's first digitation originates on the first rib, and dysfunction of the first rib can affect clavicular movements and shoulder girdle movements.

Elbow Joint

Rule out the elbow joint through the history-taking, observations, and active functional tests of elbow flexion, extension, radioulnar pronation, and supination with overpressure (Fig. 3-20, *A* and *B*).

Elbow problems can also affect the shoulder, especially with the two-joint muscles (biceps and triceps).

Elbow dysfunction in the humeroradial or humeroulnar joints can affect humeral function above.

Thoracic Outlet Problems

Adson Maneuver (Figs. 3-21 and 3-22)

Palpate the radial pulse on the affected side.

Instruct the athlete to take a deep breath and hold it, extend his or her

This test determines if a cervical rib or a reduced interscalene triangle is compressing the subclavian artery. The compression of the subclavian artery is determined by the decrease in or absence of the radial pulse.

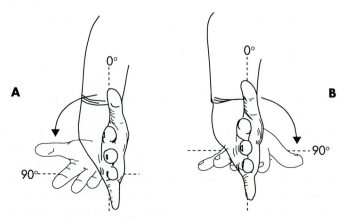

Fig. 3-20 A, Active radioulnar supination. **B,** Active radioulnar pronation.

ASSESSMENT

INTERPRETATION

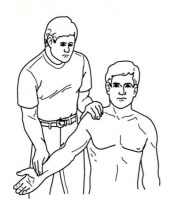

Fig. 3-21 Adson maneuver 1.

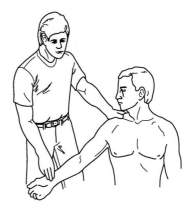

Fig. 3-22 Adson maneuver 2.

neck, and turn the head toward the affected side.

Apply downward traction on the extended shoulder and arm while palpating the radial pulse.

The pulse may diminish or become absent. In some athletes a greater effect on the subclavian artery is exerted by turning the head to the opposite side.

Costoclavicular Syndrome Test

Instruct the athlete to stand in an exaggerated military stance with the shoulders thrust backward and downward.

Take the radial pulse before and during the shoulder retraction position.

Hyperabduction Test (Fig. 3-23)

Instruct the athlete to fully abduct the shoulder or to repeatedly abduct the shoulder.

Take the radial pulse before and after the prolonged or repeated abduction. Symptoms will develop in less than 1 minute if compression is significant.

This test is most effective when the interscalene triangle is occluded by the anterior scalene muscle, which pulls tight during the cervical extension and rotation.

This test causes compression of the subclavian artery and vein by reducing the space between the clavicle and first rib. Callus formation on a previous clavicular fracture can reduce the space. Poor upper quadrant posture can also affect the size of the space.

A modification or obliteration of the radial pulse indicates that a compression exists.

If this test causes the symptoms that are the athlete's major complaint, a compression problem is at fault.

A dampening of the pulse can occur even in a healthy athlete with an anatomical predisposition for this problem but who does not have the symptoms because he or she does not assume this position repeatedly or for long periods of time. Pain or tingling can also occur while performing this test.

Repeated or prolonged positions of hyperabduction can cause a reduction in the size of the costoclavicular space of the thoracic outlet.

This position is often assumed in sleep, while performing certain activities (i.e., painting, sweeping chimneys) and during certain sports (i.e., volleyball spiker, tennis serve).

The subclavian vessels can be compressed at two locations: (1) between the pectoralis minor tendon and the coracoid process or (2) between the clavicle and the first rib.

ASSESSMENT

INTERPRETATION

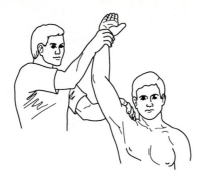

Fig. 3-23 Hyperabduction test.

Pain or a diminishing of pulse indicates that a compression exists.

Systemic Conditions

Systemic conditions that affect the shoulder must be ruled out with a thorough medical history, injury history, and observations of the athlete.

A systemic disorder can exist with any of the following responses or findings:

- bilateral shoulder pain and/or swelling
- several joints inflamed or painful
- the athlete's general health is not good, especially when the injury flares up
- painful soft tissue lesion does not respond to conventional therapy
- there are repeated insidious onsets of the problem

The following systemic disorders can affect the shoulder:

- rheumatoid arthritis
- psoriatic arthritis
- ankylosing spondylitis
- osteoarthritis
- gouty arthritis
- neoplasm
- infection (systemic, bacterial, viral)

Test the joint involved, but if a systemic disorder is suspected, send the athlete for a complete medical checkup with the family physician, including blood work, x-rays, and urine testing.

Rheumatoid arthritis occurs in the shoulders but rarely in both joints at once. Other signs and symptoms include night pain and pain at the end of range in all directions at first, after which a capsular pattern sets up. Pain can also spread into the forearm and it can last for 4 to 6 months; other joints can flare up (inflame) also.

Psoriatic arthritis can occur in the shoulder joints—usually the affected athlete has psoriatic nail (ridging) and skin lesions.

Ankylosing spondylitis can cause shoulder discomfort but primarily the sacroiliac joint changes occur first, then changes occur in the spine and finally in the other joints.

Osteoarthritis at the shoulder is usually symptom free. The athlete is aware of crepitus or grating. Trauma or overuse can lead to joint inflammation that in turn can lead to further osteoarthritic changes and the pain that is associated with these changes.

Gouty arthritis at the shoulder can be confirmed by laboratory findings of uric acid in the synovial fluid or the tissues surrounding the joint or through elevated levels of serum uric acid.

A neoplastic invasion of the upper humerus or glenoid labrum will cause shoulder joint and muscle pain. Bone tumors are fairly common in the proximal humerus. They may be benign or malignant. If malignant, this is usually the secondary site and the primary source must be determined. Boney point tenderness, excessive pain, and extreme weakness may be other signs of the presence of a neoplasm.

Bacterial and viral infections can cause joint stiffness, muscle pain, and weakness. Usually, several joints are affected and fever is associated with the presence of infection.

ASSESSMENT   INTERPRETATION

Tests in Sitting

With the athlete seated in a high-back chair, the scapula is stabilized so that each side can be tested easily.

These tests can be done when the athlete is supine, if:
- the shoulder injury is acute or painful
- the athlete is stronger than you are
- the athlete has trapezius muscle spasm
- the athlete is anxious because of the testing
- the athlete can not relax the shoulder joint or surrounding muscles

Active Glenohumeral Forward Flexion (180°) (Fig. 3-24)

The athlete raises the arms forward and overhead as far as possible.

Demonstrate the action for the athlete.

Put your hand on the athlete's other shoulder to stabilize the scapula and to prevent body lean.

The shoulder should move through a full range of motion.

Pain, weakness, or loss of range of motion can be caused by an injury to the muscles or their nerve supply.

The prime movers are:
- Anterior deltoid—axillary N. (C5, C6)
- Corocobrachialis—musculocutaneous (C6, C7)

The accessory movers are:
- Deltoid (middle fibers)
- Pectoralis major (clavicular)
- Biceps brachii

Pain at the end of range of motion can come from a capsular stretch if the capsule is damaged or from the coracoclavicular or coracohumeral ligaments.

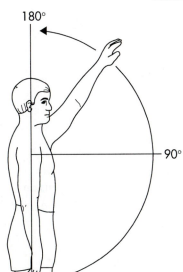

Fig. 3-24 Active glenohumeral forward flexion.

ASSESSMENT

INTERPRETATION

Passive Glenohumeral Forward Flexion (Overstretch; 180°) (see Fig. 3-24)

Have one hand over the athlete's medial clavicle and scapula to stabilize him or her while the other hand is under the elbow joint. Lift the athlete's extended arm through the full range of motion until an end feel is reached.

The end feel should be a soft tissue stretch. Pain at end of range of motion can be caused by:
- tightness or adhesion of the shoulder joint capsule
- coracoclavicular or coracohumeral (posterior band) ligament sprain
- tightness or injury to the shoulder adductors
- an impingement syndrome

Resisted Glenohumeral Forward Flexion

The athlete flexes the glenohumeral joint forward at an angle of about 30° with his or her palm facing downward.

Stabilize the scapula with one hand over the clavicular region while the other hand is on the distal forearm or elbow and resists forward flexion. The athlete attempts forward flexion against your resistance.

The athlete's palm should be face down to rule out testing biceps.

Pain and/or weakness can be caused by an injury to the muscles or their nerve supply (see Active Glenohumeral Forward Flexion).

The anterior deltoid is often contused and will elicit pain here also.

Active Glenohumeral Extension (50° to 60°) (Fig. 3-25)

The athlete extends the arm backward as far as possible.

Stabilize that shoulder to eliminate shoulder elevation.

The athlete must not lean forward.

Pain, weakness, and/or limitation of range of motion can be caused by an injury to the muscles or their nerve supply.
- Latissimus dorsi—thoracodorsal N. (C6, C7, C8)
- Posterior deltoid—axillary N. (C5, C6)
- Teres major—inferior subscapular N. (C5, C6)

The accessory movers are:
- Triceps brachii (long head)
- Teres minor muscles

Pain at the end of range of motion can come from the coracohumeral ligament.

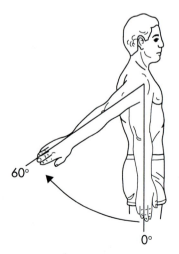

Fig. 3-25 Active glenohumeral extension.

60°

0°

ASSESSMENT

INTERPRETATION

Passive Glenohumeral Extension (60°)

Move the arm backward with one hand above the elbow and the other hand stabilizing the clavicle and scapula on that side.

Pain could be caused by an injury to the shoulder flexors or an injury to the coracohumeral ligament (anterior band).

The end feel should be bone on bone with the greater tubercle of the humerus butting the acromion posteriorly.

An end feel of tissue stretch can occur in the biceps brachii with the shoulder and elbow extended.

Resisted Glenohumeral Extension

Resist shoulder extension in midrange by resisting at the distal forearm or above the elbow with one hand and stabilizing the shoulder with the other hand.

Weakness and/or pain can be caused by an injury to the muscles or their nerve supply (see Active Glenohumeral Extension).

Active Shoulder Girdle Abduction (180°) (Fig. 3-26)
Anterior View

The athlete abducts the arms as far as possible while the therapist observes the movement in the anterior view.

Pain, weakness, and/or limitation of range of motion can be caused by an injury to the muscles or their nerve supply (Fig. 3-26).

The prime movers are:
- Deltoid (middle fibers—axillary or circumflex N. (C5, C6)
- Supraspinatus—scapular N. (C5)

The accessory movers are:
- Deltoid (anterior and posterior)
- Pectoralis major (when the arm is at an angle that is greater than 90°)
- Trapezius (to elevate the clavicle and rotate the scapula)
- Serratus anterior (for scapular rotation and fixation)
- Infraspinatus
- Teres minor (for external rotation of humerus)

If the athlete is unable to abduct the arm and is experiencing no pain, it could be caused by a ruptured supraspinatus tendon. This condition can come on insidiously (slow tendon degeneration) or can be caused by a strain or fall on the shoulder. The deltoid alone cannot act as an abductor at an angle that is below 90° without the supraspinatus muscle.

Neural problems to the long thoracic nerve, which serves the serratus anterior, limits active abduction to an angle of 90°. Neuritis or nerve palsy to the spinal accessory nerve, which innerves the trapezius, limits abduction to an angle of 10°.

A painful arc (see Fig. 3-26) occurs when there is pain at angles between 60° and 120° of abduction; the pain disappears above and below this range. This arc can be felt on the way up, the way down, actively, or passively.

Abduction of the arm occurs in the glenohumeral joint and scapulothoracic articulation in a 2:1 ratio. For every 3° of abduction, 2° of motion occur at the glenohumeral joint and 1° occurs at the scapulothoracic articulation (scapular rotation).

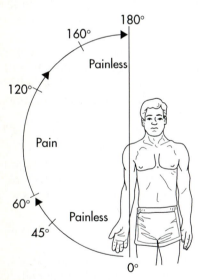

Fig. 3-26 Active glenohumeral abduction—painful arc.

ASSESSMENT

INTERPRETATION

To fully understand the scapulohumeral rhythm, the component joint actions during abduction must be understood. During shoulder abduction of 180° the following movements occur: glenohumeral abduction of 120°, glenohumeral external rotation between 70° to 90°, clavicular backward rotation of 30° to 50°, clavicular elevation between 30° to 60°, and scapular upward rotation between 30° to 60°. Some extension and side bending can occur in the thoracic spine to increase the range beyond 180°.

According to Nirschle, a weakness or injury to the rotator cuff causes an upward migration of the humeral head during abduction, causing subacromial impingement and its related problems (biceps and supraspinatus tendonitis, subacromial bursitis).

Between angles of 0° to 30° of abduction, the glenohumeral joint moves 30° and the clavicle elevates 15°.

Between angles of 30° to 90° of abduction the glenohumeral joint moves 30°, the scapula rotates upward (movement at the sternoclavicular and acromioclavicular joints) and the clavicle elevates 15°.

Between angles of 90° to 150° of abduction the glenohumeral joint moves 30° and rotates externally 70° to 90°, while the scapula rotates upward 30°. The clavicle elevates 15° to 30° and rotates backward 50°.

Between angles of 150° to 190° of abduction the glenohumeral joint moves 30° (this is sometimes referred to as adduction of the humerus because the humerus is moving toward the midline of the body) and the clavicle elevates 5° (at the acromioclavicular joint).

The humerus must externally rotate 90° or the greater tubercle of the humerus will impinge on the coracoacromial arch. Normal glenohumeral abduction is only 120° within the glenoid fossa, then motion is blocked by impingement of the surgical neck of the humerus on the acromion of the scapula and the coracoclavicular ligament.

To achieve full abduction, there must be scapular rotation upward.

A reverse scapulohumeral rhythm means that the scapula moves more than the humerus and is a sign of a major shoulder girdle dysfunction. It can be caused by:
- "frozen shoulder" syndrome (adhesive capsulitis)
- rotator cuff lesion
- severe impingement problem at the glenohumeral joint
- severe instability problem at the glenohumeral joint

Posterior View (Fig. 3-27)

SCAPULOHUMERAL RHYTHM

Stand behind the athlete to assess scapulohumeral rhythm. The glenohumeral joint allows the first 20° of

If the glenohumeral joint is frozen or not moving freely, the athlete will shrug his or her shoulder upward and may be able to attain 90° of abduction with pure scapulothoracic motion.

ASSESSMENT   INTERPRETATION

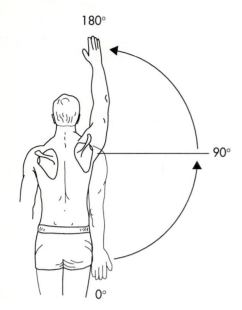

Fig. 3-27 Active shoulder girdle abduction (combined glenohumeral, scapulothoracic, and clavicular motion).

movement, then the scapula and humerus should move together.

To determine if the glenohumeral joint is not moving, you can stabilize the scapula with your hand over the acromion while the other hand elevates the humerus. You can tell whether the movement for abduction is purely scapular or glenohumeral. If the athlete cannot abduct his or her arm without lifting the shoulder, the movement is scapulothoracic motion. This inability to abduct using the glenohumeral joint indicates significant glenohumeral dysfunction (i.e., frozen shoulder, adhesive capsulitis, severe impingement problem, supraspinatus tear).

Painful Arc

A painful arc is caused by impingement of a structure under the subacromial arch, according to Kessel and Watson, and Cyriax (Fig. 3-28). The structure is pinched when the humeral greater tuberosity passes under the acromial arch at an angle of 80° of abduction.

The pain is elicited more on active then passive movement and is usually greater through the arc upward than downward. The pain usually ceases at 90° to 120° of abduction. The athlete will attempt to abduct the arm by bringing the humerus forward not in true abduction. Causes of a painful arc are discussed in the following paragraphs.

SUPRASPINATUS TENDONITIS

Supraspinatus tendonitis is the most common cause of a painful arc. There is point tenderness near or at the point of insertion of the supraspinatus on the greater tuberosity (Fig. 3-29). Pain on passive abduction at an angle of approximately 60° to 90° is a positive impingement sign.

A strain, scarring, calcification, or rupture of the tendon are

ASSESSMENT   INTERPRETATION

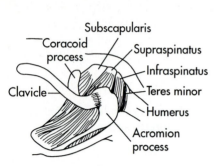

Fig. 3-28 Superior view of the rotator cuff muscles impinged with a painful arc syndrome.

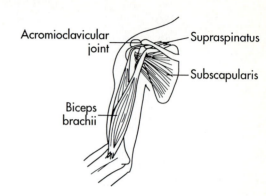

Fig. 3-29 Anterior shoulder muscles that can elicit a painful arc.

all possible causes. In the case of a strain or scarring the active abduction power is full, yet resisted abduction is painful. A calcification will show on x-rays and it is very painful. A tendon rupture will cause an inability in initiating abduction.

SUBACROMIAL BURSITIS

An acute bursitis can elicit pain before the arc is reached. No resisted tests hurt except the resisted abduction test, which compresses the bursa. This helps to distinguish it from others. If the therapist gently applies joint traction during abduction, the painful arc may go away if the problem is bursitis or capsulitis since the joint space is opened and the bursa or capsule is not compressed.

INFRASPINATUS TENDONITIS

Signs and symptoms of infraspinatus tendonitis are a painful arc, pain on resisted lateral rotation, and point tenderness at the uppermost point of insertion on the humeral tuberosity.

SUBSCAPULAR TENDONITIS

Subscapular tendonitis has a painful arc, pain on resisted medial rotation, and point tenderness at the point of insertion of the lesser tuberosity.

BICEPS TENDONITIS

In this condition the athlete experiences pain with resisted supination of the forearm and flexion of the elbow. The long head of the biceps is impinged.

OTHERS

Other less common causes of a painful arc include:
- sprain of the inferior acromioclavicular ligaments—marked by point tenderness and pain on cross-flexion
- osteoarthritis or degenerative changes of the acromioclavicular joint

ASSESSMENT

INTERPRETATION

- metastasis in the acromion—characterized by tenderness of the bone itself (neoplasm) and localized warmth
- glenohumeral capsular laxity—after dislocation or sprain, the capsular laxity may allow momentary subluxation of the head of the humerus. From a subluxed position in full abduction, as the arm moves toward the horizontal, it clicks back into place at about 80°of abduction.
- cervical disc lesion

Passive Shoulder Girdle Abduction (180°)

Lift the arm through the full range of motion.

Once above an angle of 90°, the humerus must be externally rotated to reach the end of range of motion.

The athlete must be relaxed and must not try to assist you.

Determine the end feel, the quality of the movement (crepitus, grating, smooth), any difference between active and passive abduction, and if it hurts and when.

If pain begins before the extreme range is reached and has a soft end feel, subacromial bursitis is possible.

If full range of motion is present but all extremes of range hurt and have a hard end feel, a capsular lesion is probably the cause.

If the pain is felt at the extreme of abduction only, the capsule is probably at fault.

Chronic bursitis, chronic tendonitis, and acromioclavicular joint sprains can all cause pain at the extreme of abduction but the end feel is the same as in a normal joint.

Pain and limitation can also come from an abductor muscle strain.

Pain at the acromioclavicular joint can indicate an acromioclavicular ligament sprain or degenerative changes.

The normal end feel can be tissue approximation with the arm against the head or a boney end feel with the greater tuberosity on the coracoacromial arch.

The middle and inferior bands of the glenohumeral ligament become taut with abduction.

Fine crepitus during the movement can indicate a calcium deposit in the bursa or joint.

Grating during the movement can indicate osteoarthritic changes of the surface.

Resisted Shoulder Girdle Abduction

Resist abduction with one hand on the athlete's distal forearm or elbow. The other hand rests over the shoulder to stabilize the scapula and to prevent shrugging.

Resist in midrange (not above 90°) with his or her palm down for the middle fibers of deltoid.

To test supraspinatus the shoulder is resisted at angles from 0° to 5° of abduction.

Weakness and/or pain can be caused by an injury to the muscles or to their nerve supply (see Active Shoulder Girdle Abduction).

Painless weakness of the deltoid muscle can be the result of an axillary nerve compression, which can result from damage caused by the head of the humerus when it dislocates or from direct trauma. This boney displacement may be only momentary; hence there may be no clear history of dislocation. Weakness of the deltoid, biceps, supraspinatus, and infraspinatus muscles is a clear sign of a C5 nerve root problem.

A painful arc and pain in resisted abduction suggests a supraspinatus muscle injury.

Painful weakness of the supraspinatus muscle can be caused by a tendonitis or partial rupture.

ASSESSMENT

INTERPRETATION

Weakness of the supraspinatus and infraspinatus muscle can be caused by a neuritis of the suprascapular nerve. According to Cyriax, this neuritis causes constant pain that lasts approximately 3 weeks and is felt in the scapula area and upper arm. Movements of the neck, scapula, and other upper limbs are pain free. The suprascapular nerve injury can be traumatic, caused by severe traction on the arm. It can also be caused when the suprascapular nerve is caught in the suprascapular notch. A poor postural position of a forward shoulder and forward head will put the suprascapular nerve on stretch, making it susceptible to an overstretch injury or chronic attenuation.

Subacromial bursitis can be painful with resisted abduction because of the pinching of the bursa when the deltoid contracts. Often, there is rebound pain with a bursitis (pain on release of the isometric contraction).

Active Glenohumeral Adduction (45°) (Fig. 3-30)

The athlete moves his or her arm across in front of the body.

Pain, weakness, and/or limitation of range of motion can be caused by an injury to the muscles or to their nerve supply.

The prime movers are the:
- Pectoralis major—lateral and medial pectoral N. (C5, C6, C7, C8, and T1 respectively)
- Teres major—inferior subscapular N. (C5, C6)
- Latissimus dorsi—thoracodorsal N. (C6, C7, C8)

The accessory movers are:
- Triceps (long head)
- Coracobrachialis
- Biceps brachii (short head)

Passive Glenohumeral Adduction

Carry the arm through the range and then apply a gentle overpressure at the end of the active range until an end feel is reached.

The range of the glenohumeral joint can be limited by pain if an inflamed subacromial bursa exists or if there is a tear in the rotator cuff (especially in the supraspinatus muscle).

Limitation can come from tightness in the posterior capsule.

The normal end feel is one of tissue approximation when the upper arm makes contact with the trunk.

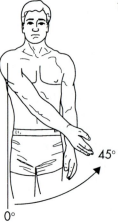

Fig. 3-30 Active glenohumeral adduction.

ASSESSMENT

INTERPRETATION

Resisted Glenohumeral Adduction

The athlete abducts the arm about 20°, then attempts to adduct it against your resistance. Resist adduction with one hand on the distal medial forearm and stabilize the shoulder with the other hand.

Pain and/or weakness can be caused by an injury to the muscles or their nerve supply (see Active Glenohumeral Adduction).

To determine if pectoralis major is at fault, test resisted cross-flexion (horizontal adduction), adduction, and internal rotation.

To determine if latissimus dorsi is involved, resist shoulder extension.

Weakness in adduction is found in seventh cervical root palsy as a result of the weakness of the latissimus dorsi.

Active Glenohumeral Lateral Rotation (90°) (Fig. 3-31)

The athlete flexes the elbow at an angle of 90° with the forearm in midposition.

The athlete's elbow must remain next to his or her side.

The athlete then turns the forearm out as far as possible with the rotation occurring at the glenohumeral joint.

Rest one hand on the athlete's shoulder to prevent shoulder elevation and the other hand keeps the athlete's elbow at his or her side.

Pain, weakness, and/or limitation of range of motion can be caused by an injury to the muscles or to their nerve supply.

The prime movers are:
- Infraspinatus—suprascapular N. (C5, C6)
- Teres minor—axillary N. (C5, C6)

The accessory mover is the posterior deltoid muscle.

Passive Glenohumeral Lateral Rotation (Overpressure; 90°)

As in active glenohumeral lateral rotation but while one hand is supporting the elbow, the other hand holds the palmar aspect of the athlete's forearm.

Then move the forearm to carry the glenohumeral joint through the full range of motion until an end feel is reached.

Pain and/or limitation at the end of range is caused by:
- injury to the middle and proximal capsule or capsular ligaments (Ferrari)
- injury to the middle of the glenohumeral ligament, when an abduction is between 60° and 90° of abduction (Ferrari)
- muscle injury to the medial rotators (tightness)
- sprain of the coracohumeral ligament, if injured with the shoulder below 60° of abduction
- anterior capsule scar from a previous shoulder dislocation
- subacromial bursitis
- subacromial bursitis that results in limited lateral rotation when the shoulder is abducted to an angle of 90° and then rotated

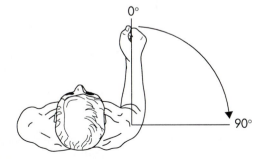

Fig. 3-31 Active glenohumeral lateral rotation.

ASSESSMENT

INTERPRETATION

Resisted Glenohumeral Lateral Rotation

The athlete flexes the elbow at an angle of 90° with the elbow next to their side and the forearm in midposition.

Resist with one hand on the distal dorsal aspect of the forearm and the other hand on the distal lateral humerus for stabilization.

The athlete attempts to laterally rotate his or her shoulder and to move the forearm outward.

The athlete must laterally rotate the glenohumeral joint only and not abduct the shoulder.

Weakness and/or pain can be caused by an injury to the muscles or to their nerve supply (see Active Glenohumeral Lateral Rotation).

Weakness and/or pain in lateral rotation and adduction suggests an injury to the teres minor muscle.

Weakness and pain in joint lateral rotation only is evidence of an infraspinatus injury.

A painless weakness in lateral rotation suggests a rupture of the infraspinatus muscle, which is rare.

A painful arc with abduction and pain with resisted lateral rotation suggests the presence of an infraspinatus tendonitis.

Active Glenohumeral Medial Rotation (90°) (Fig. 3-32)

The athlete takes the arm to full lateral rotation with the elbow flexed at an angle of 90°. Active medial rotation involves returning the forearm close to the abdomen.

The athlete's elbow must be tucked into the side of the body to prevent the athlete from adducting the arm.

Pain, weakness, and/or limitation of range of motion can be caused by an injury to the muscles or their nerve supply. The prime movers are:

- Subscapularis—superior and inferior subscapular N. (C5, C6)
- Pectoralis major—lateral and medial pectoral N. (C5, C6, C7, and C8, T1 respectively)
- Latissimus dorsi—thoracodorsal N. (C6, C7, C8)
- Teres major—inferior subscapular N. (C5, C6)

The accessory mover is the anterior deltoid muscle.

Passive Glenohumeral Medial Rotation (Fig. 3-33)

This is the same as in active glenohumeral medial rotation but hold the athlete's elbow next to their body with one hand while the other hand holds the athlete's wrist and carries their forearm from full lateral rotation to full medial rotation.

Apply an overstretch by moving the athlete's forearm behind their back.

Pain and/or limitation can be caused by tightness or injury of the shoulder lateral rotators.

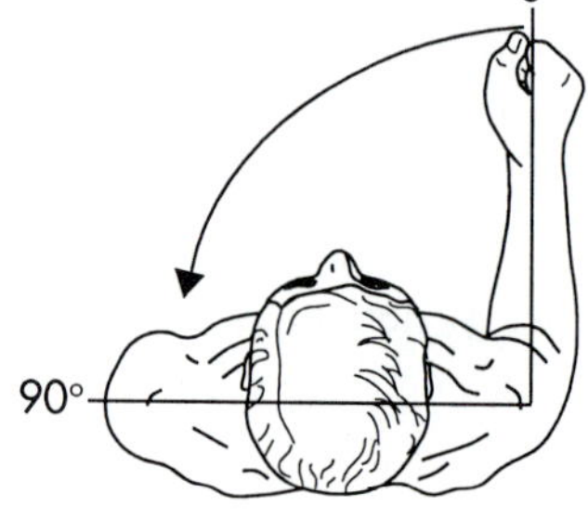

Fig. 3-32 Active glenohumeral medial rotation.

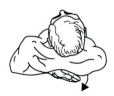

Fig. 3-33 Position for passive glenohumeral medial rotation.

ASSESSMENT

INTERPRETATION

Stabilize the athlete's elbow next to their back while passively moving the forearm away from the athlete's back until a stretch at the front of the glenohumeral joint limits range of movement.

Resisted Glenohumeral Medial Rotation

The athlete has their elbow flexed to an angle of 90° and their forearm in midposition with the elbow next to the side.

Resist with one hand just above the wrist on the palmar surface of the forearm and the other hand resting on the distal humerus and stabilizing the shoulder joint. The athlete should attempt medial rotation of the glenohumeral joint only; not adduction.

Pain and/or weakness with adduction and medial rotation can be an injury to the muscles or their nerve supply (see Active Glenohumeral Medial Rotation).

If medial rotation and cross-flexion hurt, then suspect a pectoralis major lesion.

If medial rotation and extension hurt, then suspect a latissimus dorsi lesion.

Pain and weakness with just medial rotation suggests a subscapularis injury.

If there is a painful arc and pain with resisted medial rotation only, there is probably a lesion at the tenoperiosteal junction of the subscapularis (tendonitis or strain).

Resisted Elbow Flexion with Supination (Fig. 3-34, A)

The athlete flexes the elbow to an angle of 90°.

Resist elbow flexion with one hand on the distal palmar aspect of the forearm (forearm supinated) while the other hand stabilizes the shoulder. The athlete attempts elbow flexion against your resistance.

Pain and/or weakness can be caused by an injury to the muscle or its nerve supply.

The prime mover is the biceps brachii—musculocutaneous N. (C5, C6).

Weakness in flexion with supination and weakness of the extensors of the wrist suggests a sixth cervical root compression from C5-C6 disc herniation or prolapse. Along with these elbow and wrist signs the athlete's cervical spine will display dysfunction and must be tested (see Cervical Spine Assessment, Chapter 2). However, shoulder and scapular movements will be pain free.

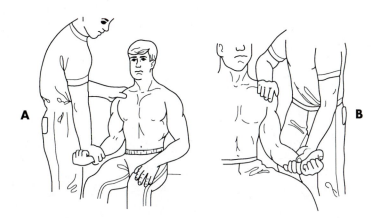

Fig. 3-34 A, Resisted elbow flexion. **B,** Resisted elbow extension.

ASSESSMENT

INTERPRETATION

Resisted Elbow Extension (Fig. 3-34, B)

The athlete flexes the shoulder slightly with the elbow in midrange. Resist at the distal dorsal aspect of the forearm with one hand while the other hand stabilizes the humerus. The athlete attempts elbow extension against your resistance.

Pain and/or weakness can be caused by an injury to the muscle or its nerve supply.

The prime mover is triceps brachii—radial N. (C7, C8).

The accessory mover is the anconeus muscle.

Weakness in elbow extension and wrist flexion suggests a seventh cervical root compression caused by C6-C7 disc prolapse or herniation.

If a disc lesion here is involved, the neck movements usually cause thoracic pain while shoulder and scapular movements have full strength. The cervical spine must then be assessed fully (see Cervical Spine Assessment, Chapter 2).

Active Shoulder Lateral Rotation, Abduction, and Flexion (Apley's Scratch Test)

The athlete reaches over their head to touch the spine of the opposite scapula, or lower, if possible.

This analyzes the combined movements of the joint. See the Interpretation Section for limits on lateral rotation and muscles of active abduction.

This is a functional movement pattern that is carried out daily to comb one's hair or close a zipper, as well as during sporting activities (e.g., tennis serve) and therefore helps determine the athlete's functional restrictions.

Active Shoulder Medial Rotation, Adduction, and Extension (Fig. 3-35)

The athlete reaches behind their back to touch the inferior angle of the opposite scapula, or higher, if possible.

This analyzes the combined movements of the joint as above. See the Interpretation Section for limits on medial rotation and muscles for active adduction.

This is functional position used when putting a belt through a belt loop and an arm into a sweater or coat sleeve. Limitations here indicate the functional restrictions the athlete may have.

SPECIAL TESTS

Shoulder Girdle Movements

The following tests can be done before the glenohumeral tests to rule out scapulothoracic articulation problems.

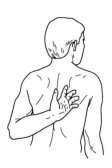

Fig. 3-35 Active shoulder medial rotation, adduction, and extension.

ASSESSMENT INTERPRETATION

Active Shoulder Girdle Elevation (Shoulder Shrug) (Fig. 3-36, A)

The athlete raises both shoulders toward the ears.

Pain, weakness, and/or limitation of range of motion can be caused by an injury to the muscles or their nerve supply.

The prime movers are:
- Levator scapulae—cervical N. (C3, C4) and dorsal scapular N. (C4, C5)
- Trapezius—spinal accessory N. and cranial nerve XI (C2-C4)

The accessory movers are the rhomboids major and minor.

Pain at the end of range of motion can be caused by:
- sprain of the costoclavicular ligament
- injury to the shoulder girdle depressors
- sprain of the coracoclavicular or acromioclavicular ligaments

Resisted Shoulder Girdle Elevation

Stand behind the athlete. The athlete elevates his or her shoulders while you attempt to push the shoulders downward.

Pain and/or weakness can be caused by an injury to the muscle or its nerve supply (see section on active shoulder girdle elevation). Painless weakness can come from a C2 or C3 nerve root problem.

Active Shoulder Girdle Depression (Fig. 3-36, B)

The athlete lowers the shoulders bilaterally.

Pain, weakness, and/or limitation of range of motion can be caused by an injury to the muscles or their nerve supply.

The prime movers are:
- Latissimus dorsi—thoracodorsal N. (C6, C7, C8)
- Pectoralis major—lateral and medial pectoral N. (C6, C7, and C8, T1 respectively)
- Pectoralis minor—medial pectoral N. (C7, C8, T1)

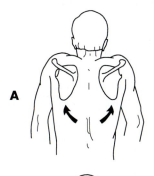

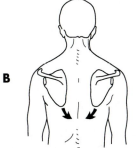

Fig. 3-36 A, Active shoulder girdle elevation. **B,** Active shoulder girdle depression.

ASSESSMENT   # INTERPRETATION

Any injury to the shoulder elevators may cause pain or weakness at the end of range of motion.

Thoracic outlet syndromes may cause referred pain down the arms during the depression motion.

An acromioclavicular separation can also cause pain during the depression movement.

A first rib syndrome (a fixed first rib) can cause pain in the supraspinatus fossa and down into the C8, T1 dermatome of the arm.

Active Shoulder Girdle Retraction (Fig. 3-37, A)

The athlete retracts the scapula when asked to stand at attention.

Stand behind and instruct the athlete to pinch his or her finger when it is placed between the scapulae.

Pain, weakness, and/or limitation of range of motion can be caused by an injury to the muscles or their nerve supply.

The prime movers are:
• Rhomboids major—dorsal scapular N. (C5)
• Rhomboids minor—dorsal scapular N. (C5)
The accessory muscle is the trapezius.

Pain at the end of range of motion can come from a conoid ligament sprain or tear and tension in the shoulder girdle protractors.

A spinal accessory neuritis can weaken the middle fibers of the trapezius muscle. With this neuritis, active abduction of the shoulder shows 10° of limitation while passive elevation goes through the full range of motion.

Active Shoulder Girdle Protraction (Fig. 3-37, B)

The athlete rolls the shoulders forward. The scapula slides forward on the thorax.

Pain, weakness, and/or limitation of range of motion can be caused by an injury to the muscles or their nerve supply.

The prime mover is the serratus anterior—long thoracic N., (C5, C6, C7).

Full abduction of the arm cannot occur without the long thoracic nerve supply to serratus anterior.

Scapular winging indicates a weak serratus anterior muscle. If the athlete does a push-up against the wall the scapula will wing even further. Painless weakness of the serratus anterior

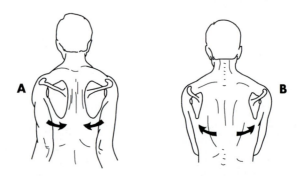

Fig. 3-37 A, Active shoulder girdle retraction. **B,** Active shoulder girdle protraction.

ASSESSMENT   INTERPRETATION

can be caused by a long thoracic nerve neuritis (palsy). With a long thoracic nerve palsy, patients suffer 2 or 3 weeks of constant aching in the scapular region and upper arm.

This pain is unaffected by movement.

This neuritis can also develop painlessly. Occasionally the palsy follows trauma—either direct or caused by lateral traction of the scapula. Sometimes it occurs after a viral infection.

Partial weakness of serratus anterior can be caused by a cervical disc lesion that involves the sixth cervical root. Bilateral weakness indicates myopathy.

Biceps Tests—Biceps Tendon Instability

Yergason's Test

Have one hand at the palmar aspect of the distal forearm and the other above the athlete's elbow, holding it in place.

With the athlete's elbow flexed at an angle of 90° and stabilized next to the athlete's thorax, give resistance while the athlete flexes and supinates the elbow while externally rotating the shoulder.

Resist yet allow the movement (isotonic muscle contraction) to occur.

If the test elicits pain or the biceps tendon (long head) subluxes, the test is positive. As a result of the rupture of the transverse humeral ligament, the biceps tendon slips out of the upper end of the groove. The athlete may describe symptoms of a snapping shoulder.

Booth and Marvel's Test (Fig. 3-38)

The athlete's shoulder is abducted and externally rotated with the elbow flexed.

Palpate the bicipital groove.

Internally rotate the arm while palpating the tendon in the groove for snapping and subluxing.

An audible or palpable snap can indicate a tear of the transverse humeral ligament, which allows tendon dislocation.

Lippman's Test

Attempt to displace the biceps tendon while the athlete's elbow is flexed at an angle of 90°.

Pain or laxity during palpation can indicate bicipital laxity or bicipital tendonitis.

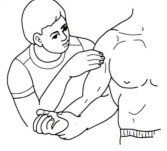

Fig. 3-38 Biceps tendon instability test (Booth and Marvel's test).

ASSESSMENT

INTERPRETATION

Ludington's Test

The athlete is asked to clasp hands (palms down) on his or her head and then contract the biceps.

While the athlete contracts and relaxes the biceps, palpate the biceps tendon below the acromion deep to the pectoralis major muscles.

Any sharp pain in the bicipital area indicates a tendonitis or strain.

If you are unable to palpate the biceps tendon during the biceps contraction and relaxation it may mean that the long head of the biceps is ruptured.

Hawkins and Kennedy's Test, or Speed's Sign

The athlete attempts forward flexion of the shoulder joint with the elbow extended and the forearm supinated.

Resist the movement with one hand on the distal volar aspect of the forearm and the other hand stabilizing the shoulder.

A positive test causes pain at the bicipital groove.

If there is pain in the biceps tendon, a biceps strain or biceps tendonitis may exist.

Drop Arm Test (Rotator Cuff Tear) (Fig. 3-39)

The athlete abducts the arm fully and then slowly lowers it to his or her side.

If there are any tears in the rotator cuff, the arm will drop from an angle of 90° of abduction to the athlete's side.

The athlete will not be able to lower the arm slowly no matter how hard he or she tries.

If the athlete can sustain abduction, a gentle tap on the forearm will cause the arm to drop to the side if the rotator cuff is torn.

When the athlete cannot lower the arm smoothly from the abducted position to the side, there is a rotator cuff tear. This is most apparent when there is a tear of the supraspinatus muscle.

Apprehension Sign (Anterior Shoulder Joint Instability or Dislocation) (Fig. 3-40)

To test for chronic shoulder joint instability or previous dislocation, place the athlete's shoulder at an angle of 90°

This test places the shoulder in a vulnerable position for dislocating so the athlete shows apprehension and will try to prevent further movement if he or she has had a previous anterior

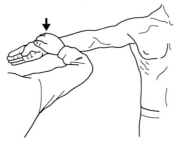

Fig. 3-39 Drop arm test (rotator cuff tear).

ASSESSMENT   INTERPRETATION

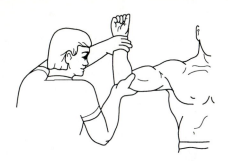

Fig. 3-40 Apprehension sign (anterior shoulder dislocation).

of abduction and externally rotate the shoulder slightly with the elbow flexed. When you attempt further external rotation, the athlete will show apprehension and prevent further rotation.

dislocation or anterior subluxation problem. According to Jobe et al., pain during this, which is difficult to localize, can indicate shoulder impingement or rotator cuff problems also.

Anterior-Posterior Glenohumeral Instability

To test for this instability, have the athlete sit in a chair. The therapist grasps the humeral head through the deltoid muscle and attempts to glide it anteriorly and posteriorly (Fig. 3-41, *A* and *B*).

The athlete must relax the shoulder musculature for an accurate test.

The amount of instability is determined by the degree of humeral head movement under the acromion. Excessive anterior instability is graded mild, moderate, and severe. Posterior instability is considered excessive when more than 50% of the head can be shifted posteriorly off the glenoid cavity.

Posterior Glenohumeral Dislocation Test (Neer and Welsh)

The athlete is sitting or lying supine with the shoulder flexed at an angle of 90° and internally rotated with the elbow flexed at an angle of 90°.

Apply a force at the elbow to push the humerus backward.

The test is repeated at various degrees of shoulder flexion and internal rotation.

This tests the amount of glenohumeral instability in a posterior direction. If there is laxity, it may be congenital or from a previous dislocation.

Impingement Signs

These tests impinge the subacromial structures as the greater tuberosity jams against the anterior-inferior acromion surface.

Hawkins and Kennedy's Test (Fig. 3-42)

With the athlete lying supine, the glenohumeral joint is forward flexed at

The greater tuberosity contacts the coracoacromial ligament. If the athlete has an impingement problem with the supraspina-

ASSESSMENT

INTERPRETATION

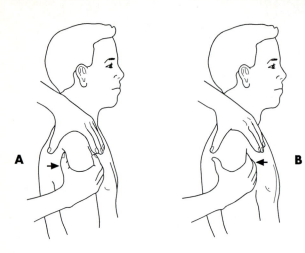

Fig. 3-41 Anterior-posterior glenohumeral instability. A, Anterior movement. B, Posterior movement.

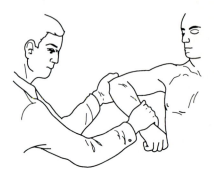

Fig. 3-42 Impingement sign (Hawkins and Kennedy).

an angle of 90°, then internally rotated.

This jams the greater tuberosity under the acromion.

A positive result occurs when the athlete feels pain in the subacromial area. The pain increases with further flexion or internal rotation.

This test is highly reliable.

Neer and Welsh Test

With the athlete lying supine, the humerus is brought into full forward flexion.

Empty Can Test (Fig. 3-43)

The athlete is asked to abduct the shoulder to 90°, cross-flex it to 30° (horizontal adduction), then medially rotate the humerus (i.e., pretending to hold a can full of liquid and then emptying its contents).

Infraspinatus Test (Fig. 3-44)

In the seated position, have the athlete abduct, cross-flex, then internally rotate the shoulder with the elbow flexed. The therapist then resists external rotation of the athlete's arm in that position. Resistance is applied at the athlete's wrist.

tus, the biceps tendon, or the related structures (subacromial bursitis, infraspinatus), this can elicit pain.

The athlete will feel discomfort when the injured structure is impinged against the anterior third of the acromion.

If the athlete experiences pain in the anterior of the shoulder joint, there may be a supraspinatus impingement problem.

This tests for infraspinatus tendonitis or impingement. It helps the therapist determine if the athlete's impingement discomfort is coming from infraspinatus or another impinged structure (supraspinatus, biceps, subacromial bursa). This test is positive when the contraction is painful and weak.

ASSESSMENT

INTERPRETATION

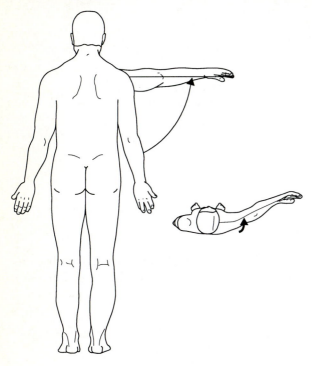

Fig. 3-43 Empty can test.

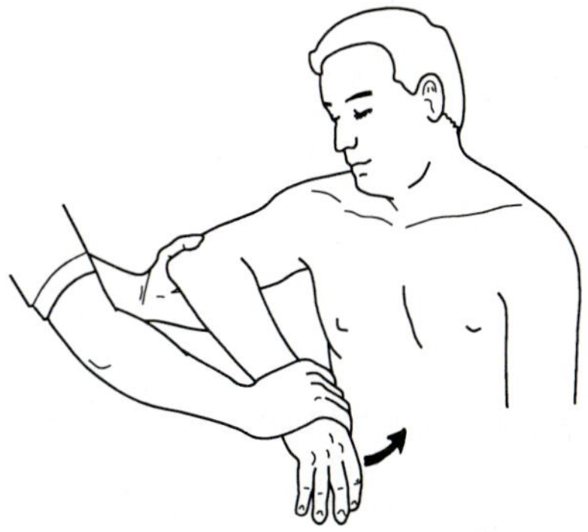

Fig. 3-44 Infraspinatus test.

Active Glenohumeral Cross-flexion (Horizontal Adduction; 120°-130°) (Fig. 3-45)

The athlete abducts the arm to an angle of 90° then brings it straight across the body with the elbow extended.

Pain, weakness, and/or limitation of range of motion can be caused by an injury to the muscles or their nerve supply.

The prime movers are:

- Pectoralis major—lateral and medial pectoral N. (C5, C6, C7 and C8, T1 respectively)
- Anterior deltoid—axillary N. (C5, C6)

The accessory movers are the biceps brachii and the coracobrachialis.

Horizontal adduction can also be painful at the end of range with a posterior capsule lesion or posterior deltoid, infraspinatus, or teres minor injury.

There will be pain and limitation of movement if there is an acromioclavicular sprain or degenerative joint changes.

Passive Glenohumeral Cross-flexion (Horizontal Adduction)

Move the arm through cross-flexion until an end feel is reached. One hand is on the back of the elbow joint while the other hand stabilizes the shoulder.

Pain and/or limitation of range of motion is caused by:

- injury of the shoulder extensors
- tightness in or a lesion of the posterior capsule
- acromioclavicular joint problems
- lesion of the posterior deltoid

The normal end feel is tissue approximation when the arm contacts the chest.

ASSESSMENT INTERPRETATION

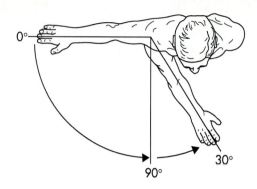

Fig. 3-45 Active glenohumeral cross-flexion (horizontal adduction).

Resisted Glenohumeral Cross-flexion (Horizontal Adduction)

The athlete cross-flexes to midrange. Resist the athlete's arm with one hand on the medial elbow or the palmar surface of the distal forearm.

With your other arm, stabilize the shoulder.

Pain and/or weakness can come from an injury to the muscles or their nerve supply (see Active Glenohumeral Cross-flexion).

Active Glenohumeral Cross-extension (Horizontal Abduction; 30° to 45°) (Fig. 3-46)

The athlete abducts the arm to an angle of 90° and extends it backward as far as possible (in the horizontal plane).

Pain, weakness, and/or limitation of range of motion can be caused by an injury to the muscles or their nerve supply.

The prime mover is the posterior deltoid—axillary N. (C5, C6).

The accessory movers are the infraspinatus and the teres minor.

Passive Glenohumeral Cross-extension (Horizontal Abduction)

Carry the arm to 90° of abduction, then cross-extend the shoulder until an end feel is reached.

Pain and/or limitation of range of motion comes from:
- injury of the pectoralis major or the anterior deltoid muscle
- lesion of the anterior glenohumeral capsule or its ligaments.

Resisted Glenohumeral Cross-extension (Horizontal Abduction)

The athlete abducts the arm to 90° then cross extends the shoulder to 30°.

Resist the athlete's arm at the dorsal aspect of the elbow or the distal dorsal aspect of the forearm as the athlete attempts to cross-extend.

With your other arm, stabilize the shoulder joint.

Pain and/or weakness can be caused by an injury to the muscles or their nerve supply (see Active Glenohumeral Cross-extension).

ASSESSMENT   INTERPRETATION

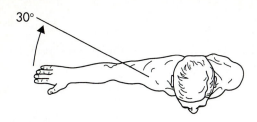

Fig. 3-46 Active glenohumeral cross-extension (horizontal abduction).

Acromioclavicular Joint Stability

Glide of the Acromion

With the athlete seated, cup the acromion with one hand while the other hand holds the clavicle.

Attempt gentle movement of the clavicle anteriorly and posteriorly.

If the acromioclavicular joint can be moved more on one side than on the other and is painful during the test, there is a laxity in the acromioclavicular ligaments or a sprain of these ligaments.

If the normal joint play is not present, glenohumeral elevation will be limited.

Superior-Inferior and Anterior-Posterior Glide of the Lateral Clavicle

Fix the acromion with one hand and attempt superior-inferior and anterior-posterior glide of the lateral clavicle.

If there is damage to the acromioclavicular or coracoclavicular ligaments (conoid or trapezoid), the mobility of the clavicle will be excessive.

If there is grating or crepitus during clavicular movement, the chronic acromioclavicular instability may have caused joint degeneration or osteoarthritis.

Traction

Apply long-axis traction on the upper humerus with one hand while the other hand palpates the acromioclavicular joint for opening.

Gapping or pain indicates a positive test.

Gapping and/or pain can indicate a significant sprain or separation of the acromioclavicular joint. Large gapping can indicate a significant separation involvement of the coracoclavicular ligaments (conoid and trapezoid).

Cranial Glide

With the athlete's elbow flexed at an angle of 90° and with the shoulder in the resting position, push upward on the athlete's elbow while palpating the acromioclavicular joint.

Gapping or pain indicates a positive test.

The humerus pushes the acromion upward and will elicit pain if the acromioclavicular joint is injured.

Compression

Ask the athlete to cross-flex (horizontally adduct) to the end of range and then internally rotate the humerus to compress the joint. Pain indicates a positive test.

The athlete will experience pain when the joint is compressed.

ASSESSMENT

INTERPRETATION

Sternoclavicular Joint Stability

Ask the athlete to elevate, depress, protract, and retract the shoulder girdle and to perform circumduction while you palpate the sternoclavicular joint.

Any excessive movement of the sternoclavicular joint indicates laxity here or a previous dislocation.

Superior-Inferior and Anterior-Posterior Glide of the Medial Clavicle

With the athlete lying supine, the therapist's thumb is positioned under the caudal surface of the clavicle about 3 cm lateral to the sternoclavicular joint; the other thumb is placed on top of the other. The therapist then applies a superior movement to the clavicle. Then an inferior motion is attempted with the thumbs on the upper surface of the clavicle and the therapist standing at the head of the athlete. The therapist's two thumbs then gently push the clavicle posteriorly to determine instability. For anterior instability testing, the therapist must grip around the clavicle with a pincer-type grasp and pull the medial aspect of the clavicle anteriorly.

If there is increased mobility of the medial clavicle, the anterior sternoclavicular, posterior sternoclavicular, or costoclavicular ligaments may be lax or torn. If there is clicking during the muscle movements or during the glide movements, the articular disc may be damaged. Hypomobility will limit glenohumeral forward flexion and abduction.

Neurological Testing

Upper Limb or Brachial Tension Test (ULTT) (Elvey Test) (See Fig. 2-50)

The athlete is lying supine with the limb being tested over the edge of the plinth, with the glenohumeral joint in slight extension. The therapist faces the athlete with his or her left hand holding the athlete's hand on the involved side while the therapist's right hand holds the athlete's elbow with slight posterior depression. The athlete's arm is then abducted 110° in the frontal plane by the therapist's right hand. The glenohumeral joint is laterally rotated until there is resistance and the athlete is asked if there is any pain (Fig. 2-50, A). A constant depression force must be maintained on the shoulder girdle in this position, then the forearm supination is added (Fig. 2-50, B). Symptoms elicited are noted. The elbow is now extended, maintaining the previous

This test should be done only when the pain in the shoulder area is vague and the therapist is unsure if the pathology is at the cervical spine, thoracic spine, brachial plexus, shoulder, or arm. If the cervical spine was not ruled out, this test may also be necessary.

The ULTT is contraindicated if:
- area of discomfort is acute or inflamed
- athlete had an instability or discomfort achieving 110° of abduction and full lateral rotation of the glenohumeral joint
- athlete has cervical spine disc pathology or degeneration
- athlete has dizziness related to vertebrobasilar insufficiency
- athlete has a history of spinal cord injury
- athlete has worsening neurological symptoms (a cervical and neurological examination should be done first)

Normal responses expected from the ULTT are:
- gentle anterior shoulder or cubital fossa tissue stretch
- tingling in the thumb and first three fingers

The shoulder abduction stretches the C5, C6, and C7 nerve roots in their foramen. The shoulder girdle depression is essen-

ASSESSMENT

positions (Fig. 2-50, *C*). Symptoms are noted and then the therapist extends the wrist and fingers (Fig. 2-50 *D*). An alternative approach extends the wrist and fingers first, then the elbow. With the component positions maintained, the symptoms are recorded. The athlete is then asked to side bend away from the involved side and the symptoms are noted.

The key to successful ULTT is maintenance of each component position before moving to the next position.

INTERPRETATION

tial. If nerve root symptoms occur at this point, a cervical nerve root irritation is confirmed. The brachial plexus is under tension also, and plexus entrapment may be indicated.

The shoulder lateral rotation's effect on the nervous system is not explained and may even decrease tension on the plexus.

The supination and elbow extension components stretch the radial and median nerves. This is important for differentiating local trauma from neural involvement (e.g., carpal fracture versus median nerve entrapment or lateral epicondylitis versus radial nerve involvement or C6 involvement). The ulnar nerve is slackened.

If wrist, hand, or elbow extension alters the neck symptoms, an injury anywhere along the nerve trunk, roots, or nerves may be responsible.

Wrist and finger components of the test stretch the ulnar and median nerves and slacken the radial nerve. This is important to distinguish local pathology from neural involvement (e.g., medial epicondylitis versus ulnar nerve or C8-T1 involvement).

The side bending away increases the tension in the plexuses and also the long thoracic nerve and axillary nerve.

Side bending toward the involved side releases the neural network.

A positive tension test (pain reproduced) can indicate:
- cervical nerve root irritation or impingement
- cervical nerve or brachial plexus impingement
- cervical dura or meningeal scarring
- cervical dural ligaments that could be irritating the posterior longitudinal ligament
- greater occipital nerve problem at base of skull
- cranial dural problem or previous cerebrovascular accident
- thoracic nerve root syndromes
- suprascapular nerve entrapment or injury
- posterior interosseous nerve impinged in the arches of Frohse
- brachial plexus damage or impingement in the thoracic outlet
- axillary nerve damage or impingement
- radial nerve damage or impingement in the radial groove of the humerus
- median nerve damage or impingement at the elbow or wrist (carpal tunnel)
- ulnar nerve damage or impingement at the elbow or wrist (tunnel of Guyon)

In general, any time a nerve is damaged through direct trauma, impingement, or overstretch, the ULTT can elicit discomfort when the nerve is put under tension (during healing or in the chronic stage).

ASSESSMENT

INTERPRETATION

Reflex Testing

These reflexes should be evaluated if a cervical nerve root irritation is suspected.

The tests should be compared bilaterally. Several taps may be necessary to elicit a response.

To test the reflex fatigability, 5 to 10 repetitions can be done. On occasion, root signs that are just developing may have a fading reflex response and it can be detected only by repeating the tendon tapping.

Biceps Reflex (C5) (Fig. 3-47)

The athlete's forearm is placed over your forearm so that the biceps is relaxed.

Place your thumb on the biceps tendon in the cubital fossa (flex elbow with resistance to make sure you are over the tendon).

Tap your thumb nail with a reflex hammer, held in the other hand. The biceps should jerk slightly, the elbow may flex, and the forearm supinate slightly.

The arm must be relaxed.

The tendon should be tapped several times.

Although the biceps is innervated by the musculocutaneous nerve at neurological levels C5 and C6, its reflex action is largely from C5. If there is a slight muscle response, the C5 neurological level is normal.

If, after several attempts, there is no response, there may be a lesion anywhere from the root of C5 to the innervation of the biceps muscle.

An excessive response may be the result of an upper motor neuron lesion (cardiovascular attack, stroke); a decreased response can be indicative of a lower motor neuron lesion.

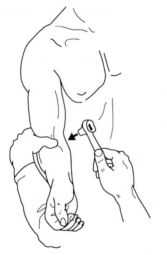

Fig. 3-47 Biceps reflex (C5).

ASSESSMENT

INTERPRETATION

Brachioradialis Reflex (C6) (Fig. 3-48, A)

Using the flat edge of the reflex hammer, tap the brachioradialis muscle tendon at the distal third of the radius.

The athlete's forearm should be supported and the forearm should be in a neutral position.

Repeat several times.

Although the brachioradialis muscle is innervated by the radial nerve via the C5 and C6 neurological levels, its reflex is largely a C6 function. A decreased response can indicate a C6 nerve root irritation. An excessive response can indicate an upper motor lesion; a decreased response can indicate a lower motor neuron lesion.

Triceps Reflex (C7) (Fig. 3-48, B)

Keep the arm as above but tap the triceps tendon where it crosses the olecranon fossa with a reflex hammer. You should see or feel a repeated slight jerk as the triceps muscle contracts.

This reflex is mainly a function of the C7 neurological level. A decreased response can indicate a C7 nerve root irritation. Upper or lower motor neuron lesions can increase or decrease the response respectively.

Dermatomes—Cutaneous Nerve Supply (Fig. 3-49 and 3-50)

The sensations are tested bilaterally with the athlete's eyes closed or looking away.

Each dermatome or cutaneous nerve supply area is pricked with a pin, in approximately 10 locations, while asking athlete if the pinprick can be felt (see figures). Ask the athlete if the sensation is sharp or dull.

The cutaneous nerve supply of the local peripheral nerves (see figure) may vary from person to person but they tend to be more consistent than dermatomes.

These tests determine if cervical segmental nerve root irritation exists and affects the involved dermatome.

The cutaneous nerve supply, especially the brachial plexus or peripheral nerves, can also be damaged by local trauma.

The axillary (circumflex) nerve can often be damaged secondary to a shoulder dislocation, causing anesthesia on the lateral aspect of the deltoid muscle.

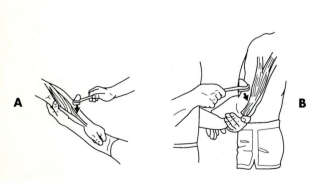

Fig. 3-48 A, Brachioradialis reflex (C6). **B,** Triceps reflex (C7).

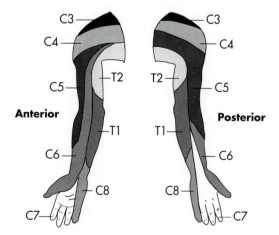

Fig. 3-49 Dermatomes of the upper limb.

ASSESSMENT	INTERPRETATION

The dermatomes vary in each individual and the boundaries are different or can overlap. The dermatomes shown in the figures are adapted from *Gray's Anatomy* and are approximations.

Then prick the opposite side, asking the athlete if the sensation feels the same on each side.

Hot or cold test tubes or cotton balls can be touched to the skin to see if sensation is affected, especially if the athlete had difficulty feeling the pin.

Determine if there is:
- decreased sensation (hypoesthesia)
- increased sensation (hyperesthesia)
- absent sensation (anesthesia)

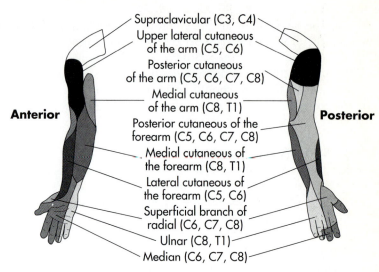

Anterior   **Posterior**

Supraclavicular (C3, C4)
Upper lateral cutaneous of the arm (C5, C6)
Posterior cutaneous of the arm (C5, C6, C7, C8)
Medial cutaneous of the arm (C8, T1)
Posterior cutaneous of the forearm (C5, C6, C7, C8)
Medial cutaneous of the forearm (C8, T1)
Lateral cutaneous of the forearm (C5, C6)
Superficial branch of radial (C6, C7, C8)
Ulnar (C8, T1)
Median (C6, C7, C8)

Fig. 3-50 Cutaneous nerve supply of the upper limb.

Maitland Quadrant Test (Fig. 3-51)

With the athlete lying supine, grasp the elbow joint with one hand while the other hand stabilizes the scapula.

To stabilize the scapula, your hand is under the athlete's shoulder, holding the spine of the scapula and the trapezius down firmly.

Then abduct the shoulder (in the horizontal plane or slightly below) while holding the athlete's elbow.

The shoulder movement is carried on toward the head until the humerus "rolls over" and reaches full abduction.

The quadrant position is at the top of the roll.

This test should be pain free in the normal glenohumeral joint. Pain, crepitus, or limitation of range of motion indicates glenohumeral joint dysfunction. Clicking can indicate a glenoid labrum tear, while crepitus usually indicates osteoarthritic joint changes.

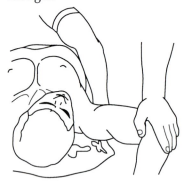

Fig. 3-51 Maitland quadrant test.

Maitland Locking Test (Fig. 3-52)

With the athlete lying supine, grasp the elbow joint with one hand and stabilize the scapula with the other (as above).

Then abduct and extend the humerus but this time maintain the humerus in medial rotation.

The humerus will abduct but then will lock at an angle of about 90°.

When the quadrant is locked, further lateral rotation can not be done.

This test should not be painful; if pain is experienced, it means that the glenohumeral joint has some dysfunction.

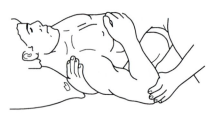

Fig. 3-52 Maitland locking test.

ASSESSMENT

INTERPRETATION

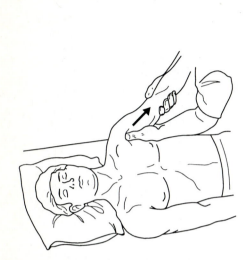

Fig. 3-53 Glenohumeral inferior glide (caudal).

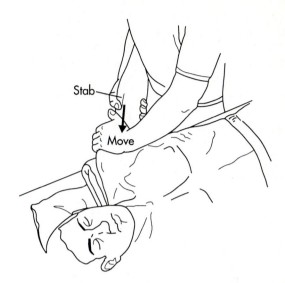

Fig. 3-54 Glenohumeral posterior glide.

ACCESSORY MOVEMENT TESTS

These accessory movements are very small but any limitations in motion can cause drastic limits in the joint's normal physiologic function.

These joint play movements must be fully restored to rehabilitate and re-achieve full joint ranges.

Inferior Glide (Fig. 3-53)

The athlete is lying supine with the glenohumeral joint abducted at an angle of about 55°.

Place one hand in the axilla to stabilize the scapula.

Your opposite hand applies a caudal traction on the humerus, pulling gently at the athlete's elbow.

The joint should move down equally on both sides without pain. Pain or decreased range of motion can be present when there is a glenohumeral problem or a muscle spasm protecting the joint.

Any hypomobility of the shoulder here can result in a compromised subacromial space (according to Tank et al.).

Full inferior glide is necessary for full abduction to be possible.

Posterior Glide (Fig. 3-54)

The athlete is lying supine with the shoulder abducted slightly and over the edge of the plinth. Ensure that the scapula and glenoid labrum are supported on the edge of the table and the

This joint play is necessary for full glenohumeral internal rotation and flexion.

Hypomobility will restrict these movements (according to Maitland).

ASSESSMENT   INTERPRETATION

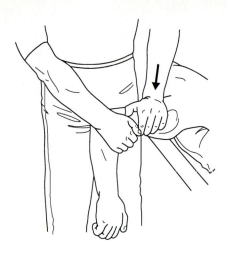

Fig. 3-55 Glenohumeral anterior glide.

humeral head is just over the edge of the table.

Stand beside the plinth, between the athlete's arm and body.

With your outer hand, support the athlete's arm by holding the elbow joint and tucking the forearm, wrist, and hand next to your side. With your other hand, gently grasp the proximal humerus.

A folded towel can be placed under the athlete's scapula to stabilize it.

Use joint traction, then lean forward and push slightly downward with the heel of your left hand over the proximal humerus.

Only the glenohumeral joint should move gently posteriorly, not the whole shoulder girdle.

Anterior Glide (Fig. 3-55)

With the athlete lying prone, stand between the athlete's arm and body.

The athlete's arm is abducted at an angle of 90° (or slightly less if impingement problems exist) and externally rotated slightly. The athlete's humerus is over the side of the plinth with the glenoid area on the edge of the plinth.

Grasp the athlete's distal humerus to hold the weight of the athlete's arm with your outer hand. Apply joint trac-

Any anterior capsule problems will elicit pain and any restriction will cause restricted abduction and external rotation.

Hypermobility will be present with athletes who sublux or dislocate anteriorly. A Bankhart lesion or Hill-Sach lesion may also be present.

ASSESSMENT

INTERPRETATION

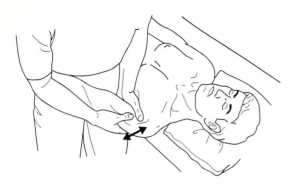

Fig. 3-56 Glenohumeral lateral distraction.

tion with this hand. Use the heel of the mobilizing opposite hand on the upper most aspect of the humerus and push gently downward to achieve an anterior glide of the humeral head.

Just the glenohumeral joint, not the entire shoulder girdle, should be moved.

If the joint is tender, both of your hands can hold the upper humerus and gently distract the head of the humerus out of the labrum and then gently glide the head anteriorly.

Lateral Distraction (Fig. 3-56)

With the athlete lying supine, stand between the athlete's body and arm.

Place one hand on the lateral aspect of the athlete's elbow and the other hand on the athlete's proximal humerus as high as possible in the axilla (an alternate placement can have the stabilizing hand on the lateral upper humerus).

Turn your body slightly away from the athlete to move the humeral head slightly out of the glenoid labrum.

Pain or decreased range of motion indicates a glenohumeral problem, often with associated spasm, and will result in all shoulder ranges of motion being decreased.

Scapular Movements

The athlete is in a side-lying position with his or her injured shoulder upward.

Face the athlete with your hands on the inferior angle and spine of the scapula.

Any pain or hypomobility indicates a decrease in scapulothoracic mobility. This mobility can be lost whenever the glenohumeral joint has been immobilized or when active forward flexion or abduction has been limited.

ASSESSMENT   INTERPRETATION

Then gently elevate, depress, and rotate the athlete's scapula on the thoracic wall.

PALPATION

Palpate areas for point tenderness, temperature differences, swelling, adhesions, calcium deposits, muscle spasms, decreased muscle tone, and muscle tears. Palpate for muscle tenderness, lesions, and trigger points.

According to Janet Travell, trigger points in muscle are activated directly by overuse, overload, trauma, or chilling and are activated indirectly by visceral disease, other trigger points, arthritic joints, or emotional distress.

Myofascial pain is referred from trigger points, which have patterns and locations for each muscle.

Trigger points are a hyperactive spot usually in a skeletal muscle or the muscle's fascia that are acutely tender on palpation and evoke a muscle twitch.

These points can evoke autonomic responses (i.e., sweating, pilomotor activity, local vasoconstriction).

Anterior Structures (Fig. 3-57)

Boney
Sternoclavicular Joint

This joint can suffer sprain or dislocation. The clavicle has potential for anterior, superior, inferior, or posterior displacement, or any combination of these. The joint and its ligaments will also be point tender.

First Costosternal Joint and First Rib

Palpate this area during breathing to ensure there is movement of the first

If the joint is hypomobile, problems of the entire shoulder girdle can develop. If there is dysfunction, there is also point tenderness.

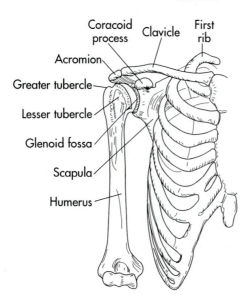

Fig. 3-57 Anterior boney structures of right shoulder.

ASSESSMENT   INTERPRETATION

rib. Palpate for a cervical rib if a thoracic outlet syndrome is present.

Pain can be elicited from a fixed first rib by postero-anterior pressure on the rib itself or on the costotransverse joint.

Costochondral Junctions (Under Pectoralis Major)

Costochondritis can develop at these junctions, causing local point tenderness. Direct trauma or coughing can irritate these junctions.

Ribs

Costochondral pathology or fixed upper ribs can lead to pain in the anterior chest or sternum and can affect normal shoulder girdle functions.

Clavicle

The clavicular fracture site is usually in the lateral one third, at the S-shaped curve of the bone. A malaligned healed clavicle can affect glenohumeral function especially during abduction and forward flexion. A large clavicle callus can occlude the thoracic outlet.

Coracoid Process

The conoid and trapezoid (coracoclavicular) ligaments hold the clavicle down and can be painful if they are sprained with an acromioclavicular joint injury. If these ligaments are tender, it is a moderate to severe sprain with major acromioclavicular ligament damage. Avulsion fractures of the coracoid process can occur from pectoralis minor or sometimes the biceps and pectoralis tendons.

Acromioclavicular Joint

A sprain, separation, or dislocation can occur here and cause exquisite point tenderness over the joint and its ligaments. A fracture or crack of the acromion process can occur, and boney point tenderness will be present.

Glenohumeral Joint

A sprain or dislocation can occur here and the location of the head of the humerus must be determined if this is suspected.

Because of the deep nature of the joint it is difficult to palpate.

Any heat or redness to the joint indicates an inflammatory process and the cause must be determined.

The humeral head, neck, or proximal humeral shaft can be fractured.

Bicipital Groove

Biceps tendonitis occurs commonly in the athlete with tendon subluxation or in the athlete who irritates the tendon through overuse (e.g., swimmers).

ASSESSMENT

INTERPRETATION

Soft Tissue (Fig. 3-58)
Biceps Brachii

The belly of the biceps muscle can rupture, contuse, or strain. Tenderness in the bicipital groove can indicate a subluxing tendon or biceps tendonitis.

According to Travell and Simons, trigger points are usually found in the distal part of the muscle with referred pain in the anterior deltoid and cubital fossa (Fig. 3-59)

Subscapularis Muscle Insertion

The subscapularis tendon insertion is the usual location for tendonitis from overuse mechanisms.

According to Travell and Simons, trigger points are acutely tender in the axilla and underside of the scapula. Pain is referred over the posterior aspect of the shoulder mainly, but can extend over the scapula and down the arm to the elbow (Fig. 3-60).

A band of pain may also exist around the wrist, especially on the dorsal aspect.

Supraspinatus Muscle Insertion

The supraspinatus tendon often develops tendonitis at its point of insertion. This occurs from an impingement mechanism and causes point tenderness at its insertion.

In athletes over the age of 40 the tendon can rupture.

Coracoacromial Ligament

Point tenderness of the ligament can accompany a severe acromioclavicular ligament sprain. According to Cuillo, point tenderness between the acromion and coracoid process is an indication of a shoulder impingement problem.

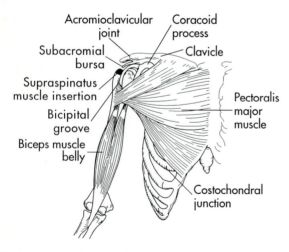

Fig. 3-58 Anterior muscle structures of the right shoulder.

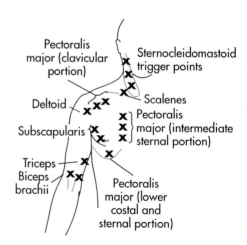

Fig. 3-59 Anterior myofascial trigger points (Travell and Simons).

ASSESSMENT   INTERPRETATION

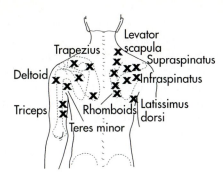

Fig. 3-60 Posterior myofascial trigger points (Travell and Simons).

Subacromial Bursa

It is debatable if the bursa can be palpated. Hoppenfeld believes it can be palpated under the acromion with the shoulder extended.

Bursitis is a frequent cause of shoulder pain, although the pain is often referred down the arm to the lower deltoid area.

Subcoracoid Bursa

Bursitis can occur here, but this is a rare occurrence.

Deltoid Muscle

This muscle can develop deltoid atrophy from axillary nerve damage or posterior glenohumeral dislocation. and

Deltoid contusions are quite common.

According to Travell and Simons, the trigger points are in the anterior pectoral axilla for the anterior deltoid, which can refer pain into the anterior and middle deltoid muscles areas (see Fig. 3-59).

The trigger points in the posterior deltoid are in the midbelly location with referred pain down the posterior and middle deltoid muscle areas.

Sternocleidomastoid Muscle

Protective spasm of the muscle can denote cervical spine dysfunction. It also attaches to the clavicle and any injury to the clavicle may cause protective muscle spasm as well. Enlarged lymph nodes near its anterior and posterior border can indicate infection. Myofascial trigger points are often present with shoulder girdle pathology (see Cervical Spine Palpation, Soft Tissue SCM) (see Fig. 3-59).

A sternoclavicular joint sprain (or dysfunction) and problems with the first costosternal joint can also cause spasming of this muscle.

Pectoralis Major Muscle

Strain can occur at the bicipital groove or in the muscle belly of the pectoralis muscle.

ASSESSMENT

INTERPRETATION

According to Travell and Simons, there are several trigger points in the midbelly area of the clavicular, sternal, and intermediate sections of the muscle (see Fig. 3-59). Referred pain from the clavicular portion projects into the anterior deltoid and through the clavicular portion of the muscle.

Trigger points in the middle section of the muscle refer pain to the anterior chest and down the inner aspect of the arm to the medial epicondyle. With further radiation, the pain pattern can extend into the ulnar aspect of the forearm and hand.

Trigger points closer to the sternum can also refer pain over the sternum without crossing the midline. Additionally, trigger points in the sternal lower fibers of the muscle can cause breast pain (see Fig. 3-59).

Scalenes Muscle

Muscle spasm of the scalenes muscles can occur and cause thoracic outlet problems or respiratory problems.

According to Travell and Simons, trigger points located in the anterior (see Fig. 3-59), medial, or posterior scalenes muscles can refer pain anteriorly to the chest wall, laterally to the upper extremity, and posteriorly to the vertebral scapular border. Pain can also be referred into the pectoral region, the biceps and triceps muscles, the radial forearm, and the thumb and index fingers. Because of all these referred patterns, the scalenes muscles must be palpated for trigger points that refer to these areas.

Posterior Structures

Boney
Scapula

Several muscle trigger points from shoulder problems and cervical lesions are located around the scapula (Janet Travell's work) (see Fig. 3-60). It is important to be familiar with the trigger points for the levator scapulae, trapezius, supraspinatus, infraspinatus, rhomboids, teres minor, and latissimus dorsi muscles because they refer pain around the scapula.

The spine of the scapula may feel contused and point tender on palpation.

The suprascapular notch is also an acupuncture point or trigger point for shoulder pain and any damage to the suprascapular nerve can elicit pain here.

The scapula can be fractured by a direct blow but this is rare in sporting events.

Soft Tissue (Fig. 3-61)
Rhomboid Muscles

These muscles can suffer postural strain or acute strain. They have many trigger points and referred pain occurs mainly along the vertebral border of the scapula. According to Yanda, they have a tendency to develop weakness with time.

ASSESSMENT   INTERPRETATION

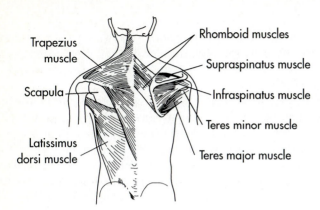

Trapezius muscle

Scapula

Latissimus dorsi muscle

Rhomboid muscles

Supraspinatus muscle

Infraspinatus muscle

Teres minor muscle

Teres major muscle

Fig. 3-61 Posterior muscles of the shoulder girdle.

Trapezius Muscles

These muscles can suffer postural strain or acute strain. Yanda's work shows that the upper fibers of trapezius have a tendency to develop muscle tightness and the middle and lower fibers tend to develop inhibitory weakness. This tendency can be augmented by poor posture (i.e., forward head posture, rounded shoulders) and by injury. Palpate these muscles to determine their tonus. The upper fibers are often in spasm if shoulder or cervical pathology exists.

According to Travell and Simons, the upper fibers of the trigger points of the trapezius muscles refer pain unilaterally along the posterolateral neck and head (Fig. 3-61).

The middle fibers of the trapezius have a trigger point on the midscapular border of the muscle. Pain is referred toward the spinous process of C7 and T1.

A trigger point can sometimes be found distal to the acromion, causing pain to the acromion process or top of the shoulder.

The lower fibers of the trapezius have a trigger point midbelly and it can refer pain to the cervical paraspinal area, the mastoid process, and the acromion. It can also refer a tenderness to the suprascapular area.

A trigger point over the scapula below the scapular spine can refer a burning pain along the scapula's vertebral border.

Supraspinatus Muscle

Any point tenderness suggests strains, tears, or tendonitis. The supraspinatus can be ruptured near its point of insertion. The supraspinatus muscle is often overused in sport and can develop fatigue muscle discomfort or tendon impingement problems. It is often injured in the overhand throw motion.

According to Travell and Simons, trigger points are present along the muscle and its tendon and pain is referred most intensely to the mid-deltoid region. The pain can also radiate down the lateral upper arm to the lateral epicondyle of the elbow (see Fig. 3-61).

ASSESSMENT

INTERPRETATION

Infraspinatus Muscle

Any point tenderness suggests strains, tears, or tendonitis. Because the infraspinatus decelerates the glenohumeral joint during the follow-through of throwing, it often develops overuse problems.

According to Travell and Simons, trigger points are in the muscle just below the scapular spine and on the middle of the vertebral border of the scapula (see Fig. 3-61). Pain is referred intensely to the anterior shoulder and deep in the shoulder joint in most cases and therefore can be confused with supraspinatus tendonitis. This pain can project from here down the anterolateral aspect of the arm, the lateral forearm, and the radial aspect of the hand and even fingers occasionally.

Teres Major Muscle

According to Travell and Simons, the trigger points are located on the inferior angle of the scapula and the axilla.

These trigger points refer pain to the posterior deltoid region, over the long head of the triceps, and occasionally to the dorsal forearm.

Teres Minor Muscle

Any point tenderness suggests strains, tears, or tendonitis. This muscle can be injured during the throwing motion.

According to Travell and Simons, the trigger point is in the midbelly location and the pain is very sharp and deep there (see Fig. 3-61).

Latissimus Dorsi Muscle

This muscle can develop atrophy and strain. It is often overused and develops point tenderness in athletes who medially rotate the glenohumeral joint along with shoulder extension (i.e., paddlers, gymnasts, swimmers). Its trigger points are in the axilla and at the axillary border of the inferior border of the scapula. Referred pain can extend to the back of the shoulder and down the medial forearm and hand (see Fig. 3-61).

Levator Scapulae Muscle

This muscle can develop strain, especially at the point of insertion. Muscle spasm here often denotes cervical or shoulder dysfunction. It tends to develop muscle tightness with time (Yanda).

There are often trigger points in this muscle when shoulder girdle dysfunction exists; these trigger points are located at the angle of the neck and is experienced locally there; it also projects down the vertebral border of the scapula (Travell and Simons) (see Fig. 3-61).

ASSESSMENT

INTERPRETATION

Lateral Structures

Boney
Acromion

Acromioclavicular separation and dislocation can occur and the joint and its ligaments will be exquisitely point tender. Palpate for heat, which indicates an inflammatory process. Acromioclavicular joint degeneration may also cause point tenderness in the area.

Soft Tissue
Upper Trapezius Muscle

Upper trapezius muscle spasm is common with neck or shoulder pathology. See trigger points in the section on Posterior Structures.

Deltoid Muscle (Middle Fibers) (Fig. 3-62)

Contusion and exostosis (calcium in deltoid muscle or at the point of insertion) can develop. The area will be point tender and a hard mass is often palpable if an exostosis is or has developed. See trigger points in the section on Anterior Structures.

Triceps Muscle (Fig. 3-62)

Contusion, strain, and deposition of calcium can occur in muscle. The area is point tender and the calcium is palpable. See trigger points in the section on Posterior Structures of the Elbow.

Supraspinatus Tendon

This tendon can develop tendonitis. See trigger points in the section on Posterior Structures.

Scalenes Muscle

Spasm or hypertrophy can lead to thoracic outlet impingement problems that can refer pain to the shoulder. See trigger points in the section on Anterior Structures.

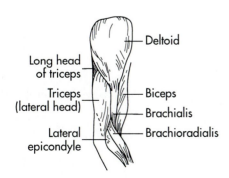

Fig. 3-62 Lateral muscles of the shoulder and upper arm.

ASSESSMENT

INTERPRETATION

Axilla (Fig. 3-63)

Soft Tissue
Latissimus Dorsi Muscle

This muscle can become strained or overused. It will be point tender in the axilla and into its insertion on the humerus. Its trigger points are in the axilla (see section on Posterior Structures).

Pectoralis Major Muscle

Strain and tendonitis can affect this muscle and cause point tenderness. Occasionally this muscle can be torn.

Teres Major Muscle

Strain can develop in this muscle and cause point tenderness.

Teres Minor Muscle

There are trigger points in the axilla (see section on Posterior Structures). This muscle can strain or tear.

Biceps Brachii Muscle

Strain and tendonitis can develop in this muscle and cause point tenderness.

A rupture of the biceps tendon may cause axillary and arm pain. A palpable lump may be felt in the biceps muscle when the athlete is asked to contract the biceps.

Serratus Anterior Muscle

The medial wall is made up of ribs 2 to 6 and the serratus anterior muscle lies over them. A lesion of this muscle may cause point tenderness here. According to Travell and Simons, its trigger points are located midmuscle and pain is referred to the midchest area and can project down the axilla and the ulnar aspect of the arm, forearm, and hand.

Lymph Nodes

Infection of tumors can cause enlargement of these nodes. Any suspicious nodes require further examination by a physician.

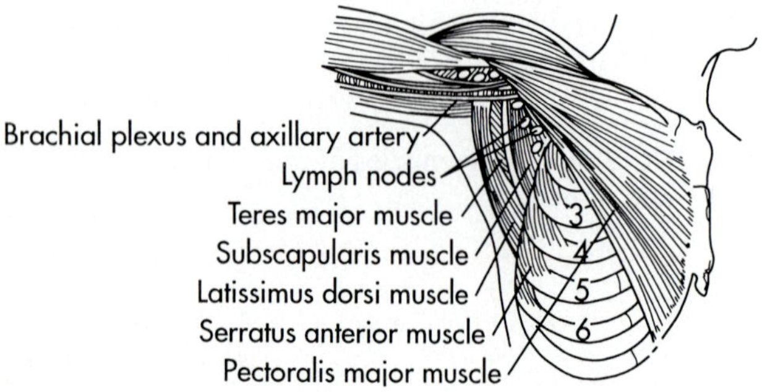

Brachial plexus and axillary artery
Lymph nodes
Teres major muscle
Subscapularis muscle
Latissimus dorsi muscle
Serratus anterior muscle
Pectoralis major muscle

Fig. 3-63 Soft tissue structures in the axilla.

ASSESSMENT

INTERPRETATION

Brachial Plexus and Axillary Artery

The brachial plexus and axillary artery run deep in the center of the axilla. The axillary pulse can be palpated in the axilla if a circulatory deficiency is suspected. The brachial plexus is difficult to palpate but if tingling occurs down the limb with deep palpation in this area, neural problems may be implicated.

BIBLIOGRAPHY

Alderink G and Kuck D: Isokinetic shoulder strength of high school and college-aged pitchers, J Orthop Sports Phys Therapy 7:4, 1986.

Allman F: Fractures and ligamentous injuries of the clavicle and its articulations, J Bone Joint Surg 49A:774, 1967.

Anderson JE: Grant's atlas of anatomy, Baltimore, 1983, Williams & Wilkins.

Anderson JR et al: Glenoid labrum tears related to the long head of biceps, Am J Sports Med 13:337, 1985.

Andrews JR et al: Musculotendinous injuries of the shoulder and elbow in athletes, Athletic Training, The Journal of the NATA Association 2:68, 1976.

APTA Orthopaedic Section Review for Advanced Orthopaedic Competencies Conference, lecture by Sandy Burkart, "The Shoulder," Chicago, Aug 8, 1989.

Baker C, Uribe J, and Whitman C: Arthroscopic evaluation of acute initial anterior shoulder dislocations, Am J Sports Med 18(1):25-8, 1990.

Booher JM and Thibodeau GA: Athletic injury assessment, Toronto, 1985, Times Mirror/Mosby College Publishing.

Booth RE and Marvel JP: Differential diagnosis of shoulder pain, Orthop Clin North Am 6:353, 1975.

Bowers DK: Treatment of acromioclavicular sprains in athletes, Phys Sports Med 11(1):79, 1983.

Braatz J and Gogia P: The mechanics of pitching, Orthop Sports Phys Therapy 9(2):56, 1987.

Butler DS: Mobilization of the nervous system, New York, Churchill Livingstone, 1992.

Cain P et al: Anterior stability of the glenohumeral joint, Am J Sports Med 15(2):144, 1987.

Cailliet R: Shoulder pain, ed 3, Philadelphia, FA Davis, 1991.

Cuillo J: Swimmer's shoulder, Clin Sports Med 5:115-136, 1984.

Cyriax J: Textbook of orthopedic medicine: diagnosis of soft tissue lesions, vol 1, London, 1978, Bailliere Tindall, 1978.

Davies GJ et al: Functional examination of shoulder girdle: The Physician and Sportsmedicine 9(6):82, 1981.

Donatelli R: Physical therapy of the shoulder, New York, Churchill Livingstone, 1987.

Donatelli R and Greenfield B: Case study: rehabilitation of a stiff and painful shoulder: a biomechanical approach, J Orthop Sports Phys Therapy 118-126, Sept 1987.

Donatelli R and Wooden M: Orthopaedic physical therapy, New York, Churchill Livingstone, 1989.

Donoghue DH: Subluxing biceps tendon in the athlete, Sports Med 20-29, March/April 1973.

Einhorn A: Shoulder rehabilitation: equipment modifications, Orthop Sports Phys Therapy 6(4):247, 1985.

Edmond S: Manipulation mobilization extremity and spinal techniques, Toronto, Mosby-Yearbook Inc., 1993.

Engle R and Canner G: Posterior shoulder instability approach to rehabilitation, J of Orthopaedic and Sports PT 10:488-494, 1989.

Ferrari D: Capsular ligaments of the shoulder: anatomical and functional study of the anterior superior capsule, Am J Sports Med 18(1):20-24, 1990.

Fukuda K et al: Biomechanical study of the ligamentous system of the acromioclavicular joint, J Bone Joint Surg 434, 1986.

Garth W et al: Occult anterior subluxations of the shoulder in noncontact sports, Am J Sports Med 15(6):579, 1987.

Glick JM et al: Dislocated acromioclavicular joint: follow-up study of 35 unreduced acromioclavicular dislocations, Am J Sports Med 5(6):265, 1977.

Goodman C and Snyder T: Differential diagnosis in physical therapy, Toronto, WB Saunders Co., 1990.

Gould JA and Davis GJ: Orthopaedic and sports physical therapy, Toronto, 1985, The CV Mosby Co.

Gowan I et al: A comparative electromyographic analysis of the shoulder during pitching, Am J Sports Med 15(6): 586, 1987.

Grana W et al: How I manage acute anterior shoulder dislocations, The Physician and Sportsmedicine 15(4):88, 1987.

Grant R: Physical therapy of the cervical and thoracic spine, New York, 1988, Churchill Livingstone.

Hawkins R and Abrams J: impingement syndrome in the absence of rotator cuff tear (stages 1 & 2), Orthop Clin North Am 18:373-382, 1987.

Hawkins RJ and Kennedy JC: Impingement syndrome in athletes, Am J Sports Med 8:151, 1980.

Henry J and Genung JA: Natural history of glenohumeral dislocation—revisited, Am J Sports Med 10(3):135, 1982.

Hoppenfield S: Physical examination of the spine and extremities, New York, 1976. Appleton-Century Crofts.

Jackson D: Chronic rotator cuff impingement in the throwing athlete, Am J Sports Med 4(6):231-240, 1976.

Jobe FW and Jobe CM: Painful athletic injuries of the shoulder, Clin Orthop 1173:117, 1983.

Jobe FW et al: Rotator cuff function during golf swing, Am J Sports Med 14(5):388, 1986.

Kaltenborn F: Mobilization of the extremity joints, ed 3, Oslo: Universitetsgaten, 1980, Olaf Norlis Bokhandel.

Kapandji IA: The physiology of the joints, vol 1, Upper limb, New York, 1983, Churchill Livingstone.

Kellgren J: On the distribution of pain arising from deep somatic structures with charts of segmental pain areas, Clin Sci 4:35, 1939.

Kendall FP and McCreary EK: Muscles testing and function, Baltimore, Williams & Wilkins, 1983.

Kennedy JC et al: Orthopaedic manifestations of swimming, Am J Sports Med 6(6):309-322, 1978.

Kessel L and Watson M: The painful arc syndrome, J Bone Joint Surg 59B:82, 1977.

Kessler RM and Hertling D: Management of common musculo-skeletal disorders, Philadelphia, 1983, Harper and Row.

Kulund D: The injured athlete, Toronto; 1982, JB Lippincott.

Kummel BM: Spectrum of lesions of the anterior capsular mechanism of the shoulder, Am J Sports Med 7(2):111, 1979.

Lippman, RK: Frozen shoulder: periarthritis—bicipital tenosynovitis, Arch Surg 47:283, 1943.

Lombardo S et al: Posterior shoulder lesions in throwing athletes, Am J Sports Med 5(3):106,1977.

Ludington NA: Rupture of the long head of the biceps flexor cubiti muscle, Arch Surg 77:358, 1923.

Magee DJ: Orthopedics conditions, assessments, and treatment, vol 2, Alberta, 1979, University of Alberta Publishing.

Magee DJ: Orthopaedic physical assessment, Toronto, 1987, WB Saunders Co.

Maitland GD: Peripheral manipulation, Toronto, 1977, Butterworth & Co.

Mannheimer JS and Lampe GN: Clinical transcutaneous electrical nerve stimulation, Philadelphia, 1986, FA Davis Co.

McLaughlin HL: Recurrent anterior dislocation of the shoulder II: a comparative study, Joint Trauma 7:191, 1967.

McMaster WC: Anterior glenoid labrum damage: a painful lesion in swimmers, Am J Sports Med 14(5):383, 1986.

McMaster WC: Painful shoulder in swimmers: a diagnostic challenge, Phys Sports Med 14(12):108, 1986.

Nash H: Rotator cuff damage: reexamining the causes and treatments, Phys and Sports Med 16(8):129, 1988.

Neer CS II: Impingement lesions, Clin Orthop 173:70-77, 1983.

Neer CS II and Welsh RP: The shoulder in sports, Orthop Clin North Am 8:583, 1977.

Nirschl RP: Shoulder tendonitis AAOS Symposium on the upper extremity in sports, St Louis, 1986, The CV Mosby Co.

Nitz A et al: Nerve injury and grades II and III sprains, Am J Sports Med 13(3):177, 1985.

Nuber GW et al: Fine wire electromyography analysis of muscles of the shoulder during swimming, Am J Sports Med 14(1):7, 1986.

O'Donaghue D: Treatment of injuries to athletes, Toronto, 1984, WB Saunders Co.

Pappas AM et al: Symptomatic shoulder instability due to lesions of the glenoid labrum, Am J Sports Med 11:279, 1983.

Perry J: Anatomy and biomechanics of the shoulder in throwing, swimming, gymnastics, and tennis, Clin Sports Med 2:247, 1983.

Pettrone FA and Nisch RP: Acromioclavicular dislocation, AM J Sports Med 6(4):160, 1978.

Priest JD and Nagel DA: Tennis shoulder, Am J Sports Med 4(1):28, 1976.

Rathbun JB and McNab I: The microvascular pattern of the rotator cuff, Bone Joint Surg 52B:540, 1970.

Reid DC: Functional anatomy and joint mobilization, Alberta, 1970, University of Alberta Press.

Reid DC: Sports Injury Assessment and Rehabilitation, New York, Churchill Livingstone, 1992.

Ringel S et al: Suprascapular neuropathy in pitchers, Am J Sports Med 18(1):80-86, 1990.

Rowe CR: Factors related to recurrences of anterior dislocation of the shoulder, Clin Orthop 20:40, 1961.

Ryu RKN et al: Am J Sports Med 16(5):481-485, 1988.

Salter EG Jr et al: Anatomical observations on the acromioclavicular joint and supporting ligaments, Am J Sports Med 15(3):199, 1987.

Schenkman M and Cartaya V: Kinesiology of the shoulder complex, J Orthop Sports Phy Therapy, March 1987.

Simon E: Rotator cuff injuries: an update, J of Orth and Sports PT pp. 394-398, April 1989.

Slocum DB: The mechanics of some common injuries to the shoulder in sports, Am J Surg 98:394, 1959.

Smith MJ and Stewart MJ: Acute acromioclavicular separations—a 20-year study, Am J Sports Med 7(1):62, 1979.

Taft T et al: Dislocation of the acromioclavicular joint, J Bone Joint Surg 69A(7):1045, 1987.

Tank R and Halbach J: Physical therapy evaluation of the shoulder complex in athletes, J Orthop Sports Phy Therapy 1982, pp. 108-119.

Thein L: Impingement syndrome and its conservative management, J Orthop Sports Phy Therapy 11(5):183-191, November 1989.

Tomberlin JP et al: The use of standardized evaluation forms in physical therapy, J Orthop Sports Phy Therapy 1984, pp. 348-354.

Torg J: Athletic injuries to the head, neck, and face, Philadelphia, 1982, Lea & Febiger

Travell J and Simons D: Myofascial pain and dysfunction: the trigger point manual, Baltimore, 1983, Williams & Wilkins.

Tullos HS and King JW: Throwing mechanism in sports, Orthop Clin North Am 4:709, 1973.

Welsh P and Shepherd R: Current therapy in sports medicine 1985-1986, Toronto, 1985, BC Decker.

Williams L and Warwick R: Gray's Anatomy, New York, 1980, Churchill Livingstone.

Yanda V: Muscles and cervicogenic pain syndromes in Grant R: Physical therapy of the cervical and thoracic spine.

CHAPTER 4
Elbow Assessment

The elbow complex is a central link in the upper extremity kinetic chain and is crucial to hand movements. This kinetic chain includes the cervical spine, shoulder, elbow, forearm, wrist, and hand. any dysfunction or pathology in one of the joints can have an effect on the others. For example, if elbow flexion is limited, the wrist and hand cannot function normally for combing the hair or to eat. If shoulder extension is limited, the elbow will not flex and extend during normal walking. Man's prehensile skill depends on the integrity of the elbow joint, as well as the whole upper kinetic chain (upper quadrant).

The elbow is composed of three articulations (Fig. 4-1):
- humeroulnar joint
- humeroradial joint
- radioulnar joint

The humeroradial and humeroulnar joints allow flexion and extension and both are considered to be uniaxial diarthrodial hinge joints with one degree of freedom of motion. The humeroulnar joint is formed by the articulation between the trochlea of the humerus and the trochlear notch of the ulna. The humeroradial joint is formed by the articulation between the capitellum of the humerus and the head of the radius.

During elbow extension there is:
- proximal (superior) glide of the ulna in the trochlea
- pronation and abduction of the ulna on the humerus
- distal movement and pronation of the radius on the humerus

During elbow flexion there is:
- distal (inferior) glide of the ulna in the trochlea
- supination and adduction of the ulna on the humerus
- proximal movement and supination of the radius on the humerus

The radioulnar joints are uniaxial pivot joints and are composed of two articulations:
- proximal radioulnar joint
- distal radioulnar joint

The proximal radioulnar joint is formed by the articulation of the head of the radius in the radial notch of the ulna with the annular ligament holding the head in place. The distal radioulnar joint is formed by the articulation of the ulnar notch of the radius, the articular disc, and the head of the ulna. The proximal and distal radioulnar joints function together, producing pronation and supination, and are considered diarthrodial uniaxial pivot joints. The humeroulnar, humeroradial, and proximal radioulnar joints are enclosed in one capsule. During forearm pronation and supination the head of the radius spins, rolls, and slides (glides) in the radial notch.

The close-packed position of the humeroulnar joint is extension and supination; the capsular pattern is more limited in terms of flexion than extension. The resting, or loose-packed, position of the humeroulnar joint is elbow flexion of approximately 70° with the forearm supinated to an angle of 10°.

The close-packed position of the humeroradial joint is the elbow flexed at an angle of 90° and the forearm supinated at an angle of approximately 5°. The capsular pattern of the humeroradial has more limitation of flexion than extension. The resting, or loose-packed, position of the humeroradial joint is with the elbow extended and the forearm supinated.

The close-packed position for the radioulnar joints is at 5° of supination. The radioulnar capsular pattern has equal limitation of supination and pronation at the end of the range of motion. The resting, or loose-packed, position for the proximal radioulnar joint is with the forearm supinated at an angle of approximately 35° and the elbow flexed at an angle of 70°. The resting, or loose-packed, position for the distal radioulnar joint is the forearm supinated approximately 10°.

The majority of the close-packed, resting positions and capsular patterns are taken from Kaltenborn's work.

Make certain that the athlete's problem originates at the elbow and not at the cervical spine, shoulder joint, wrist, or brachial plexus. The elbow

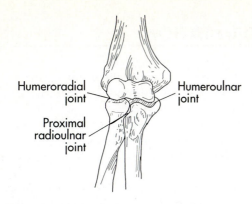

Fig. 4-1 Three articulations at the elbow joint, anterior aspect.

Humeroradial joint

Humeroulnar joint

Proximal radioulnar joint

joint is largely derived from C6 and C7 and therefore it can be the site of referred pain from other structures of the same segmental derivation.

When it is injured, the elbow joint can develop neurovascular problems from the structures damaged or from secondary complications, especially swelling. For this reason it is important to assess and reassess the neurovascular systems by examining the athlete's circulation, strength, sensation, swelling, and pulses. The patient should be informed of what neurovascular problems to watch for and to seek medical assistance immediately if a problem develops.

ASSESSMENT	INTERPRETATION

HISTORY

Mechanism of Injury

Direct Trauma (Fig. 4-2)
   Was it direct trauma?

Contusion
   • near boney structures
   • in soft tissue
   • to ulnar nerve

Falling on the tip of the elbow often results in an olecranon contusion and this can be associated with an abrasion. The boney prominences of the lateral condyle and radial head are also frequently contused. The medial condyle is closer to the body and is thus more protected, being injured less frequently than the exposed lateral structures. Contusions of the soft tissue of the biceps and triceps are common, especially in contact sports. Repeated blows to these muscles can result in myositis ossificans if the injured site is not protected. The ulnar nerve is subject to direct trauma because of its exposed position in the ulnar groove. Trauma can cause transient paresthesia, which usually subsides quickly or within several hours. Prolonged paresthesia or ulnar palsy can result if the trauma causes significant bleeding that results in adhesion formation within the nerve itself.

Fracture
   • distal humerus, proximal ulna, and/or proximal radius

Fractures about the elbow usually occur in children and adolescents because their epiphyseal plates are not closed and the

ASSESSMENT

- supracondylar
- olecranon process
- head of the radius

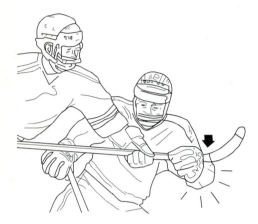

Fig. 4-2 Direct blow to the elbow.

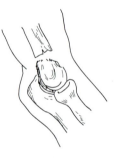

Fig. 4-3 Supracondylar fracture—hyperextension mechanism.

INTERPRETATION

ligament structures are stronger than the cartilaginous epiphyseal plates. Condylar and epicondylar fractures occur especially on the medial aspect of the elbow.

Fractures are often associated with a dislocation. Fractures of the distal humerus, proximal ulna, and/or proximal radius can also occur. These can range from simple avulsions to more complicated fractures.

The medial epicondylar fractures are usually avulsion fractures from excessive force on the ulnar collateral ligament or the common flexor origin.

The lateral epicondylar fracture is also often an avulsion fracture through a growth center and is usually the result of excessive force through the common extensor origin.

Condylar and transcondylar fractures can occur in the skeletally more mature athlete with closed epiphyseal plates. These fractures may be undisplaced or displaced and require immobilization and transportation to the nearest medical facility.

With all fractures of the elbow, the possibility exists of disruption of the arterial supply causing Volkmann's ischemic contracture, which constitutes a medical emergency.

A supracondylar fracture usually occurs in children and is a very serious injury because of possible damage to the blood vessels that supply the forearm and hand, especially the brachial artery and the median nerve. The mechanism involves falling on the outstretched hand or forced elbow hyperextension (where dislocation does not result) (Fig. 4-3). Such falls are common in gymnastics, cycling, and horseback riding. The distal fragment of the humerus is pushed forward and then backward by the force and is maintained in that position by spasm of the triceps muscle. The forearm appears shortened and there is severe bleeding and soft-tissue damage.

A direct blow to the flexed elbow can fracture the tip of the olecranon process but this is rare. A direct blow to the olecranon can cause a fracture separation of the olecranon epiphysis in a child. The ossification center can vary from a small flake to up to 25% of the olecranon. In the adult, this fracture can be displaced and may require open reduction and fixation if unstable.

A fracture of the ulna just distal to the olecranon, along with a dislocation of the radial head, is called a Monteggia fracture-dislocation. It is the result of a fall on the outstretched arm. When the arm is extended to break the athlete's fall, the head of the radius may fracture as it takes the force that is transmitted up the forearm. If more than one third of the articular surface is damaged or if there is more than 30° angulation, an open reduction may be necessary. This can occur in the child but it usually causes an epiphyseal separation and angulation deformity. Traction manipulation or surgery may be necessary.

ASSESSMENT   # INTERPRETATION

Osteochondritis of the Capitellum (Panner Disease)

Direct trauma or inadequate circulation through the elbow joint has been associated with osteochondritis of the capitellum (aseptic or avascular necrosis of the capitellum), primarily in the adolescent male. It can occur in younger athletes but is rarely seen before the age of 5 years. Possible causes of this condition include:

- bacterial infection
- fracture
- heredity
- vascular insufficiency

According to Reid and Kushner, repeated minor trauma may account for this condition in young baseball pitchers, gymnasts, and javelin throwers (see Overuse, Pitching Act).

Bursitis
- olecranon
- radiohumeral

The olecranon bursa lies between the tip of the olecranon and the overlying skin (Figs. 4-4 and 4-5). A fall on the tip of the elbow or a direct blow to the olecranon can cause swelling into the bursa, resulting in olecranon bursitis. Chronic olecranon bursitis results from mismanagement of the acute bursitis or from repeated blows to the olecranon. Repeated trauma such as in hockey and football or weight-bearing forces to the olecranon, as in wrestling, can also cause bursitis and, eventually, chronic bursitis. Cartilaginous or, occasionally, calcified nodules may also develop in the bursa.

The radiohumeral bursa lies directly under the extensor aponeurosis and over the radial head. Bursitis in this area is not to be confused with lateral epicondylitis. A direct blow or extensor muscle overuse can inflame this bursa.

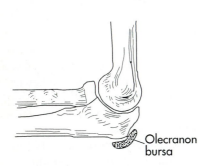

Fig. 4-4 Olecranon bursa.

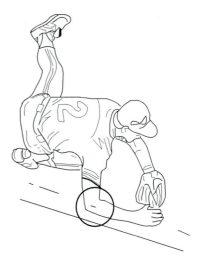

Fig. 4-5 Falling on the elbow.

ASSESSMENT

INTERPRETATION

Make sure that the bursitis is not caused by infection, since this needs prompt medical attention. This is particularly important in football players who hit the bursa on the field and may have also abraded the injury site. Such an infection often occurs in the wrestler who abrades the site while wrestling on an unclean wrestling mat.

Overstretch

Was it an overstretch?

Elbow Joint Hyperextension
FALLING ON THE OUTSTRETCHED ARM

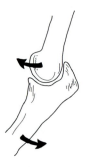

Fig. 4-6 Hyperextension injury mechanism.

Fractures of the upper humerus can occur with this mechanism, especially in sports that involve excessive force (e.g., horseback riding, wrestling, or football).

Elbow joint hyperextension injuries usually result from falling on an outstretched arm with the elbow extended and the forearm supinated. The force is transmitted through the ulna to the olecranon process, which is levered against the humerus, forcing the ulna backward and the humerus forward (Fig. 4-6). The structures that can be injured with this force are:

- The biceps brachii can be strained at its point of insertion on the neck of the radius or ruptured if the force is severe.
- The brachialis can be strained at its point of insertion on the ulna.
- The brachioradialis can be strained if the hyperextension force occurred while the forearm was in slight pronation.
- The anterior portion of the medial (ulnar) and/or lateral (radial) collateral ligaments of the elbow can be sprained or torn—the medial collateral ligament is injured more often because of the valgus position of the joint.
- The elbow capsular and collateral ligaments can be sprained or even ruptured depending on the forces involved—they can also avulse a piece of the condyle (most commonly the medial epicondyle).

If the hyperextension force carries on, it could tear both the collateral ligaments, and the elbow can then sublux or dislocate. In the dislocated elbow the olecranon usually dislocates posteriorly with a resulting tear of the capsule and ligament. A dislocated elbow is very serious because of the possibility of damage to the blood vessels (brachial artery) or the nerves (usually the median nerve). Fractures frequently accompany the dislocation, especially in the adolescent. The epicondyles, the olecranon, and the coronoid process or radial head can all be avulsed or fractured directly. In the adolescent, the medial epicondyle epiphysis avulsion fracture is most common.

The ulnar nerve is not usually injured in a hyperextension mechanism unless the medial epicondyle is fractured.

ASSESSMENT

INTERPRETATION

With any injuries caused by hyperextension, whether it is in the capsular ligaments or the collateral ligaments, it is possible for the capsule to ossify later. This ossification can lead to a chronic loss of elbow range, which can occur in the anterior capsule around the coronoid process of the ulna or in the posterior capsule around the olecranon process.

In the child or young adolescent, the forces of hyperextension usually cause a supracondylar fracture.

The older athlete tends to fracture the ulnar or radius when excessive force goes through the elbow joint.

Elbow hyperextension problems are very common in female gymnasts because of the nature of the sport and because of the hypermobility required, particularly during vaulting and floor exercises. Elbow hyperextension injuries are also common in wrestling because of the nature of the holds and joint levering required to gain an advantage over an opponent.

Falling on the outstretched arm can cause the athlete to slowly flex the elbow to dissipate the force, and, on occasion, the eccentric contraction of the triceps can tear the tendon or, less frequently, the belly of the triceps muscle.

Elbow Joint Hyperflexion

Flexion of the elbow joint is normally limited by the tissue approximation but if the elbow is passively forced into greater flexion the posterior capsule can be sprained or torn. If the elbow is forced into flexion with the shoulder fully flexed also, the triceps muscles can be strained.

Elbow Joint
VALGUS/VARUS (FIG. 4-7, A AND B)
Elbow extended
Elbow flexed to midrange

A valgus force of the extended elbow will cause a medial collateral ligament sprain or tear, especially of the anterior oblique portion, with damage to the anterior capsule (Fig. 4-8; see Fig. 4-7, A). In the adolescent the epicondyle can be avulsed by this force.

A valgus force with the elbow flexed to midrange will also damage the medial collateral ligament but without any capsular or boney involvement. According to Reid et al, acute medial collateral ligament ruptures are often associated with ulnar nerve paresthesia.

A varus force of the extended or midrange elbow can damage primarily the anterior capsule or the joint articular surfaces and secondarily the lateral (radial) collateral ligament (see Fig. 4-7, B).

Radioulnar Joint
PRONATION/SUPINATION

During pronation and supination the proximal and distal radioulnar joints allow the movement to take place.

ASSESSMENT   INTERPRETATION

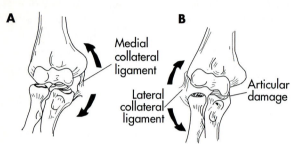

Fig. 4-7 Elbow joint damage. **A,** Valgus overstretch. **B,** Varus overstretch.

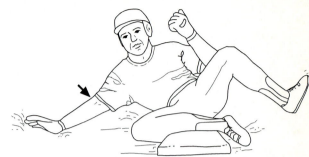

Fig. 4-8 Elbow joint valgus overstretch mechanism.

The quadrate ligament at the proximal radioulnar joint can be injured with an overstretch in either direction.

Forced pronation can cause a posterior subluxation of the ulnar head; the posterior capsule and triangular ligament of the distal radioulnar joint can also be sprained.

Forced supination can sprain the annular ligament or the lateral (radial) collateral ligament (anterior fibers) of the elbow. The anterior ligament or capsule at the distal radioulnar joint can be sprained. The pronating muscles (especially the pronator teres) give the greater restraint and therefore can be strained.

Radial Head
JOINT DISTRACTION (PULLED ELBOW)

In the adult, the soft-tissue resistance to distraction is mainly the anterior capsule with slight involvement of the collaterals.

The radial head can be pulled out of the annular ligament in a child between the ages of 2 and 4 because of incomplete radial head development and the immaturity of the annular ligament. This can occur when the child is pulled too forcibly by the hand or swinging a child by the hands. With radial head displacement the arm will hang limply at the child's side with the forearm in pronation. This must be reduced and full function regained because an inadequate reduction results in deformity and disability of the elbow joint at a later time.

Overcontraction
Acute Muscle Strain
- Common flexor origin
- Common extensor origin
- biceps
- triceps

A forceful muscle contraction against too great a resistance can cause a muscle strain (Fig. 4-9). The most frequent sites are the common extensor tendon (lateral epicondyle) and the common flexor tendon (medial epicondyle). These occur with a strong contraction where the resistance is too great and muscle is on stretch (eccentrically loaded). Often these muscles are decelerating the wrist joint during a fall or following a tennis backhand. The tendon can be strained or, on occasion, avulsed or ruptured.

ASSESSMENT

INTERPRETATION

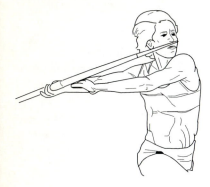

Fig. 4-9 Forceful muscle contraction while on stretch.

The biceps or triceps muscles, because they cross two joints, are also susceptible to strain and occasionally to rupture. These strains occur most frequently at the musculotendinous junction and occasionally in the muscle belly. The biceps tendon can be strained or ruptured at the tenoperiosteal insertion. The biceps injury can result from the deceleration forces at the elbow on the follow-through of the throwing motion to prevent elbow hyperextension.

The triceps can be strained, avulsed, or ruptured when they decelerate the elbow joint due to a fall on the outstretched arm or decelerating the shoulder girdle on the follow-through of a throw.

Overuse

Was it an overuse mechanism?
Wrist extensor-supinator

Wrist extensor-supinator overuse can cause the following:
- lateral epicondylitis or periostitis where the extensor aponeurosis inserts
- tendonitis or strain of any of the wrist extensors, particularly the extensor carpi radialis brevis at its point of origin
- radiohumeral bursitis
- microtears of the common extensor tendon resulting in subtendinous granulation
- radial head fibrillation
- radial tunnel syndrome (or posterior interosseous entrapment)
- annular ligament inflammation

Rule out the possibility of the following:
- cervical radiculopathy—C6 nerve root dysfunction can lead to weakness in the wrist extensors, leaving the athlete prone to these overuse conditions. Test the cervical spine fully if suspected (see Cervical Spine Assessment)
- radial tunnel syndrome (posterior interosseous nerve entrapment)

When the posterior interosseous nerve is entrapped the signs may appear the same as lateral epicondylitis, but the entrapment causes:
- tenderness over the supinator muscle (distal to the lateral epicondyle)
- pain on resisted finger extension
- significant pain on resisted supination

ASSESSMENT

INTERPRETATION

- tenderness over the radial nerve
- pain radiating along the nerve

Racquet sports where incorrect wrist motion occurs are the most frequent cause for wrist extensor-supinator injuries in sport. For example, the tennis player who does not keep the wrist locked during the backhand stroke can have the extensor tendons pulled away from the origin because the wrist gives (flexes) as the racquet contacts the ball. With repeated backhands, microtrauma to the eccentrically loaded tendon can occur. Several factors can add to this problem, for example:

- weak wrist extensors
- incorrect grip on the racquet
- an incorrect grip size on the racquet
- racquet that is strung incorrectly, too heavy, or too stiff
- player who is out of position
- inadequate warmup or training
- hitting the ball too hard

Age-related tissue changes can also contribute to injury. With aging there is a loss of the mucopolysaccharide chondroitin sulfate that makes the tendon less extensible and more susceptible to injury. Most extensor carpi radialis brevis tendonitis problems occur in the athlete who is over the age of 35.

Incorrect wrist motion or overuse of the wrist extensors during badminton, squash, and racquetball can also lead to any of the above injuries—these problems are commonly referred to as "tennis elbow."

Wrist Flexion With a Valgus Force at the Extending Elbow

Medial epicondylitis, sometimes called "Little League elbow," occurs readily in throwing or pitching sports (e.g., baseball, softball, javelin) where the elbow is extending with a severe valgus force and the wrist is flexing.

Pitching Act (Fig. 4-10)

Each pitcher or thrower has a unique pitching style. During windup, the thrower attempts to contract all the antagonist muscles to place the body in a position so that each muscle, joint, and body part can summate their forces synchronously for a powerful release of energy during the pitch. The pitcher initiates the windup by stepping backward with the left leg. The pitcher then shifts body weight by flexing the left hip and knee backward and upward while rotating the trunk to the right. The right foot acts as the pivot point. The pitcher continues to turn to the

The cycle of pitching begins with a cocking phase, two acceleration phases, and a follow-through phase.

ASSESSMENT   INTERPRETATION

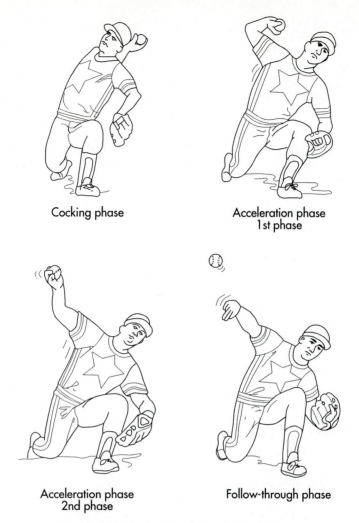

Cocking phase

Acceleration phase
1st phase

Acceleration phase
2nd phase

Follow-through phase

Fig. 4-10 Mechanics of the pitching act.

right until the shoulders and hips are perpendicular to the strike zone at an angle of 90°. At the height of the coiling movement and knee lift, the hands separate and the early cocking phase begins.

WIND-UP PHASE

EARLY COCKING PHASE

The hip on the coiled limb begins to extend and abduct as the pelvis and trunk begin to turn toward the plate with the body pivoting over the right

Few, if any, injuries occur during this phase.

ASSESSMENT

INTERPRETATION

leg with the knee slightly flexed. The ball is lowered in front of the body. The pelvis, hip, and trunk uncoil explosively to the left with the entire right side of the pelvis driving forward with hip and knee extension.

LATE COCKING PHASE

This begins as the stride leg contacts the ground. The shoulder of the throwing arm is at an angle of 90° of abduction and approximately 100° to 120° of external rotation, with about 30° of horizontal abduction (or cross-extension). Experienced pitchers develop anterior capsule laxity and the ability to stretch the soft tissue to allow extreme ranges of external rotation. The posterior deltoid muscle brings the humerus into horizontal abduction while the supraspinatus, infraspinatus, and teres minor muscles must stabilize the head of the humerus. The internal rotators are stretched. The scapular stabilizers contract to maintain a solid base for the glenohumeral movement. The elbow is flexed approximately 90° with the forearm supinated and the wrist in neutral or in a position of slight extension. The body moves forward, leaving the shoulder and arm behind. The lumbar spine then moves into a hyperextended position and force is generated from the trunk, pelvis, and spine into the upper extremity.

ACCELERATION—FIRST PHASE

The primary phase of acceleration begins with a powerful internal rotation of the shoulder musculature and the forward motion of the ball. According to Perry, the anterior capsule recoils like a spring with the force reversal of internal rotation with incredible torque. The subscapularis, pectoralis major, latissimus dorsi, and teres major muscles contract concentrically while in a lengthened muscle stretch position. The serratus anterior muscle abducts the scapula.

COCKING PHASE

The athlete prepares for this phase by turning the body away from the direction of the throw and shifting the center of gravity backward.

The shoulder comes into play with the shoulder externally rotated, abducted, and cross-extended (horizontally abducted).

There are valgus forces placed on the medial elbow but this evokes pain only if there is an existing medial soft-tissue injury.

The body then rotates and weight is transferred forward. The shoulder is then fully externally rotated and the elbow is flexed as the trunk moves forward.

ASSESSMENT

INTERPRETATION

ACCELERATION—SECOND PHASE

During the second part of the acceleration phase, the shoulder internal rotation continues while the elbow moves from an angle of 25° to 30° of extension. The trunk continues rotating to the left while the shoulder joint cross-flexes (horizontally adducts). There are significant valgus and extension forces through the elbow joint during this period. The biceps work eccentrically to decelerate elbow extension and the ball is released before full elbow extension while the forearm moves from a supinated to a pronated position.

The shoulder is then internally rotated vigorously, which puts an extreme valgus stress on the elbow as the forearm lags behind while the humerus internally rotates. The elbow is usually injured during the second acceleration phase from the extreme valgus and extension. Repetition of this action can result in:

- wrist flexor strains
- medial epicondylitis
- medial (ulnar) collateral ligament attenuation, sprains, or ruptures
- traction spurs at the medial epicondyle
- avulsion fracture of the medial epicondyle (especially the epiphyseal plate in the young athlete)
- traction spurs of the ulnar coronoid process
- compression fractures of the radial head or capitellum (as the cubital valgus deformity progresses)
- osteophytes on the posteromedial aspect of the olecranon fossa
- chondromalacia on the medial aspect of the olecranon fossa
- articular cartilage roughening and degeneration
- ulnar nerve traction problems
- osteochondritis of the capitellum

The extreme valgus position stretches the medial structures and compresses the lateral structures.

Damage because of the valgus and extension load on the elbow can be permanent if the epiphyseal plates of the young baseball pitcher are not closed (the medial and lateral epicondyle epiphysis close at the age of 16 years in males and 14 to 15 years in females).

FOLLOW-THROUGH

The left stride foot is important because once it is planted it starts the deceleration forces of the body. The trunk forward bends and rotates left with a gradual deceleration dissipation of torque. Once the ball is released, powerful deceleration muscle contractions are necessary to slow the upper limb motion. The posterior rotator cuff muscles and posterior deltoid muscle contract eccentrically to prevent the humerus from being pulled out of the glenoid fossa. The scapular stabilizing muscles must contract to control the forward motion of the entire shoulder girdle. The biceps brachii contracts vigorously to decelerate elbow extension

The entire shoulder girdle then follows through ballistically in the direction of the throw, with the elbow flexors contracting eccentrically to decelerate the elbow joint. If the extension is not slowed, olecranon impaction syndrome can occur, which can result in damage to the olecranon articular cartilage or the bone.

ASSESSMENT   INTERPRETATION

and pronation. The shoulder girdle forces are gradually dissipated as the glenohumeral joint adducts and the scapula protracts in a cross-body motion.

Repeated Elbow Extension with a Valgus Force (Fig. 4-11)

With professional baseball pitchers the damage to the elbow from this repeated valgus and extension stress can progress further and result in:

- olecranon fossa and lateral compartment loose bodies
- ulnar nerve problems (entrapment and/or dislocation) such as neuritis and neuropathy
- trochlear fractures
- biceps flexion contracture
- anterior capsule contracture
- medial collateral ligament attenuation
- bone spurs
- radial head degeneration
- avascular necrosis

Additionally, compression forces on the lateral aspect of the joint due to the valgus stress may eventually result in osteochondral fractures of the capitellum.

During the follow-through, the triceps forcefully extends the elbow and these extension forces can result in:

- olecranon avulsion fracture
- triceps strain
- olecranon hypertrophy and spurs
- humeroulnar joint or radial head degeneration
- pronator teres strain

Repeated Wrist Flexion

Golfers often have wrist flexor overuse problems at the medial epicondyle. The lower hand on the grip of the club moves from a wrist extended position to wrist flexion and overuse can lead to problems. Experienced tennis players can suffer from overuse of the wrist flexors from the overhand serve motion. This also occurs in the throwing athlete, combined with elbow

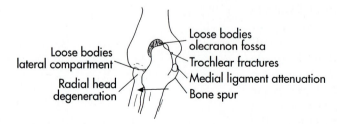

Fig. 4-11 Chronic throwing lesions, elbow joint valgus and extension stress.

ASSESSMENT

INTERPRETATION

valgus forces and pronation, as mentioned earlier (see Wrist Flexion with Valgus Force).

Repeated Elbow Flexion

Repeated elbow flexion from weight lifting or rowing can lead to ulnar neuritis because the nerve is on full stretch in the elbow flexed position.

The posterior interosseous nerve can also be irritated by repeated elbow flexion because it becomes stretched over the prominent radial head.

Reenacting the Mechanism

Can the athlete reenact the mechanism using the opposite limb?

Determine shoulder position.

Determine elbow position.

Determine hand position.

Having the mechanism reenacted by the opposite limb allows the athlete to clarify his or her explanation of what happened and allows you to determine which structures were stressed. The most common injury mechanisms are landing on the outstretched arm or tip of the elbow. Determine if the elbow was fully extended, in pronation or supination, and the position of the shoulder and hand at the time of the fall.

Force Involved

Ask for relevant information about the force of the blow or twist involved.

Ask about the forces involved in the sport.

Asking about the degree of force can help determine the amount of possible damage.

Nature of the Sport

Ask questions about the nature of the sport and its related movements, especially when an overuse injury is involved.

Asking questions about the sport (e.g., action for tennis serve, arm movements during the overhand throw) can help determine which anatomic structures have been stretched, impinged, or overused.

Pain

Location

Where is the pain located?

Can the athlete point to the pain with one finger? (Fig. 4-12)

If the athlete can point with one finger to a spot that is painful, the injury is most likely in a superficial structure and is usually less severe than if there is diffuse pain.

Superficial structures give rise to pain that the athlete can localize easily and this pain is usually perceived at the location of the lesion.

Deeper structures give rise to pain that is referred or radiated (along a myotome, dermatome, or sclerotome) and is difficult for the athlete to localize.

Local Pain

Local point tenderness can occur with:
• olecranon bursitis

ASSESSMENT   INTERPRETATION

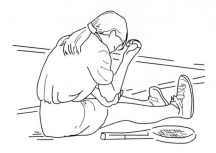

Fig. 4-12 Elbow pain.

- lateral epicondylitis
- medial epicondylitis
- muscle strains (biceps, triceps, wrist flexors, or extensors)
- ligament sprains (ulnar or radial collateral)

Ligaments are tender only when they are injured or if they support a joint that is in dysfunction (Mennell J).

Diffuse Pain

Diffuse painful areas occur with:
- referred or radiating pain in specific dermatomes or from a local cutaneous nerve supply
- joint subluxations or dislocations where multiple injuries are involved
- severe hematomas
- fractures (pain referred down the involved bone and often in the involved sclerotome)

Onset

How quickly did the pain begin?

Immediate

Pain that occurs immediately in a joint usually suggests an injury of an acute or severe nature. Such injuries include:
- hemarthroses
- fractures
- subluxations
- severe ligament or capsule sprains or tears

Gradual onset

A gradual onset of pain often occurs with overuse injuries and is associated with repeated microtrauma. Such pain could be indicative of:
- lateral or medial epicondylitis
- ulnar neuritis

ASSESSMENT   # INTERPRETATION

6 to 24 Hours

Pain 6 to 24 hours post-participation can result from a less severe injury or a chronic lesion such as:
- elbow joint synovial swelling
- muscular lactic acid buildup
- mild bursal swelling

Type of Pain

Can the athlete describe the pain?

According to Mannheimer and Lampe, different musculoskeletal structures give rise to different types of discomfort.

Sharp

Sharp pain may be experienced with an injury to the following:
- skin and fascia (e.g., lacerations)
- superficial muscle (e.g., strains common wrist flexors or extensors)
- superficial ligament (e.g., medial collateral or lateral collateral sprains)
- inflammation of a bursa (e.g., olecranon bursitis)
- periosteum (e.g., acute lateral or medial epicondylitis)

Dull Ache

Dull, aching pain may be felt with an injury to the following:
- subchondral bone (e.g., chronic epicondylitis and chondromalacia of the humerus or ulna)
- fibrous capsule (e.g., anterior capsule damage from hyperextension)
- bursa (e.g., chronic olecranon bursitis)

Tingling (Paresthesia)

A tingling sensation may be felt with the following:
- peripheral nerve damage (e.g., ulnar, median, or radial nerve)
- irritation of the nerve roots of C5, C6, C7, C8, T1 can cause tingling in the involved dermatome in the elbow area (Fig. 4-13)
- circulatory problem (e.g., with occlusion of an artery such as the brachial or median artery)

Numbness

Numbness can be caused by damage to the nerve in the area such as the ulnar, median, and radial nerve or damage to the dorsal nerve root affecting C6, C7, C8, and T1 dermatomes (see Fig. 4-13).

ASSESSMENT

INTERPRETATION

Twinges

Movement that repeats the mechanism of injury can cause twinges of pain if the injury is to the local muscle or ligament.

Severity

Is the pain mild, moderate, or severe?

The degree of pain is not a good indicator of the severity of the injury because complete ligament tears can be painless and severe pain can come from a minor periosteal irritation or a ligament sprain.

Time of pain

Is the pain worse in the morning, evening, or during the night?

Morning

Morning pain suggests that rest does not relieve the injury, which can indicate that:
- the injury is still acute
- an infection or systemic problem exists
- rheumatoid arthritis may be present

Evening

Pain that escalates as the day progresses suggests that daily activity is aggravating the injury.

During the Night

Pain that lasts all night is a sign of a more serious pathologic condition, such as:
- bone neoplasm
- local or systemic disorder (gout, rheumatoid arthritis, Reiter syndrome, ankylosing spondylitis, psoriatic disease)

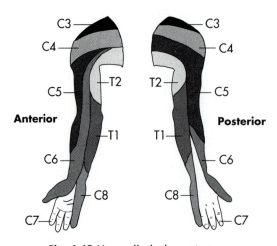

Fig. 4-13 Upper limb dermatomes.

ASSESSMENT

INTERPRETATION

Aggravating Activities

What activities aggravate the pain?

Repeating the movements involved in the mechanism will usually aggravate the condition.

Certain movements such as gripping increase the pain of an acute lateral epicondylitis.

Throwing aggravates medial compartment problems.

Repeated full elbow extension positions aggravate the humeroulnar and humeroradial joint, and repeated pronation and supination positions aggravate the radioulnar joint.

The collateral ligaments become more painful when they are stretched, and muscle strains and tendonitis become worse when the muscle is contracted or stretched.

The bursae are painful when they are pinched or compressed.

Any internal derangement (osteochondral fracture, joint mice, synovitis) is aggravated by elbow joint movements.

Periosteal pain or fractures are aggravated by vibration of the involved bone.

Alleviating Activities

What activities alleviate the pain?

Acute injuries generally feel better after rest, whereas chronic conditions improve with movement.

Overuse conditions settle down when the irritating movement is stopped.

Swelling

Location

Where is the swelling located?

Local

Common local swelling locations include the following:
- olecranon bursa and the radiohumeral bursa
- muscle strains or contusions to the tendon, belly, tenoperiosteal junction—these strains or contusions usually occur at the common extensor origin, common flexor origin, or in the biceps, triceps, and pronator teres muscles
- intracapsular effusion (Fig. 4-14)

Marked posterior joint swelling is usually olecranon bursitis, whereas anterior and posterior swelling is often an intracapsular effusion.

Synovial capsule effusion — Humerus
Annular ligament
Radius — Ulna

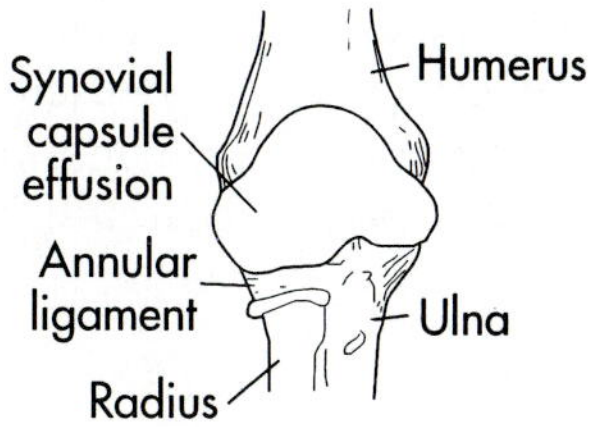

Fig. 4-14 Intracapsular effusion (anterior view).

ASSESSMENT

INTERPRETATION

Diffuse

Diffuse swelling can be caused by:
- severe hematoma
- dislocation
- fracture

Time of Swelling
How quickly did the elbow swell?

Immediately to Within 2 Hours

Swelling that occurs immediately or within the first 2 hours is an indication of damage to a structure with a rich blood supply. If swelling is associated with severe trauma, a fracture of dislocation can be suspected. Swelling that extends into the joint suggests a hemarthrosis (intra-articular fracture or severe traumatic effusion). If associated with a direct blow, the swelling can be indicative of muscular or soft tissue damage.

Within 6 to 24 Hours

Joint swelling that develops 6 to 24 hours after injury suggests a synovial irritation.
Common causes of synovitis are:
- bone chips (osteochondritis dessicans)
- capsular sprain
- ligament sprain
- joint subluxation

After Activity Only

Swelling that develops after activity only can occur with chronic bursitis or if something in the joint is irritating the synovium (e.g., a bone fragment).
Repeated trauma can keep a bursa inflamed.

Function

Range of Motion
How much range of motion did the elbow have at the time of injury?

The range of motion possible immediately after the injury occurs is indicative of the elbow joint function and the athlete's willingness to move it.
Limitations in functioning or a reluctance to move the joint immediately can be an indication of a substantial injury (e.g., second-degree ligament injury, fracture) or a strong psychologic fear of the injury on the part of the athlete.
In the case of a severe injury, immediate disability is present.
Joint effusion will limit both flexion and extension and the athlete may protect the injury by holding the elbow in flexion next to the body.

ASSESSMENT

INTERPRETATION

Locking

Is there locking?

Locking of the elbow occurs when a loose body is present in the joint following a previous elbow dislocation. This locking usually limits extension and it is usually momentary and quite unexpected.

Weakness

Is there weakness?

Immediate weakness can be caused by a reflex inhibition if there is a substantial injury.

Flexion, Extension problems

Are there problems with flexion or extension?

Problems with flexion or extension can involve the humeroulnar or humeroradial joints.

Pronation, Supination Problems

Are there problems with pronation or supination?

Problems with pronation and supination can involve the superior or inferior radioulnar joints.

Daily Function

How limited is the daily functioning of the arm, then and now?

Problems with the daily functions of the arm help determine the degree of disability the injury has caused and the best approach toward rehabilitation.

Sensations

Can the athlete describe the sensations felt at the time of injury and now?

Warmth

The presence of warmth suggests an active inflammation or infection.

Tingling, Numbness

Tingling or numbness in the upper arm, forearm, or hand can suggest:
- C5, C6, C7, or C8 nerve root compression
- thoracic outlet compression
- an injury to the medial, lateral, or posterior cutaneous nerve of the arm
- an injury to the intercostobrachial cutaneous nerve of the arm
- an injury to the medial, lateral, or posterior cutaneous nerve of the forearm
- an injury to the median, ulnar, or radial cutaneous nerve of the hand
- ulnar neuritis or neuropathy—cubital tunnel
- median neuritis or neuropathy—pronator syndrome, anterior interosseous nerve entrapment

ASSESSMENT

INTERPRETATION

- radial neuritis or neuropathy—posterior interosseous nerve entrapment

Clicking

Clicking may be indicative of a loose body in the joint. During elbow dislocations an avulsion or chipping of the epicondyles or articular surface is fairly common and will cause clicking.

Grating

Grating within the joint is a sign of osteoarthritic changes or damage to the articular surface (chondromalacia, osteochondritis, osteoarthritis).

Particulars

Has the athlete seen a physician or orthopedic surgeon?
What was the diagnosis?
Were x-rays taken?
What was his or her advice?
What was prescribed?
What treatment was carried out at the time of injury and now?
Ice (R.I.C.E. or P.I.E.R.)?
Heat?
Immobilization?
Sling?
Has this happened before?
If so, when?
Describe it fully?
What was done for it at that time?

Record the physician's diagnosis and address.
Record the x-ray results and where they were done.
Record the physician's recommendations and prescription.
The treatment at the time of injury is important to determine whether the inflammation process was controlled or increased. Ice and immobilization (in the form of a sling) can help limit the secondary edema.
If this injury is a recurrence, record all the details of the previous episode, including the following:
- date of injury
- mechanism of injury
- length of disability
- previous treatment and rehabilitation
- diagnosis
Common problems that tend to recur include:
- medial epicondylitis
- lateral epicondylitis
- biceps tendon strains
- wrist flexor and extensor strains
- olecranon bursitis

OBSERVATIONS

Gait (Fig. 4-15)

Observe as the athlete walks into the clinic or to the examining table. Observe the athlete's arm carriage and willingness to move the joint.

The arm swing should be a relaxed flexion and extension of the shoulder and elbow. The opposite leg and arm should swing rhythmically during gait. Reluctance to move the elbow with it held in flexion can be caused by a significant elbow injury. An elbow with joint effusion will be held at an angle of 70° of flexion, which allows the greatest joint space for the effusion.

ASSESSMENT   INTERPRETATION

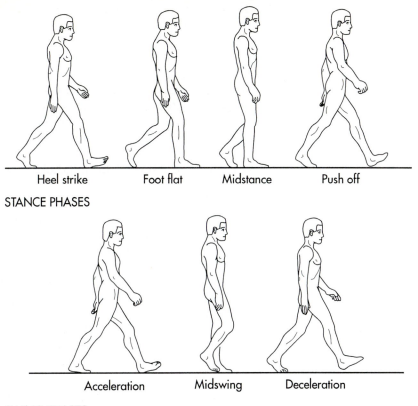

Heel strike   Foot flat   Midstance   Push off

STANCE PHASES

Acceleration   Midswing   Deceleration

SWING PHASES

Fig. 4-15 Gait.

Clothing Removal

Observe as the athlete removes his or her coat, sweater, or shirt.

During clothing removal, the wrist, elbow, and shoulder should work together in a coordinated effort—elbow discomfort will make this effort awkward and difficult. The athlete may compensate by removing the uninjured limb from the sleeve first and then carefully lifting the sleeve off the injured limb. The athlete's willingness to move the joint helps gauge the degree of disability and the best approach for the functional assessment. Problems with flexion and extension at the elbow are caused by injury to the humeroradial or humeroulnar joints. Problems with supination or pronation are caused by the superior or inferior radioulnar joints.

Standing Posture

Observe the cervical spine, ribs, clavicle, scapula, shoulder, elbow, wrist, and hand (the entire upper quadrant).

Compare bilaterally.

The athlete must be undressed

ASSESSMENT

INTERPRETATION

enough to fully expose the neck and entire upper extremity.

Anterior View
Cranial and Cervical Position
Cervical spine rotated or side bent

A cervical spine rotated or side bent may indicate compensation for cervical spine dysfunction, which can refer pain down into the upper extremity. For example, cervical problems can refer pain to the lateral epicondyle that may seem very much like lateral epicondylitis.

Facial expressions can often indicate the severity of the injury.

Shoulder Position

The glenohumeral joints, the clavicles, and the acromioclavicular and sternoclavicular joints should be level. Overdevelopment of one side of the body due to repetitive overhead movement patterns such as those during tennis serves and pitching will cause that shoulder area to drop. This drop shoulder can cause thoracic outlet syndromes that can also lead to neural or circulatory problems into the involved upper extremity.

Anterior Glenohumeral Joint

If the humerus sits anteriorly in the glenoid cavity because of tight medial rotators, previous dislocation or other shoulder pathology, the subacromial structures (subacromial bursa, biceps tendon, supraspinatus tendon) can be impinged. These impinged structures can refer pain or problems to the involved upper extremity.

Acromioclavicular and Sternoclavicular Joints

These joints should be level with one another and have normal symmetry. If the clavicle is elevated at the acromioclavicular joint or the sternoclavicular joint, the joint may be sprained or subluxed. Dysfunction in these joints can lead to dysfunction in the kinetic chain of the upper quadrant. For example, elevation of a clavicle will cause a reduction in its ability to rotate and elevate during glenohumeral abduction and flexion.

Thoracic Outlet

The brachial plexus, subclavian artery, and vein run through this outlet. If the outlet is reduced, neural and circulatory function into the limb may be affected.

Elbow Joint
Is the athlete supporting the elbow?
Is it flexed or extended?

If the elbow is supported in flexion, the injury is still acute or has suffered significant damage.

If the elbow is held in flexion, it is a sign of capsular or joint swelling because in this position the joint space is at a maximum to hold the swelling. The resting position for the elbow joint

ASSESSMENT

INTERPRETATION

with effusion is humeroulnar flexion at an angle of approximately 70° with the forearm supinated.

A biceps injury or contracture will limit extension and will be observable from this view. The biceps can develop a flexor contracture. This is commonly seen in professional baseball pitchers or in athletes with previous elbow dislocation where full range was not regained. In the acute condition the biceps can go into spasm to limit elbow extension after a hyperextension injury. Tightness in the biceps can also occur from prolonged immobilization of the elbow or from any injury that limits extension for a prolonged period of time (i.e., wearing a sling too long).

Normal Carrying Angle (Fig. 4-16)

When the elbow is extended with the palm facing forward, the angle formed is called the carrying angle. This carrying angle is necessary to allow the forearm to clear the body when carrying an object in the hand. The normal carrying angle for men is 5° to 10°; the normal carrying angle for women is 10° to 15° because of the necessity of the forearm to clear the wider female pelvis.

Cubitus Valgus (Fig. 4-16)

In cubitus valgus there is an increased carrying angle, one that is greater than 15°. This may have been caused from epiphyseal damage secondary to a lateral epicondylar fracture.

Cubitus Varus (Fig. 4-16)

Cubitus varus or "gunstock deformity" (a carrying angle less than 5° to 10°) is often caused by a supracondylar fracture in a child, where the distal end of the humerus experiences malunion or growth retardation because of damage to the epiphyseal plate.

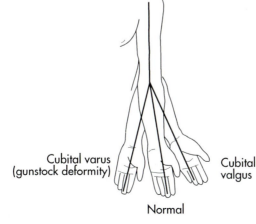

Fig. 4-16 Carrying angle.

Cubital varus (gunstock deformity)

Cubital valgus

Normal

ASSESSMENT

INTERPRETATION

Hyperextension

Hyperextension of the elbow can be caused by a shortened olecranon process or lax ligaments. Hyperextension occurs when the elbow can extend beyond 0° (up to 15° of hyperextension can exist).

Biceps Atrophy

Atrophy in the biceps is a sign of a C5 nerve root problem.

Forearm
Supinated or pronated
Muscle hypertrophy or atrophy

Any problem with the radioulnar joint will cause it to rest in the midposition or in a position of slight pronation.

The racquet sport player (or athlete who continually uses one arm more than the other) will have hypertrophy of the forearm muscles and often a dropped arm and shoulder on the dominant side.

Atrophy in the forearm can occur with C6, C7, or C8 nerve root problems.

Hand
Circulatory changes
Hand musculature atrophy

If severe injury to the elbow occurs, observe any circulatory or neural involvement (i.e., cyanosis or muscle atrophy). Redness, cyanosis, or blanching in the hand may be caused by circulatory or neural problems. Raynaud disease can also cause blanching.

Atrophy may be readily seen in the hand and can cause a decrease in the thenar or hypothenar eminence.

Posterior View
Shoulder Joint
Level

An athlete who overdevelops one shoulder or arm in a sport (e.g., fencing, baseball, javelin) may develop a drop shoulder on the well-developed side (Fig. 4-17). This can lead to thoracic outlet problems, which in turn can cause neural or circulatory problems into that arm (compressed brachial plexus, subclavian artery or vein).

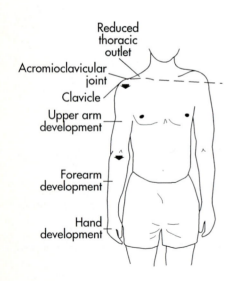

Reduced thoracic outlet
Acromioclavicular joint
Clavicle
Upper arm development
Forearm development
Hand development

Fig. 4-17 Drop shoulder.

ASSESSMENT

INTERPRETATION

Elbow Joint
   Extended or flexed

When the elbow is extended the epicondyles and the tip of the olecranon should be at the same level. If a line is drawn between the epicondyles, the olecranon should be on the center of the line. When the elbow is flexed to an angle of 90°, the tip of the olecranon lies directly distal to the line joining the epicondyles. If a line from the olecranon is drawn to each epicondyle, the three prominences and lines should form an isosceles triangle. If this triangle is abnormal, the following could exist:

- posterior elbow dislocation—the olecranon is shifted backward and upward while the elbow is fixed by muscle spasm (Fig. 4-18)
- fracture of the epicondyle—the epicondyle may be displaced and swollen
- intracondylar fracture—the epicondylar line is abnormally lengthened and the epicondyles can be squeezed together and moved independently
- fracture of the olecranon—the olecranon is enlarged

If the triangle is normal, but abnormal in relation to the shaft of the humerus, there could be a supracondylar fracture in which the three boney landmarks are displaced posteriorly (Fig. 4-19).

Lesion Site

Swelling

It is important to record whether swelling is intracapsular or extracapsular, intramuscular or intermuscular.

Swelling in the joint will limit elbow extension; it is held at an angle of 70° of flexion. The earliest sign of joint effusion is filling in of the capsule around the olecranon or epicondyles. In the flexed elbow the hollows may be totally filled in. If swelling progresses once the hollows are filled in, areas around the radiohumeral joint and above and below the annular ligament can become swollen.

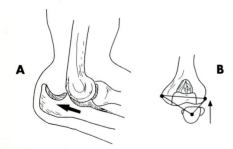

Fig. 4-18 A, Posterior elbow dislocation. **B,** Posterior view, boney alignment.

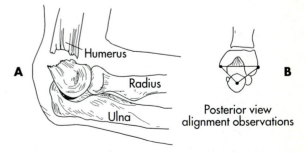

Fig. 4-19 A, Supracondylar fracture. **B,** Posterior view boney alignment.

ASSESSMENT   INTERPRETATION

Joint Deformity and Boney Contours

Gross swelling or joint deformity is present in a severe injury such as supracondylar fracture or elbow dislocation. If deformity is present and a severe boney injury is suspected, immobilize the joint and transport the patient immediately, making sure to monitor pulses and sensations.

Boney Exostosis

Hypertrophy of the lateral or medial epicondyle can develop from epicondylitis. This is particularly common for the medial epicondyle in the young thrower who overtrains or the throwing athlete who has avulsed the medial epicondyle.

Hypertrophy of the olecranon can be caused by a posterior impingement syndrome of the elbow, sometimes called boxer's elbow. This syndrome is caused by repeated elbow extension during punching in the boxer or repetitive throwing in pitchers. There is repetitive compression of the olecranon in the fossa, resulting in synovitis, articular cartilage damage, and eventual degenerative changes.

Muscle Atrophy/Hypertrophy

Muscle atrophy occurs from a significant muscle injury or damage to the nerve root or local nerve supply for that muscle.

Hypertrophy occurs when the athlete uses these muscles excessively and overdevelops the muscle fibers of that muscle group.

Skin Condition

Always observe the skin for abrasions or lacerations in the elbow area. Infections are a common secondary complication to elbow injuries.

Observe the skin for signs of inflammation or circulatory problems at the lesion site and distally.

SUMMARY OF TESTS

FUNCTIONAL TESTS
   Rule Out
      Cervical spine
      Shoulder joint
      Thoracic outlet
      Wrist joint
      Systemic conditions
   Humeroulnar and humeroradial joints
      Active elbow flexion
      Passive elbow flexion
      Resisted elbow flexion
      Active elbow extension
      Passive elbow extension
      Resisted elbow extension

ASSESSMENT   INTERPRETATION

Forearm—radioulnar joint
   Active radioulnar pronation
   Passive radioulnar pronation
   Resisted radioulnar pronation
   Active radioulnar supination
   Passive radioulnar supination
   Resisted radioulnar supination
Wrist Joint
   Active wrist flexion
   Passive wrist flexion
   Resisted wrist flexion
   Active wrist extension
   Passive wrist extension
   Resisted wrist extension

SPECIAL TESTS

Valgus stress
Varus stress
Tennis elbow test
Golfer's elbow test
Tinel sign—ulnar nerve
Elbow flexion test
Pinch test
Reflex testing
   Biceps reflex
   Brachioradialis reflex
   Triceps reflex
Sensation testing
Circulatory testing

ACCESSORY MOVEMENT TESTS

Humeroulnar joint
   Traction
   Medial (ulnar) glide
   Lateral (radial) glide
Humeroradial joint
   Traction
Radioulnar joint
   Proximal radioulnar joint dorsal and volar glide
   Distal radioulnar joint dorsal and volar glide

Rule Out

Cervical Spine

Active cervical side bending, forward bending, back bending, and rotation with overpressures (Fig. 4-20).

If any active movements or overpressure indicate limitation and/or pain, a full cervical assessment is necessary to clear the cervical spine. The reason for this is because there are cervical

ASSESSMENT   INTERPRETATION

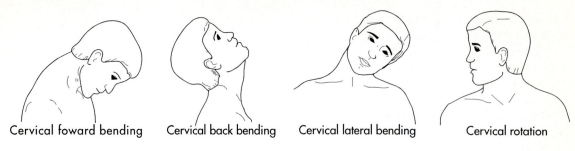

Cervical foward bending   Cervical back bending   Cervical lateral bending   Cervical rotation

Fig. 4-20 Active movements of the cervical spine.

Do *not* overpressure backbending if the range is full or painful.

conditions that refer pain to the elbow areas. For example:
- C5 nerve root injury can cause weakness or pain during resisted elbow flexion.
- C6 nerve root injury can cause weakness or pain during resisted radioulnar supination and resisted wrist extension.
- C7 nerve root injury can cause weakness or pain during resisted elbow extension and wrist flexion.
- A trigger point for C6 cervical dysfunction often refers pain to the lateral epicondyle.

Shoulder Joint

Active shoulder girdle forward flexion and abduction with overpressures (Fig. 4-21).

If either of the active movements or their overpressure indicate limitation and/or pain, a full shoulder assessment is necessary because:
- Severe subacromial bursa can refer pain to the elbow or even into the forearm or hand.
- Injury to the humerus can refer pain along the involved sclerotome and into the epicondyles or elbow joint.

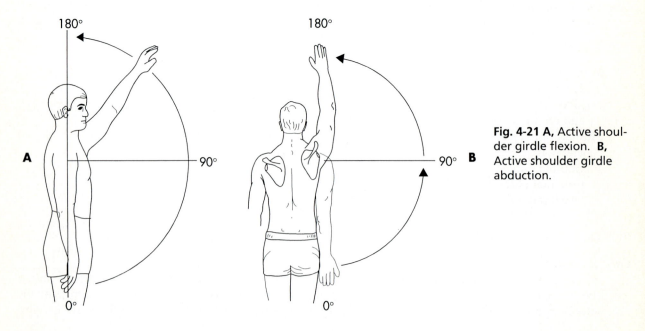

Fig. 4-21 A, Active shoulder girdle flexion. **B,** Active shoulder girdle abduction.

ASSESSMENT

INTERPRETATION

Thoracic Outlet

If there is neural or circulatory involvement, thoracic outlet syndrome tests should be done.

Adson Maneuver (Fig. 4-22 and 4-23)

Palpate the radial pulse on the affected side.

Instruct the athlete to take a deep breath and hold it, extend his or her neck, and turn the head toward the affected side.

Apply downward traction on the extended shoulder and arm while palpating the radial pulse.

The pulse may diminish or become absent.

In some athletes a greater effect on the subclavian artery is exerted by turning the head to the opposite side.

This test determines if a cervical rib or a reduced interscalene triangle is causing compression of the subclavian artery. The compression of the artery is determined by the decrease or absence of the radial pulse during the test.

Costoclavicular Syndrome Test

Instruct the athlete to stand in an exaggerated military stance with the shoulders thrust backward and downward.

Take the radial pulse before and while the shoulders are being held back.

This test causes compression of the subclavian artery and vein by reducing the space between the clavicle and the first rib. A modification or obliteration of the radial pulse indicates that a compression exists. Pain or tingling can also occur. If this test causes the symptoms that are the athlete's major complaint, a compression problem is at fault. A dampening of the pulse may occur even in healthy athletes who do not have these symptoms because they do not assume this position repeatedly or for long periods of time.

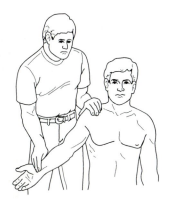

Fig. 4-22 Adson maneuver I.

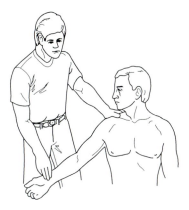

Fig. 4-23 Adson maneuver II.

ASSESSMENT

INTERPRETATION

Hyperabduction Test (Fig. 4-24)

The athlete is instructed to fully abduct the shoulder or to repeatedly abduct the shoulder.

Measure the athlete's radial pulse before and after the prolonged or repeated abduction.

Repeated or prolonged positions of hyperabduction can compress the structures in the outlet. This overhead position is often assumed in sleep, in certain occupations (painter, chimney sweep), and in the course of certain sports (volleyball spiker, tennis serve). The subclavian vessels can be compressed in two locations: (1) between the pectoralis minor tendon and the coracoid process or (2) between the clavicle and first rib. Pain or a diminished pulse can indicate that a compression exists.

Wrist Joint

Active wrist flexion and extension with overpressure.

If the active movements or overpressures indicate limitation and/or pain, a full wrist assessment is necessary. Pain or limitations of the wrist joint can cause elbow dysfunction. For example:

- an inferior radioulnar joint can refer pain into the superior radioulnar joint or the elbow joint
- wrist flexors and extensors originate on the medial and lateral epicondyles of the humerus and may cause local pain where the muscle and tendon meet.
- wrist carpal injury can affect the function of the ulna and radius and in turn cause dysfunction at the elbow joint

Systemic Conditions

Systemic conditions that can affect the elbow must be ruled out with a complete medical history, injury history, and observations of the athlete.

A systemic disorder can exist with any of the following responses or findings:

- bilateral elbow pain and/or swelling
- several joints inflamed or painful

- Rheumatoid arthritis rarely occurs first in the elbow joints but does show up there with time. Other signs include morning joint stiffness, pain and swelling, and the presence of subcutaneous nodules.
- Ankylosing spondylitis can have elbow involvement but this is usually seen in the more advanced cases.
- Psoriatic arthritis can affect the elbow early during its course and frequently develops in this joint. Other signs of this condition include ridging of the finger nails and psoriatic skin lesions.

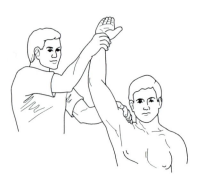

Fig. 4-24 Hyperabduction test.

ASSESSMENT

- athlete's general health is not good, especially during injury flare-ups
- repeated insidious onsets

The systemic disorders that can affect the elbow include:

- rheumatoid arthritis
- ankylosing spondylitis
- psoriatic arthritis
- osteoarthritis
- gout
- Reiter syndrome
- neoplasm tumor (rare)
- hemophilia
- local or systemic bacterial or viral infections

If a systemic problem is suspected, test the joints involved but refer the athlete to his or her family physician for a complete checkup that includes x-rays, urine and blood tests, and a test of the serum uric acid level.

INTERPRETATION

- Osteoarthritis from repeated elbow trauma can occur in athletes who engage in repetitive throwing. Other signs include local joint pain, tenderness, and crepitus.
- Gout is rare in the elbow except in severe cases.
- Reiter syndrome only involves the elbow when the condition is widespread.
- Tumors are rare but should be looked for by x-ray in chronic nonresponsive joints.
- Hemophilia is most common in the knee joint but the second most common location is the elbow.
- Local infections of the elbow joint can occur and the inflammation should be palpated for, especially if local abrasions are seen. Viral infections and systemic bacterial infections can also cause muscle and joint pain.

Humeroulnar and Humeroradial Joints—Elbow

Active Elbow Flexion (135° to 150°)

The athlete is sitting with arms at the side. The athlete is asked to bring his or her hand to the shoulder through the full range of elbow flexion.

Pain, weakness, or limitation of range of motion can be caused by an injury to the elbow flexors or their nerve supply.

The prime movers (Fig. 4-25) are:

- Biceps brachii—musculocutaneous N. (C5, C6)
- Brachialis—musculocutaneous N. (C5, C6)
- Brachioradialis—radial N. (C5, C6)

If the biceps and the brachialis muscles are weak, as in a mus-

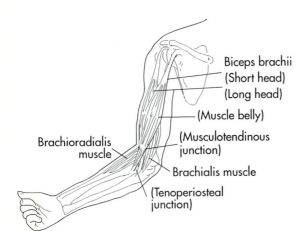

Biceps brachii
(Short head)
(Long head)

(Muscle belly)

(Musculotendinous junction)

Brachioradialis muscle

Brachialis muscle

(Tenoperiosteal junction)

Fig. 4-25 Elbow joint flexors. Biceps lesion sites (tendon, belly, musculotendinous junction, tenoperiosteal junction).

ASSESSMENT

INTERPRETATION

culocutaneous nerve lesion, the athlete will pronate the forearm before flexing the elbow.

The humeroulnar joint capsular pattern has more limitation in flexion than in extension (10° limited extension; 30° limited flexion) while pronation and supination will be full.

The close-packed position of the humeroradial joint is 80° of flexion with the forearm in midposition. This position is the resting position of the humeroulnar joint.

Passive Elbow Flexion (160°)

Lift the athlete's forearm to carry the elbow joint through full flexion until an end feel is reached. Assess the quality of the movement through the entire range (crepitus, grating, etc.).

The end feel should be soft-tissue approximation of the forearm and upper arm musculature.

Swelling in the humeroulnar joint will limit passive flexion. More range of flexion can occur passively if the forearm and upper arm muscular development is not excessive. In this case the end feel can be the radial head in the radial fossa and the coronoid process into the coronoid fossa.

Pain or limitation of range can be caused by:
- posterior capsule tightness or sprain
- triceps or anconeus injury

To test the triceps specifically, the elbow and shoulder can both be passively flexed to stretch the triceps at its outer range.

Resisted Elbow Flexion (Fig. 4-26)

The athlete flexes an elbow 90° with the forearm in the positions mentioned below. Resist flexion with one hand proximal to the wrist joint on the palmar side while the other hand stabilizes the shoulder joint.

The forearm can be supinated to test the biceps brachii, pronated to test the brachialis, and in midposition to test the brachioradialis muscles.

Weakness or pain can come from the elbow flexors or their nerve supply (see Active Elbow Flexion). Weakness or pain on flexion and supination is indicative of a lesion of the biceps brachii. There are four sites for this lesion and its associated pain (Fig. 4-25). These are as follows:
1. Long head of the biceps—point tenderness is in the bicipital groove.
2. Biceps belly—muscle fibers tear at the posterior aspect of the muscle belly and point tenderness can be elicited by pinching the deep aspect of the muscle belly.

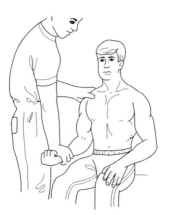

Fig. 4-26 Resisted elbow flexion.

ASSESSMENT

INTERPRETATION

3. Lower musculotendinous junction—point tenderness occurs where the muscle and tendon meet.
4. Tenoperiosteal junction—pain is local and distinct and it can radiate into the forearm as far as the wrist; there may also be pain on full passive pronation.

Weakness can occur from a cervical spine compression or impingement at the C5 or C6 nerve root. The C5 nerve root will also cause shoulder abduction weakness; C6 nerve root will also cause wrist extension weakness.

Weakness or pain with flexion and pronation comes from an injury to the brachialis muscle.

Weakness or pain with elbow flexion in the midposition suggests a brachioradialis injury.

Active Elbow Extension (0° to -5°)

The athlete starts with the gleno-humeral joint and the elbow flexed, then fully extends the elbow joint.

The elbow can hyperextend up to -10° in hypermobile athletes, especially in women (Fig. 4-27).

Pain, weakness, or limitation of range of motion can be caused by an injury to the elbow extensors or their nerve supply.

The prime movers are:
- Triceps brachii—radial N. (C6, C7,C8, T1)
- Anconeus—radial N. (C6, C7, C8, T1)

Passive Elbow Extension (0° to -5°)

Place one hand under the athlete's distal humerus while the other hand is on the dorsal aspect of the athlete's forearm.

Carry the forearm from a fully flexed elbow position to complete elbow extension, or until an end feel is reached.

The end feel should be bone on bone (olecranon process in olecranon fossa).

A soft end feel suggests joint swelling.

A springy end feel suggests a biceps flexor contracture, anterior capsule contracture, or a loose body of cartilage or bone in the joint.

During passive extension, note any joint crepitus. Crepitus can indicate articular surface degeneration.

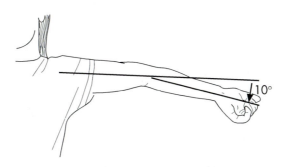

Fig. 4-27 Hyperextension of the elbow joint, anterior view.

ASSESSMENT

INTERPRETATION

If an end feel is not reached with full elbow extension, lift up gently on the humerus to hyperextend the joint until the end feel is reached.

Pain or limitation of range of motion can be caused by:
- medial ulnar collateral ligament sprain or tear
- lateral radial collateral ligament sprain or tear
- anterior capsule tightness or sprain
- biceps tendonitis or biceps strain
- brachialis strain

Full extension is the close-packed and most stable position for the humeroulnar joint and the loose-packed and least stable position for the humeroradial joint.

The brachialis muscle can be damaged by a supracondylar fracture or a posterior dislocation of the ulna on the humerus. If this occurs the brachialis muscle can develop scar tissue or myositis ossificans that can limit elbow extension permanently.

Resisted Elbow Extension (Fig. 4-28)

With the athlete's elbow flexed at an angle of 90° and the forearm supinated, place one hand on the dorsal aspect of the distal forearm and the other hand on the anterior surface of the upper humerus to stabilize the shoulder joint.

The athlete attempts to extend the elbow joint.

Pain or weakness can come from the elbow extensors or their nerve supply (see Active Elbow Extension).

The usual injury to the triceps is a contusion. Strains of the triceps are uncommon—if this muscle is affected, the usual site is at the musculotendinous junction.

Pain felt near the shoulder on resisted elbow extension can occur when the triceps contract and pull the head of the humerus into the glenoid cavity; this can result in impingement and compression of the subacromial structures (especially the subacromial bursa, the supraspinatus tendon, or the long head of the biceps tendon). Weakness can also be caused by radial palsy or a C7 nerve root problem.

Radial palsy is due to pressure in the axilla and can come from improper crutch usage or sleeping with the inner side of the arm draped over a couch or arm rest—"Saturday-night palsy." There will also be weakness with wrist extension and thumb abduction. This palsy is often painless.

A C7 nerve root irritation can come from a C6 cervical disc herniation—the triceps may be found weak alone or in conjunction with the wrist flexors. Cervical movements usually cause local neck and scapular pain. Often the pain is severe and the weakness is slight.

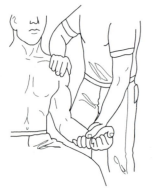

Fig. 4-28 Resisted elbow extension.

ASSESSMENT

INTERPRETATION

Radioulnar Joint—Forearm

Active Radioulnar Pronation (80° to 90°) (Fig. 4-29)

The athlete's forearm is in midposition and should rest on a plinth to prevent humeral movements. The athlete has the elbow flexed and then turns the palm down from midposition so that it faces the floor.

The measurement may be easier if the athlete holds a pencil clasped in the hand (perpendicular to the fingers) during this movement and you watch the pencil range.

Pain, weakness, or limitation of range of motion can come from the radioulnar pronators or their nerve supply.

The prime movers are:
- Pronator teres—median N. (C6, C7)
- Pronator quadratus—median N. (C7, C8, T1)

Pain may come from the radioulnar joint when there is a fractured radial head or a dislocation of the radius from the annular ligament. Limitation of range of motion can come from dysfunction of the proximal, middle, or distal radioulnar joints.

In a capsular pattern, both pronation and supination show pain and limitation at the extremes.

Passive Radioulnar Pronation (90°)

Grasp the athlete's distal forearm above the wrist joint with one hand and stabilize the elbow with the other hand.

Your hand pronates the forearm until the athlete's palm faces downward and an end feel is reached.

The end feel should be a tissue stretch.

Pain or limitation or range of motion can be caused by:
- dorsal radioulnar ligament sprain or tear
- ulnar collateral ligament sprain or tear
- dorsal radiocarpal ligament sprain or tear
- fracture or osteoarthritis of the radial head
- biceps strain at the tenoperiosteal junction
- quadrate ligament sprain or tear at the proximal radioulnar joint
- interosseous ligament sprain
- triangular ligament sprain or tear (of the distal radioulnar joint)

Resisted Radioulnar Pronation

Stabilize the elbow joint to prevent shoulder abduction and internal rotation.

The resisting hand is placed against the volar surface of the distal end of the radius. Use the entire hand and the thenar eminence.

Weakness or pain can come from the radioulnar pronators or their nerve supply (see Active Radioulnar Pronation). A common cause of pain is a pronator teres injury at the medial epicondyle. If this is the cause, pain will also exist on resisted wrist flexion; pronator quadratus is rarely injured.

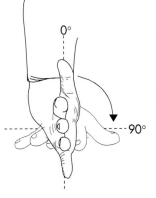

Fig. 4-29 Active radioulnar pronation.

ASSESSMENT

The fingers wrap around the ulna.

The athlete is asked to attempt forearm pronation from a midposition so that the palm turns downward.

Active Radioulnar Supination (90°) (Fig. 4-30)

The athlete's forearm should rest on a plinth to eliminate humeral movement.

The athlete has the elbow flexed and moves the forearm from midposition until the palm faces up.

Using a pencil to measure range may help (see pencil position in Active Radioulnar Pronation).

Passive Radioulnar Supination (90°)

As above, with stabilization at the elbow, supinate the distal forearm until the palm faces upward and an end feel is reached.

Resisted Radioulnar Supination

Stabilize the elbow at the athlete's side to prevent shoulder adduction and external rotation.

Your thenar eminence of the other hand is placed on the dorsal distal surface of the athlete's radius with the fingers wrapped on the ulna.

INTERPRETATION

Pain, weakness, or limitation of range of motion can come from the radioulnar supinators or their nerve supply.

The prime movers are the:
- Biceps brachii—musculocutaneous N. (C5, C6)
- Supinator—posterior interosseous nerve (C5, C6)

The limits of supination are determined by the degree to which the radius can rotate around the ulna. Therefore rotation can be limited by radial head pathology or injury to the distal or proximal radioulnar articulation.

The end feel should be tissue stretch.

Pain or limitation of range of motion may be caused by:
- volar radioulnar ligament (the triangular ligament) sprain or tear
- annular ligament sprain or tear
- medial collateral ligament (anterior fibers) sprain or tear
- lateral collateral ligament (anterior fibers) sprain or tear
- pronator muscle strain or tear
- capsule sprain of the distal radioulnar joint

Pain or weakness can come from the radioulnar supinators or their nerve supply (see Active Radioulnar Supination).

Pain on resisted radioulnar supination and elbow flexion is a sign of a biceps brachii injury.

If supination is painful but elbow flexion is not, the supinator is injured.

To help differentiate between a biceps and supinator injury

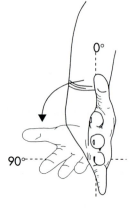

Fig. 4-30 Active radioulnar supination.

ASSESSMENT

The athlete's forearm is in midposition.

The athlete is asked to attempt to turn the forearm so that the palm faces upward while you resist the movement.

Wrist Joint

Active Wrist flexion (80° to 90°) (Fig. 4-31)

The athlete is sitting with hands over the edge of the plinth.

The forearm must be supported and stabilized.

The forearm is in pronation.

The athlete flexes his or her wrist as far as possible.

Passive Wrist Flexion (90°)

Stabilize the inferior radioulnar joint with one hand while the other hand grasps the metacarpals.

Move the wrist joint through the full range of wrist flexion until an end feel is reached.

INTERPRETATION

you can test supination with the elbow extended—this minimizes the biceps involvement.

Pain, weakness, or limitation of range of motion can come from the wrist flexors or their nerve supply.

The prime movers are:
- Flexor carpi radialis—median N. (C6, C7)
- Flexor carpi ulnaris—ulnar N. (C8, T1)

The capsular pattern for the wrist is about the same limitation of flexion as of extension. Capsular pattern limitation and pain can be caused by:
- acutely sprained joint
- carpal fracture
- rheumatoid arthritis
- osteoarthritis
- capsulitis

Range of motion can be limited by an injury to the wrist extensors or the dorsal radiocarpal ligament. If the ligament between the capitate and the third metacarpal ruptures, you can feel a depression at this point on full flexion. If the lunate-capitate ligament is sprained, pain is felt at the dorsum of the hand at the extreme of passive flexion.

Other ligament sprains are:
- radioulnate
- capitate—third metacarpal
- ulnar-triquetral

There is point tenderness over the involved ligament.

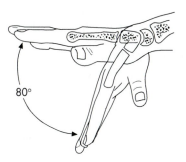

Fig. 4-31 Active wrist flexion.

ASSESSMENT

INTERPRETATION

Resisted Wrist Flexion

The athlete flexes the elbow to an angle of 90° with the forearm supinated and the wrist flexed slightly.

Stabilize the distal forearm with one hand while the other hand resists wrist flexion with pressure across the palm of the hand.

Weakness or pain can come from the wrist flexors or their nerve supply (see Active Wrist Flexion).

Pain during wrist flexion can be caused by:
- medial epicondylitis
- strain of the common wrist flexors or their tendons
- common wrist flexor periostitis
- wrist flexor tendonitis

Weakness with wrist flexion and elbow extension suggests a C7 root lesion— the triceps reflex can be sluggish. With this weakness the hand deviates radially on resisted wrist flexion.

Active Wrist Extension (70° to 90°)

The athlete is positioned as in active wrist flexion.

The athlete extends the wrist as far as possible.

Pain, weakness, or limitation of range of motion can come from the wrist extensors or their nerve supply.

The prime movers are:
- Extensor carpi radialis longus—radial N. (C6, C7)
- Extensor carpi radialis brevis—radial N. (C6, C7)
- Extensor carpi ulnaris—deep radial N. (C6, C7, C8)

An extensor muscle strain or tendonitis is the usual cause of pain.

Passive Wrist Extension (80° to 90°) (Fig. 4-32)

The athlete is positioned as in wrist flexion but you lift the metacarpals and move the wrist joint through the full range of wrist extension until an end feel is reached.

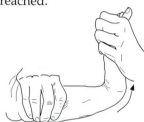

Fig. 4-32 Passive wrist extension.

Range of motion can be limited by a wrist flexor injury or a palmar radiocarpal ligament sprain or tear.

Limitation of both passive flexion and extension is a capsular pattern and can suggest:
- carpal fracture
- rheumatoid arthritis
- osteoarthritis
- chronic immobility
- synovitis

Limitation of extension only can be caused by:
- capitate subluxation
- Kienböck disease (aseptic necrosis of lunate)
- ununited fracture (especially scaphoid)

Resisted Wrist Extension

The athlete flexes the elbow to an angle of 90° with the forearm pronated and wrist in midposition.

Resist wrist extension with pressure on the dorsal aspect of the hand while the other hand stabilizes the distal forearm.

To rule out the finger extensors they may be flexed during the test.

Weakness or pain suggests an injury to the wrist extensors or their nerve supply (see Active Wrist Extension). Pain here can indicate:
- lateral epicondylitis
- a lesion of the common extensors
- strain of the common extensors or the tendon
- extensor digitorum brevis (most commonly injured)

Pain with wrist extension usually comes from the wrist joint itself, seldom from the fingers. Flexing the fingers rules out the finger extensors.

ASSESSMENT

INTERPRETATION

Painless weakness could be due to:
- radial nerve palsy
- C6 cervical nerve root irritation (with elbow flexor weakness)
- C8 nerve root irritation (the extensors and flexor carpi ulnaris become weak and when resisted wrist extension is tested, the hand deviates radially)

SPECIAL TESTS

Valgus Stress

The athlete's elbow is supinated and in slight flexion (20° to 30°) to unlock the olecranon from the fossa.

Method 1
Put a valgus stress on the elbow by stabilizing above the condyles with one hand (which acts as a fulcrum) while the other hand applies an abduction force on the distal ulna.

This is repeated with the athlete's elbow flexed to approximately 50° (Fig. 4-33).

You should determine elbow joint hypermobility, normal, or hypomobility during the test and whether the test elicits any pain. The most common form of instability at the elbow is medial joint laxity, often caused by repeated valgus stress during the pitching motion. This test determines the stability of the medial collateral ligament. The anterior oblique portion of this ligament is the major contributor to its stability. This test can detect 1st or 2nd degree sprains, or 3rd degree (tears) of the medial collateral ligament.

Method 2
Cradle the athlete's arm on your hip and, with both hands around the joint, your outside hand applies a valgus stress while the inside hand palpates the medial collateral ligament.

Repeat in flexion to approximately 50°.

With Method 2, the medial collateral ligament can be palpated for joint opening while the test is being done. The flexor muscles of the forearm restrict valgus opening and pain may be elicited if they are strained or partially torn.

The humeroradial joint compresses with valgus stress, causing it to become inflamed and painful. Any humeroradial joint dysfunction may cause pain during this test.

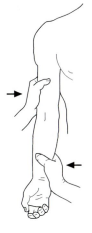

Fig. 4-33 Special test, elbow valgus stress.

ASSESSMENT

INTERPRETATION

Varus Stress

Method 1

The athlete's arm is extended and supinated. Apply an adduction force to the elbow joint with one hand on the medial humerus and the other hand on the lateral forearm just above the wrist.

According to Morrey and Kai-Nan, varus stress is resisted mainly by the anterior capsule and boney articulation, with the lateral (radial) collateral contributing only to a minor degree. Therefore if there is joint opening during this varus test the anterior capsule may be damaged and or there may be boney fracture.

Method 2

Support the athlete's arm on your hip while your hands grasp around the elbow joint. The inner hand applies a varus force while the outer hand palpates the lateral collateral ligament.

Tennis Elbow Test (Fig. 4-34) (Lateral Epicondylitis or Extensor Tendonitis)

Method 1

The athlete's elbow is extended, the forearm is pronated, and the hand is closed in a fist.

Stabilize the elbow in extension and resist wrist extension. A positive sign is an acute and sudden pain in the lateral epicondyle area.

Pain during this test can be from the following:
- lateral epicondylitis or periostitis
- a common extensor tendon strain
- extensor carpi radialis brevis tendonitis or strain (usually at the tenoperiosteal junction)
- extensor muscle belly lesion (occasionally)
- extensor carpi radialis longus tendonitis or strain
- radial tunnel compression of the posterior interosseous nerve—compression occurs between the heads of the supinator or at the canal of Frohse (fibrous arch in the supinator). The posterior interosseous nerve can also be compressed by a ganglion or fibrous band anterior to the radial head, a leash of vessels from the radial recurrent artery, or a tendinous band of extensor carpi radialis brevis.

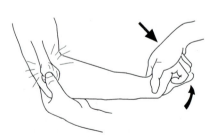

Fig. 4-34 Tennis elbow test.

ASSESSMENT

INTERPRETATION

Method 2

The athlete's elbow is extended, the forearm is pronated, and the hand is closed in a fist.

Passively flex and ulnar deviate the wrist while maintaining elbow extension.

A positive sign is lateral epicondyle pain.

As above but the extensors are stretched over the radial head and wrist, producing pain.

Golfer's Elbow Test (Medial Epicondylitis or Flexor Tendonitis)

Method 1

The athlete extends the elbow with the forearm in a supinated position. Passively extend the wrist with an overpressure while keeping the elbow extended.

Pain or weakness can be elicited if there is:
- strain of the common wrist flexor origin
- medial epicondyle periostitis
- wrist flexor tenoperiosteal strain

There is usually a full range of elbow movements.

Method 2

The athlete's elbow is extended, the forearm is pronated, and the wrist is in midposition. Resist wrist flexion while maintaining elbow extension.

Tinel Sign for the Ulnar Nerve (Fig. 4-35)

Tap the ulnar nerve in its groove between the olecranon and the medial epicondyle.

A positive sign is indicated by a tingling sensation in the ulnar nerve distribution in the forearm and hand (medial forearm, IV and V finger).

This test is designed to elicit pain caused by a neuroma within the ulnar nerve, perineural adhesions, or to detect if ulnar neuritis exists.

The nerve can be damaged or develop neuritis from the following:
- recurrent ulnar nerve subluxations or dislocation (especially with cubital valgus structural abnormality)

Repeated pitching can lead to an increased cubital valgus deformity and the resulting ulnar nerve irritation, subluxation, or dislocation problems.
- cubital tunnel compression of the ulnar nerve between the two heads of the flexor carpi ulnaris muscle
- tension through an elbow valgus deformity
- direct trauma with inflammation of the neural sheath
- repeated mild injuries or microtrauma
- friction neuritis from repeated flexion and extension motions with valgus stress
- postural habits that place the elbow in flexion for prolonged periods of time and compress the nerve (e.g., sleeping with elbows flexed and hands under head)

With neural involvement, it is important to rule out other causes:

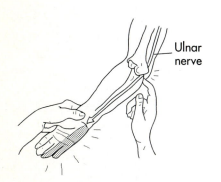

Ulnar nerve

Fig. 4-35 Tinel sign for the ulnar nerve.

ASSESSMENT

INTERPRETATION

- C7 disc protrusion with radiculopathy
- thoracic outlet syndrome
- contracture or ganglion in connection with the flexor carpi ulnaris tendon
- repeated sport or occupational neural compression
- cervical rib
- superior sulcus tumor
- compression at the Guyon canal

Elbow Flexion Test

The athlete is asked to fully flex the elbow and hold it for 5 minutes.

Tingling, paresthesia, or numbness in the ulnar nerve distribution of the forearm and hand indicate a positive test.

This test is used to determine if a cubital tunnel syndrome is present and whether it is compressing the ulnar nerve. The nerve can be trapped in the cubital tunnel between the heads of the flexor carpi ulnaris or by scar tissue in the ulnar groove.

Perineural adhesions, osteophytes, or exostosis from previous soft tissue or boney damage can also elicit ulnar nerve symptoms with this test.

Pinch Test

The athlete is asked to pinch the *tips* of the index finger and thumb together—there should be tip to tip prehension.

You can demonstrate the movement.

Pinching of the pulps of the thumb and index finger instead of the tips is a positive sign.

A positive sign is caused by an injury to the anterior interosseous nerve, a branch of the median nerve, and is called anterior interosseous nerve syndrome. Sensory and motor function both can be affected.

The anterior interosseous nerve may be trapped between the heads of the pronator teres causing functional impairment of:
- the flexor pollicis longus muscle
- the lateral half of the flexor digitorum profundus muscle
- the pronator quadratus muscle

There can be paralysis of the pollicis and indicis flexor muscles. Deep pronator teres tendonitis from excessive lifting can also entrap the anterior interosseous nerve. The median nerve can be compressed by the pronator teres muscle above the anterior interosseous nerve, causing impairment of the above plus:
- flexor carpi radialis
- flexor digitorum
- palmaris longus

Median nerve sensory deficit may also be affected.

The anterior interosseous nerve can be entrapped by other flexor muscles that include:
- flexor pollicis longus accessory head (Ganser muscle)
- flexor digitorum superficialis accessory head

Reflex Testing

Each reflex test should be repeated 10 times to check reflex fatigability.

ASSESSMENT

INTERPRETATION

Biceps Reflex (C5) (Fig. 4-36)

Place one of the athlete's arms over your forearm.

Your thumb is placed over the biceps tendon in the cubital fossa.

Tap the thumb with the tip of the hammer.

There should be a biceps contraction.

Although the biceps is innervated by the musculocutaneous nerve at the neurological levels C5 and C6, its reflex action is largely from C5.

- If there is a light response, the C5 neurological level is normal.
- If, after several attempts, there is no response, there may be a lesion anywhere from the root of C5 to the innervation of the biceps muscle.
- An excessive response may be the result of an upper motor lesion (cardiovascular attack or stroke); a decreased response can be indicative of a lower motor neuron lesion.

Brachioradialis Reflex (C6) (Fig. 4-37, A)

The athlete's arm is supported as above.

Tap the brachioradialis tendon at the distal end of the radius with the broad side of the hammer.

The muscle should contract.

Although the brachioradialis muscle is innervated by the radial nerve via the C5 and C6 neurological levels, its reflex is largely a C6 function.

The interpretation is the same as the biceps reflex above but the C6 neurological level is implicated.

Triceps Reflex (C7) (Fig. 4-37, B)

Athlete's arm is as above.

With the reflex hammer, tap the triceps tendon where it crosses the olecranon fossa.

The muscle should contract.

This reflex is mainly a function of the C7 neurological level.

The interpretation is the same as the biceps reflex above but the C7 neurological level is implicated.

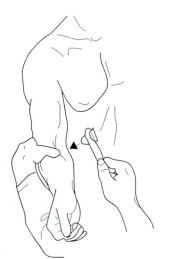

Fig. 4-36 Biceps tendon reflex (C5).

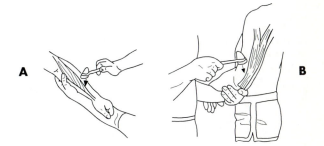

Fig. 4-37 A, Brachioradialis tendon reflex (C6). **B,** Triceps tendon reflex (C7).

ASSESSMENT

INTERPRETATION

Sensation Testing (Dermatomes and Cutaneous Nerves)

Using a pin, prick the athlete's arm in the dermatomes shown in the illustration (see Fig. 4-13). The athlete's eyes are closed or they look away.

The athlete reports on whether the sensation is sharp or dull. The test is done bilaterally so that comparison of sensation can be made.

Each dermatome should be pricked in about 10 different spots.

The C6 nerve root distribution of the lateral forearm and thumb and the sensory branches of the musculocutaneous nerve should be tested.

The C7 nerve root distribution of the posterior forearm and the hand on the dorsal or palmar aspect of the middle finger should be tested.

The C8 nerve root distribution of the medial forearm and fifth finger and the antebrachial cutaneous nerve should be tested.

The C5 nerve root distribution of the lateral arm and the sensory branches of the axillary nerve should be tested.

The T1 nerve root distribution of the medial arm and the brachial cutaneous nerve should be tested.

The cutaneous nerve supply should be tested by using the same technique, with the pin pricking in 10 locations (Fig. 4-38).

The object is to test C5, C6, C7, C8, and T1 for nerve root irritation or impingement.

Lack of sensation of the lateral arm can be traced to the:
- sensory branches of the axillary nerve
- C5 nerve root
- upper lateral cutaneous of the arm (C5, C6)
- posterior cutaneous of the arm (C5, C6, C7, C8)

Lack of sensation of the lateral forearm can be traced to the:
- sensory branches of the musculocutaneous nerve
- C6 nerve root
- lateral cutaneous of the forearm (C5, C6)

Lack of sensation of the medial forearm can be traced to the:
- antebrachial cutaneous nerve
- C8 nerve root
- medial cutaneous of the forearm (C8, T1)

Lack of sensation of the medial arm can be traced to the:
- brachial cutaneous nerve
- T1 nerve root
- medial cutaneous of the arm (C8, T1)
- medial cutaneous of the forearm (C8, T1)

Lack of sensation of the posterior upper arm can be traced to the:
- C5 or T1 nerve root
- medial cutaneous of the arm (C8, T1)
- posterior cutaneous of the arm (C5, C6, C7, C8)

Lack of sensation at the posterior forearm can be traced to:
- a C6, C7, C8, or T1 nerve root
- medial, lateral, or posterior cutaneous nerves of the forearm

Circulatory Testing

Palpate the brachial, radial, and ulnar pulses especially following fractures and compression injuries.

The brachial artery pulse can be palpated medial to the biceps brachii tendon.

The radial artery pulse can be palpated at the wrist on the distal radial creases just lateral to the flexor digitorum tendon.

The ulnar artery pulse is palpable proximal to the pisiform bone on the palmar aspect of the ulna.

Elbow joint injuries can lead to neurovascular problems because of direct damage (e.g., supracondylar fracture, elbow dislocation) or secondary complications (e.g., bleeding, swelling, tight cast); therefore the pulses need to be assessed. Diminished or absent pulses are a medical emergency and the athlete must be transported to a medical facility immediately. Volkmann's ischemic contracture can result from prolonged neurovascular occlusion to the forearm and hand. The flexor muscles develop shortening and contractures and there is ulnar and median nerve paralysis.

ASSESSMENT

INTERPRETATION

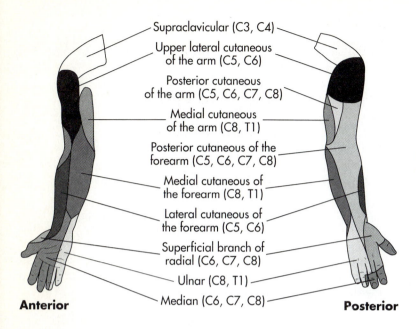

Supraclavicular (C3, C4)

Upper lateral cutaneous of the arm (C5, C6)

Posterior cutaneous of the arm (C5, C6, C7, C8)

Medial cutaneous of the arm (C8, T1)

Posterior cutaneous of the forearm (C5, C6, C7, C8)

Medial cutaneous of the forearm (C8, T1)

Lateral cutaneous of the forearm (C5, C6)

Superficial branch of radial (C6, C7, C8)

Ulnar (C8, T1)

Median (C6, C7, C8)

Anterior

Posterior

Fig. 4-38 Cutaneous nerve supply of the upper limb.

ACCESSORY MOVEMENT TESTS

Humeroulnar Joint
Traction (Fig. 4-39)

The athlete is lying supine with the elbow joint flexed to 70° and the forearm in supination.

Stabilize the athlete with one hand on the posterior aspect of the humerus while the other hand is in an overgrasp position, holding the ulna as proximally as possible.

Apply distal traction force to separate the joint surfaces.

Medial (Ulnar) Glide
Method 1 (Fig. 4-40)

The athlete is lying supine with the elbow flexed 70° and with the forearm supinated.

Stand beside the athlete, between the athlete's arm and trunk.

One hand stabilizes the distal humerus on the posterior medial aspect while the other hand holds the forearm on the radial side.

Gently push the forearm in a medial direction until an end feel is reached.

Any hypermobility can indicate joint dysfunction, with ligament or capsular laxity.

ASSESSMENT   INTERPRETATION

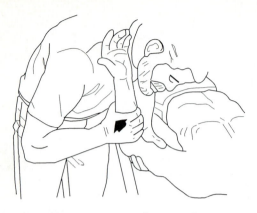

Fig. 4-39 Humeroulnar traction.

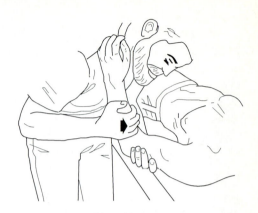

Fig. 4-40 Humeroulnar medial glide.

Method 2 (Fig. 4-41)

The athlete is lying supine with the elbow extended and forearm supinated. Apply a valgus stress to the elbow with one hand on the distal forearm and the other hand stabilizing the distal humerus.

Lateral (Radial) Glide
Method 1 (Fig. 4-42)

The athlete is lying supine with the elbow flexed at an angle of 70° and with the forearm supinated.

Stand beside the athlete, between the athlete's arm and body.

Stabilize the athlete's humerus distally and laterally with one hand while the other hand, on the athlete's medial proximal forearm, pushes the forearm laterally until an end feel is reached.

Method 2 (Fig. 4-43)

The athlete is lying supine with the elbow extended and forearm supinated.

Apply a varus stress with one hand stabilizing the distal humerus medially; the other hand is on the distal forearm, pushing the forearm medially.

Humeroradial Joint

Traction (Fig. 4-44)

The athlete is lying supine with the elbow flexed slightly and the forearm in midposition.

If the joint opens medially and is accompanied by pain, this is a sign of a medial collateral ligament tear. A small amount of medial glide is needed for full elbow flexion.

The joint opening laterally with pain is a sign of a lateral collateral ligament tear. A slight amount of lateral glide is necessary for full elbow extension.

Hypermobility can occur if the annular ligament is lax or if there has been a previous radial head dislocation.

Full movement is necessary for full elbow extension.

ASSESSMENT   INTERPRETATION

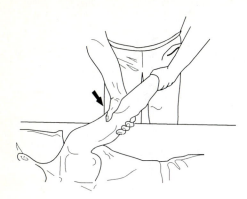

Fig. 4-41 Humeroulnar medial glide.

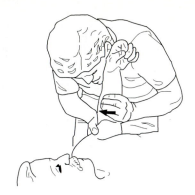

Fig. 4-42 Humeroulnar lateral glide.

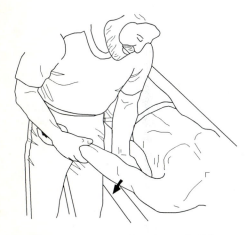

Fig. 4-43 Humeroulnar lateral glide.

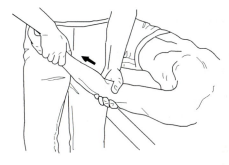

Fig. 4-44 Humeroradial traction.

Stabilize the distal humerus with one hand and hold the distal radius with the other hand (using mainly the thumb and index finger). The radius is pulled distally until an end feel is reached.

Radioulnar Joint

Proximal (Superior) Radioulnar Joint Dorsal and Volar (Palmar) Glide (Fig. 4-45)

The athlete is sitting with the elbow resting on a treatment table. The athlete's elbow is flexed to 70° and the forearm is supinated to 35°.

Stabilize the proximal ulna with one hand wrapped around the posteromedial aspect.

The other hand is around the head of

Dorsal glide is necessary for full pronation; the ventral glide is necessary for full supination.

ASSESSMENT

INTERPRETATION

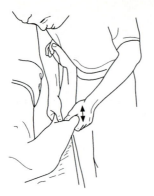

Fig. 4-45 Proximal radioulnar joint—
Dorsal and volar glide.

the radius with the fingers on the volar
aspect and the palm on the dorsal
aspect.

Gently move the radial head volarly
and dorsally with hand and finger pressure.

Distal (Inferior) Radioulnar Joint Dorsal and Volar (Palmar) Glide (see Fig. 5-53)

The athlete rests the forearm on the
plinth in a slightly supinated position.

Stabilize the distal radius with
thumb on the dorsal surface and fingers
on the palmar aspect of the radius.
Gently move the ulna dorsally and
volarly.

These dorsal and volar glides of the ulna are necessary for
full pronation and supination to occur. The dorsal glide is necessary for full supination; the volar glide is necessary for full
pronation.

PALPATION

Palpate areas for point tenderness,
temperature differences, swelling,
adhesions, crepitus, calcium deposits,
muscle spasms, and muscle tears.
Palpate for muscle tenderness, lesions,
and trigger points.

According to Janet Travell, myofascial trigger points in muscle are activated directly by overuse, overload, trauma, or chilling and are activated indirectly by visceral disease, other trigger
points, arthritic joints, or emotional distress. Myofascial pain is
referred from trigger points, which have patterns and locations
for each muscle. A trigger point is a hyperactive spot, usually in
a skeletal muscle or the muscle's fascia, that is acutely tender on
palpation and evokes a muscle twitch. These points can also
evoke autonomic responses (e.g., sweating, pilomotor activity,
local vasoconstriction).

Medial Aspect

Boney (Fig. 4-46)
Medial Epicondyle

This is frequently fractured in children, usually with a hyperextension
mechanism and especially if it causes a
posterior elbow dislocation.

Medial epicondylitis or periostitis occurs at the common flex-
or origin from overuse of these flexors in sport (e.g., mishitting a
golf ball, tennis serve, baseball pitching, javelin throwing).

Medial epicondyle fractures can occur in the young pitcher.

ASSESSMENT   INTERPRETATION

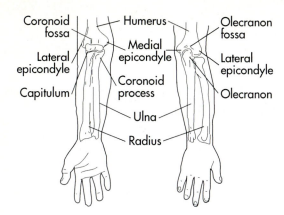

Fig. 4-46 Boney anatomy of the elbow and forearm.

This is an avulsion fracture of the epicondyle by the common flexor origin or the medial collateral ligament.

Medial Supracondylar Line of the Humerus

This is the point of origin of the pronator teres. It can be tender because of overuse (tendonitis) or from a strain of this muscle.

Soft Tissue
Ulnar Nerve

Place the athlete's elbow in a flexed position and palpate in the ulnar groove for tenderness.

Attempt to displace the ulnar nerve from the groove (gently). Tap it for the Tinel sign.

Ulnar nerve neuritis, contusion, or inflammation can cause a tingling on the medial side of the arm and into the medial aspect of the hand when the nerve is tapped. This is the Tinel sign (see Special Tests for more detail).

The ulnar nerve can be damaged by:
- direct trauma
- fractures (supracondylar or medial epicondyle)
- adhesions
- excessive cubital valgus
- repeated cubital valgus (pitcher)
- prolonged elbow flexion with ulnar nerve traction occurring between the two heads of flexor carpi ulnaris
- ulnar nerve subluxation or dislocation caused by a shallow groove or chronic overuse problems (pitcher)

Medial (Ulnar) Collateral Ligament (Fig. 4-47)

This ligament has three bands: anterior, posterior, and oblique. The anterior band is attached to the medial epicondyle of the humerus and to a tubercle on the medial margin of the coronoid process. The posterior triangle band is attached to the lower back part of the medial epicondyle and to the medial margin of the olecranon. The poorly developed oblique band runs between the olecranon fossa and the coronoid process.

The anterior segment of the ligament is a round cord that is taut in extension. The posterior segment is a weak fan-shaped

ASSESSMENT   INTERPRETATION

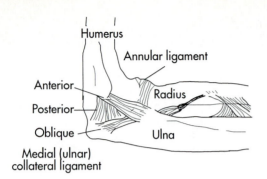

Fig. 4-47 Medial ligaments of the elbow.

structure that is taut in flexion. If it is sprained with a valgus stress, it will be point tender (especially the anterior band).

Wrist Flexors

Muscle strains can cause point tenderness usually at their origin but can occur anywhere along their length.

PRONATOR TERES

Pronator teres syndrome is an impingement of the median nerve resulting in sensory and motor loss (flexor carpi radialis, palmaris longus, and the flexor digitorum muscles can be affected). The deep head of pronator teres impinges the nerve. Impingement of the median nerve can also develop from pronator teres tendonitis and in this case the muscle may also be point tender.

The myofascial trigger points of pronator teres refer pain deeply into the forearm and wrist on the radial palmar surface.

FLEXOR CARPI RADIALIS

The myofascial trigger points are midbelly and pain can be referred to the radial aspect of the wrist crease and can extend into the hand.

PALMARIS LONGUS

The myofascial trigger point is midbelly and a prickling pain can be referred mainly into the palm of the hand, with some referred into the distal forearm.

FLEXOR CARPI ULNARIS

Pain and tenderness from the myofascial trigger point can be referred to the ulnar palmar surface of the wrist with a trigger point location midbelly.

ASSESSMENT   INTERPRETATION

FLEXOR DIGITORUM (SUPERFICIALIS AND PROFUNDUS)

The trigger point is midbelly and pain can be referred down the muscle fibers that they activate.

Posterior Aspect

Boney
Medial and Lateral Epicondyles

See the observations and the posterior view regarding the alignment of the epicondyles and the olecranon. The epicondyle surfaces can be palpated if injury is suspected. Avulsion fractures can occur at the epicondyles.

Olecranon Process

This can be palpated if a fracture or contusion occurs in that area—the olecranon process is covered by the triceps aponeurosis and bursa.

Soft Tissue (Fig. 4-48)
Olecranon Bursa

This covers the olecranon; it will feel boggy and thick if bursitis exists.

Synovial thickening or rice bodies may be palpated in the bursa from previous trauma or a chronic bursal problem.

It is important to determine if the inflamed bursa is due to infection or trauma. If the inflammation is due to infection, the athlete must be referred to a physician for antibiotic medication.

Triceps

If a muscle strain or contusion is involved in the triceps it can often be palpated as a lump or nodule at the musculotendinous junction.

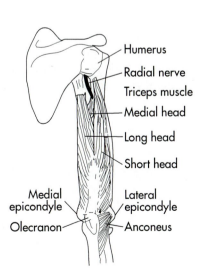

Humerus
Radial nerve
Triceps muscle
Medial head
Long head
Short head
Medial epicondyle
Lateral epicondyle
Olecranon
Anconeus

Fig. 4-48 Posterior structures of the elbow joint—muscles and boney landmarks.

ASSESSMENT

INTERPRETATION

The triceps muscle can be avulsed or ruptured but this is rare. There will be a marked defect in the muscle during palpation and considerable swelling. This should be surgically repaired as soon as possible.

A hard lump (myositis ossificans) can develop in the triceps from repeated trauma.

There are five trigger points in the triceps muscle with referred pain (Fig. 3-60).

Myofascial trigger points from the long head refer pain into the posterior arm and shoulder and sometimes to the base of the neck, according to Travell and Simons. The medial head can have pain extended to the lateral epicondyle and along the radial aspect of the forearm from the muscle's lateral border trigger point and into the medial epicondyle from the medial head's medial border trigger point. The lateral head myofascial trigger points can refer pain on the posterior aspect of the arm into the dorsum of the forearm and occasionally into the fourth and fifth fingers. (Refer to Travell J and Simons D: *Myofascial Pain and Dysfunction* for further details and illustrations.)

Triceps tendonitis can occur in weight lifters, throwers, boxers, and other sports that have repeated elbow extension activities.

Anconeus

The anconeus is rarely injured unless there is an extreme hyperextension force. Its trigger point is in the muscle belly and pain is referred to the lateral epicondyle.

Lateral Aspect (Fig. 4-49)

Boney
Lateral Epicondyle

Palpate this to diagnose lateral epicondylitis or periostitis; chronic strain of the extensor carpi radialis brevis is commonly the cause of pain at the muscle's origin into the lateral epicondyle. This occurs commonly in sports such as tennis, rowing, squash, and racquet ball. The other extensors on occasion may be involved. The lateral epicondyle can be avulsed in the young athlete.

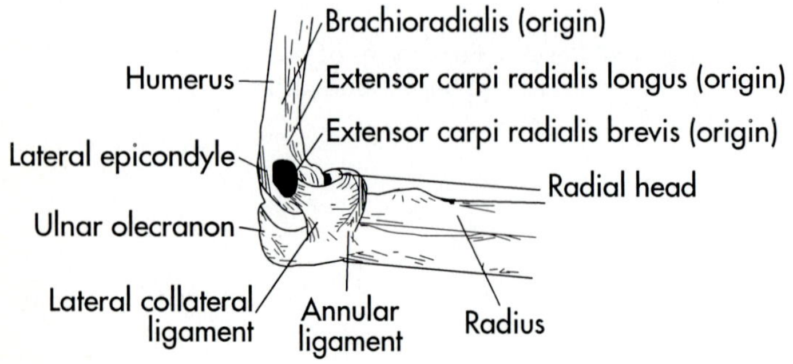

Brachioradialis (origin)
Humerus
Extensor carpi radialis longus (origin)
Extensor carpi radialis brevis (origin)
Lateral epicondyle
Radial head
Ulnar olecranon
Lateral collateral ligament
Annular ligament
Radius

Fig. 4-49 Lateral structures of the elbow joint—ligaments, boney landmarks and muscle origins.

ASSESSMENT

INTERPRETATION

Lateral Supracondylar Ridge

This is the site of the origin of extensor carpi radialis longus and brachioradialis. It may be tender from overuse or from a strain of either of these muscles.

Radial Head

Pain in and around the radial head may indicate synovitis, osteoarthritis, or a fracture. The radial head can be dislocated traumatically or because of a congenital susceptibility.

Soft Tissue (Fig. 4-50)
Brachioradialis

Palpate the muscle for strains or tears.

Wrist Extensors

Palpate form origin to insertion for strains or tears.

EXTENSOR CARPI RADIALIS LONGUS

Overuse tendonitis makes this tendon point tender just distal to its origin.

Trigger points from this muscle can refer pain and tenderness to the lateral epicondyle and dorsum of the hand (anatomical snuff box area).

EXTENSOR CARPI RADIALIS BREVIS

This is the most common site for tendonitis or tenoperiosteal problems caused by overuse of the wrist extensors (also called tennis elbow). Trigger points in the muscle can refer pain to the back of the hand and wrist.

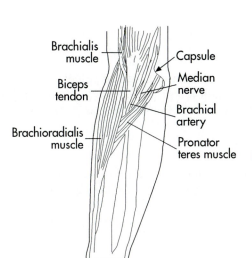

Brachialis muscle
Biceps tendon
Brachioradialis muscle
Capsule
Median nerve
Brachial artery
Pronator teres muscle

Fig. 4-50 Contents of cubital fossa.

ASSESSMENT

INTERPRETATION

EXTENSOR CARPI ULNARIS

This muscle is injured less often but can be strained—its trigger points refer pain to the ulnar side of the wrist.

Supinator

This muscle originates on the lateral epicondyle and the upper dorsal aspect of the ulna. It should be palpated for a strain or tear.

Anconeus

This muscle originates on the lateral epicondyle and refers pain to the epicondyle if the muscle is involved. It should be palpated for strains or tears.

Lateral (Radial) Collateral Ligament

This is attached to the lower part of the lateral epicondyle of the humerus and to the annular ligament and upper end of the supinator crest of the ulna.

It blends in with the supinator and extensor carpi radialis brevis origin and should be palpated for tenderness due to a sprain.

Annular Ligament

This can be damaged in the "pulled elbow" condition in children.

Radioulnar Bursa

This will be point tender if it is inflamed.

Anterior Aspect

Boney
Coronoid Process

Palpate deeply in the cubital fossa to locate this process.

Head of the Radius

The head of the radius can be palpated for fracture or dislocation—supination and pronation of the radioulnar joint during palpation may help to locate it.

Soft Tissue (see Fig. 4-50)
Biceps Brachii

Palpate the tendon and periosteal junction for a strain of this muscle. Its trigger points are usually found in the distal part of the muscle with referred pain in the anterior deltoid and cubital fossa. Biceps ruptures are rare but can occur.

Brachialis

Following severe trauma to the muscle (i.e., humeral fracture, elbow dislocation) the brachialis muscle can develop myositis

ASSESSMENT

INTERPRETATION

ossificans. Deep, gentle palpatory skills should be used to locate this muscle. Its trigger points are distal and lateral in the muscle near the cubital fossa and pain is referred to the dorsum of the thumb (carpometacarpal joint) and to the first dorsal interspace.

Cubital Fossa (see Fig. 4-50)

The cubital fossa is the triangular space below the elbow crease. It is bounded laterally by the extensor muscles (brachioradialis) and medially by the flexor muscles (pronator teres).
It contains:
- the biceps tendon
- the brachial artery
- the median nerve

Wrist Flexors
Pronator teres
Flexor carpi ulnaris
Flexor digitorum
Flexor carpi radialis
Flexor pollicis longus
Palmaris longus

See section on Palpation, Medial Aspect.

Biceps Tendon

Palpate the tendon and tenoperiosteal junction for a strain.

Brachial Artery (Ulnar and Radial Artery)

Palpate if a circulatory problem is suspected from trauma or post-dislocation. The brachial artery bifurcates to become the radial and ulnar artery just below the joint line.
Damage to this artery can cause a severe compartment syndrome called Volkmann's ischemic contracture.

Median Nerve

This nerve cannot be palpated but pressure on it can cause sensation changes in its cutaneous distribution.

Anterior Joint Capsule

This is quite deep but may be palpated for tenderness if there has been a hyperextension injury with damage to the anterior capsule. A capsule is not palpable unless it is inflamed.

Musculocutaneous Nerve

This nerve is deep to the biceps muscle over the brachialis muscle above the elbow joint line. If it is impaired, it will affect the lateral cutaneous nerve of the forearm.

BIBLIOGRAPHY

Anderson E: Grant's atlas of anatomy, Baltimore, 1983, Williams & Wilkins.

Andrews JR et al: Musculotendinous injuries of the shoulder and elbow in athletes, Athletic Training 2:68, 1976.

APTA Orthopaedic Section Review for Advanced Orthopaedic Competencies Conference, Sandy Burkhart, The Elbow, Chicago, Aug 9, 1989.

Braatz J and Gogia P: The mechanics of pitching, J Orthop Sports Phys Ther, Aug: 56-59, 1987.

Booher JM and Thibodeau GA: Athletic injury assessment, Toronto, 1985, Times Mirror/Mosby College Publishing. Injuries to the elbow, Clin Symp 22:2, 1970.

Cyriax J: Textbook of orthopedic medicine: diagnosis of soft tissue lesions, vol 1, London, 1978, Bailliere Tindall.

Daniels L and Worthingham C: Muscle testing: techniques of manual examination, Toronto, 1980, WB Saunders Inc.

Donatelli R and Wooden M: Orthopaedic physical therapy, New York, 1989, Churchill Livingstone.

Gould JA and Davis GJ: Orthopaedic and sports physical therapy, ed 2, Toronto, 1989, The CV Mosby Co.

Grana WA and Raskin A: Pitcher's elbow in adolescents, Am J Sports Med 8(5):333, 1980.

Gugenheim JJ and others: Little League survey: the Houston study, Am J Sports Med 4:189, 1976.

Hang Y: Tardy ulnar neuritis in a Little League baseball player, Am J Sports Med 9(4):244, 1981.

Hoppenfeld S: Physical examination of the spine and extremities, New York, 1976, Appleton & Lange.

Jobe F et al: Reconstruction of the ulnar collateral ligament in athletes, J Bone Joint Surg 68A(8):1158, 1986.

Josefsson P et al: Surgical versus non-surgical treatment of ligamentous injuries following dislocation of the elbow joint: J Bone Joint Surg 69A(4):605, 1987.

Kaltenborn F: Mobilization of the extremity joints, ed 3, Oslo, 1980, Olaf Norlis Bokhandel Universitegaten.

Kapandji IA: The physiology of the joints, vol 1, Upper limb, New York, 1983, Churchill Livingstone Inc.

Kendall FP and McCreary EK: Muscles testing and function, Baltimore, 1983, Williams & Wilkins.

Kessler RM and Hertling D: Management of common musculo-skeletal disorders, Philadelphia, 1983, Harper and Row.

Klafs CE and Arnheim DD: Modern principles of athletic training, ed 5, St Louis, 1981, The CV Mosby Co.

Kulund D: The injured athlete, Toronto, 1982, JB Lippincott.

Lee D: Tennis elbow: a manual therapist's perspective, J Orthop Sports Phys Ther 8(3):134, 1986.

Lesin B et al: Acute rupture of the medial collateral ligament of the elbow requiring reconstruction, J Bone Joint Surg 68A(8):1278, 1986.

Lipscomb Brant: Baseball pitching injuries in growing athletes, J Sports Med 3(1):25, 1975.

Magee DJ: Orthopaedics conditions, assessments, and treatment, vol 2, Alberta, 1979, University of Alberta Publishing.

Magee DJ: Orthopaedic physical assessment, Toronto, 1987, WB Saunders Co.

Maitland GD: Peripheral manipulation, Toronto, 1977, Butterworth & Co.

Mannheimer JS and Lampe GN: Clinical transcutaneous electrical nerve stimulation, Philadelphia, 1986, FA Davis Co.

Mennell J McM: Joint pain, Boston, 1964, Little, Brown and Co.

Morrey B and Kai-Nan A: Articular and ligamentous contributions to the stability of the elbow joint, Am J Sports Med 11(5):315, 1983.

Nirschl R and Pettrone F: Tennis elbow, J Bone Joint Surg 61A(6):835, 1979.

Nitz A et al: Nerve injury and grades II and III sprains, Am J Sports Med 13(3):177, 1985.

Norkin C and Levangia P: Joint structure and function, Philadelphia, 1983, FA Davis Co.

O'Donaghue D: Treatment of injuries to athletes, Toronto, 1984, WB Saunders Co.

Perry J: Anatomy and biomechanics of the shoulder in throwing, swimming, gymnastics, and tennis, Clin Sports Med 2:247, 1983.

Petersen L and Renstrom P: Sports injuries, their prevention and treatment, Chicago, 1986, Year Book Medical Publishers, Inc.

Priest J and Weise D: Elbow injury in women's gymnastics, Am J Sports Med 9(5):288, 1981.

Reid DC: Functional anatomy and joint mobilization, Alberta, 1970, University of Alberta Publishing.

Reid DC: Sports injury assessment and rehabilitation, New York, 1992, Churchill Livingstone.

Reid DC and Kushner S: The elbow region. In Donatelli R and Wooden M: Orthopaedic physical therapy, New York, 1989, Churchill Livingstone.

Rettig A: Stress fracture of the ulna in an adolescent tournament tennis player, Am J Sports Med 11(2):103, 1983.

Round Table Discussion: Prevention and treatment of tennis elbow, Physician Sports Med 2:33, 1977.

Roy S and Irvin R: Sports medicine: prevention, evaluation, management, and rehabilitation, Englewood Cliffs, NJ, 1983, Prentice Hall.

Sisto D et al: An electromyographic analysis of the elbow in pitching: Am J Sports Med 15(3):260, 1987.

Stover CN et al: The modern golf swing and stress, Physician Sports Med 9:43, 1976.

Tomberlin JP et al: The use of standardized evaluation forms in physical therapy, J Orthop Sports Phys Therapy, 348-354, 1984.

Travell J and Simons D: Myofascial pain and dysfunction: the trigger point manual, New York, 1983, Williams & Wilkins.

Welsh P and Shepherd R: Current therapy in sports medicine—1985-1986. Toronto, 1985, BC Decker Inc.

Williams PL and Warwick R: Gray's Anatomy, New York, 1980, Churchill Livingstone Inc.

Wilson FD et al: Valgus extension overload in the pitching elbow, AM J Sports Med 11(2):83, 1983.

CHAPTER 5

Forearm, Wrist, and Hand Assessment

Pain at the wrist or hand can be referred from the cervical spine, the shoulder joint, the thoracic outlet, the brachial plexus, the elbow joint, or the radioulnar joint. These other areas should be ruled out during the history-taking and observations. If these joints or structures cannot be eliminated as the source of the problem then they must be tested during the functional testing.

The hand and particularly the fingers are very susceptible to injury during sporting events. The mobility and dexterity of the hand depends on the movement at both the wrist and the forearm. Injuries to the fingers and hand may appear minor but are potentially very debilitating and therefore must be fully assessed and rehabilitated.

The wrist and hand must be studied as an integral part of the entire upper quadrant because:

- The hand has a great range of movement, for which it relies on full functioning of the shoulder, elbow, and wrist.
- The blood and nerve supply to the hand runs down the length of the extremity.
- Some of the muscles for the hand and wrist originate in the forearm or at the elbow joint.

The joints that will be discussed here include (Fig. 5-1):

- forearm
- wrist (see Fig. 5-1)
- hand and thumb

FOREARM

The joints of the forearm include the proximal (superior) and distal (inferior) radioulnar joints. There is also a middle radioulnar syndesmosis that may be included in this category. These radioulnar joints are uniaxial pivot joints. They allow pronation and supination and depend on normal humeroradial and humeroulnar joints to function fully.

The close-packed position of the proximal radioulnar joint and distal radioulnar joint is at an angle of 5° to 10° of supination. The resting, or loose-packed, position of the proximal radioulnar joint is when the forearm is supinated approximately 35° and the elbow is flexed 70°. The resting position of the distal radioulnar joint is at an angle of 10° of supination. The capsular pattern for both the proximal and distal radioulnar joint is equal restriction in pronation and supination (when the elbow has marked flexion and extension restrictions).

NOTE: The close-packed, resting position and capsular patterns vary in the literature. The joint positions for these patterns follow Freddy M. Kaltenborn's techniques (see bibliography for reference).

Proximal Radioulnar Joint

The proximal (superior) radioulnar joint is the articulation between the convex circumference of the head of the radius and the ring formed by the radial notch of the ulna and the annular ligament. The head of the radius will spin on the capitellum and roll and slide in the radial notch. Because of these movements of the radius, any humeroradial dysfunction will affect the radioulnar joint.

This joint allows active pronation and supination. The accessory movements that occur during pronation and supination are dorsal glide and volar (palmar) glide of the radius on the ulna.

Distal Radioulnar Joint

The distal (inferior) radioulnar joint is the articulation between the convex head of the ulna and the concave ulnar notch of the distal end of the radius.

The surfaces are enclosed in a capsule and held together by an articular disc. This triangular disc of fibrocartilage is located between the distal end of the ulna and the medial part of the lunate or triquetral bones of the wrist. When the hand is ulnar-deviated it articulates with the triquetral bone.

The radius moves over the ulna, allowing pronation and supination. The accessory movements during pronation include the distal end of the ulna moving laterally and posteriorly and during supination the distal ulna moving medially and anteriorly. Because of these ulnar movements, any humeroulnar joint dysfunction will affect the distal radioulnar joint.

Middle Radioulnar Joint

The middle radioulnar syndesmosis includes the interosseous membrane and the oblique cord between the shafts of the radius and ulna. The oblique cord is a flat cord formed in the fascia overlying the deep head of the supinator and running to the radial tuberosity—its functional purpose is minimal. The interosseous membrane is made up of fibers that slant caudally and medially from the radius to the ulna. These fibers transmit forces from the wrist or hand up into the humerus and they are tight midway between supination and pronation.

This joint serves primarily to provide surface area for muscle attachments.

WRIST (see FIG. 5-1)

Radiocarpal Joint

The radiocarpal joint, a biaxial ellipsoid joint, is the articulation between the distal end of the radius and the scaphoid and lunate carpal bones. There is an articular disc that articulates with the lunate and triquetrum that is sometimes referred to as the *ulnomeniscocarpal joint*. The disc adds stability, absorbs shock, and binds the distal radioulnar joint. The active movements of the radiocarpal joint are flexion, extension, ulnar and radial deviation, and circumduction. The accessory movements are distraction, dorsal and volar (palmar) glide, and radial and ulnar glide. The resting position is neutral with some ulnar deviation. The close-packed position is wrist extension with radial deviation. The capsular pattern has equal limitation of wrist flexion and extension.

Intercarpal Joints

These joints are the joints between the individual bones of the proximal and distal rows of carpals. There are some accessory movements with gliding between the bones (volar and dorsal glide). The resting position is slight flexion. The close-packed position is wrist extension.

Midcarpal Joints

The proximal row of carpals (lunate, scaphoid, and triquetrum) articulate with the distal row of carpals (hamate, pisiform, capitate, trapezoid, and trapezium). On the medial side, the convex heads of the capitate and the hamate articulate with the concave scaphoid, lunate and triquetral bones, and together they form a compound sellar joint. On the lateral side the trapezium and trapezoid articulate with the scaphoid forming another sellar joint.

The active movements of the midcarpal joints are the same as those of the radiocarpal joint (flexion, extension, ulnar and radial deviation, and circumduction). The accessory movements include distraction and volar (palmar) and dorsal glide.

The resting position of these joints is slight flexion and ulnar deviation and the close-packed position is wrist extension with ulnar deviation. The pisotriquetral joint is a small plane joint that allows a small amount of gliding to take place.

HAND AND THUMB

The hand is designed so that the thumb has the greatest mobility and can easily move to oppose each finger. The second and third fingers are less

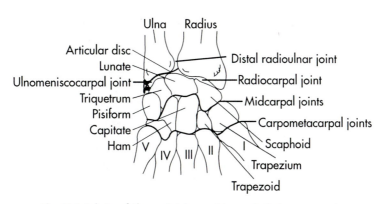

Fig. 5-1 Joints of the wrist (carpal bones). Palmer aspect.

mobile and hold the arch of the hand, as well as providing stability for tight opposition grips with the thumb. The fourth and fifth fingers are quite mobile to adapt to different surfaces and allow grasping of a variety of shapes.

Intermetacarpal Joints

The bases of the second, third, fourth, and fifth metacarpal bones articulate with one another in a gliding motion. During the grasp movement the intermetacarpal joints allow the formation of an arch in the hand and, during the release, the arch is also flattened by intermetacarpal movement.

Carpometacarpal Joints

The carpometacarpal joint of the thumb is a saddle (sellar) joint between the first metacarpal bone and the trapezium. The thumb's active movements at this joint are flexion, extension, abduction, adduction, rotation, and opposition. The accessory movements are axial rotation and distraction.

The carpometacarpal joint of the thumb has a resting position in mid flexion-extension and mid abduction-adduction. The close-packed position is one of full opposition. The capsular pattern is limited abduction and extension, while flexion is full.

The second metacarpal articulates with the trapezoid carpal bone and the third metacarpal articulates with the capitate carpal bone. The fourth and fifth metacarpals articulate with the hamate carpal bone. The movements for the second to fifth

carpometacarpal joints permit a gliding motion. The capsular pattern for the carpometacarpal joints two through five is equal limitation in all directions.

Metacarpophalangeal Joints

The first to fifth metacarpals articulate with the proximal phalanges; the second and third joints are less mobile than the fourth and fifth joints.

The active movements of these joints are flexion, extension, adduction, abduction, and circumduction. These joints allow accessory movements of rotation, dorsal and volar (palmar) glide, radial and ulnar glide, and distraction.

The resting position of these joints is one of slight flexion. The close-packed position for the second to fifth joint is full flexion. However, the close-packed position for the first metacarpophalangeal joint is full opposition and the capsular pattern is more restriction in flexion than in extension.

Interphalangeal Joints (DIP, PIP)

These uniaxial joints are the articulations between the phalanges of each digit and the active movements that occur are flexion and extension. The accessory movements are rotation, abduction, adduction, and anterior and posterior glide.

The resting position is one of slight flexion. The close-packed position is one of full extension. The capsular pattern is that flexion is more limited than extension.

ASSESSMENT

INTERPRETATION

HISTORY

Mechanism of Injury

Direct Trauma (Fig. 5-2)
Was it direct trauma?

Contusions
FOREARM AND WRIST

The boney prominences of the ulna and radius on both the palmar and dorsal aspects are susceptible to injury through a direct blow. The tendons that cross the wrist can be contused, and repeated trauma can lead to tenosynovitis. Any or all of the extensor or flexor tendons can be involved.

ASSESSMENT

INTERPRETATION

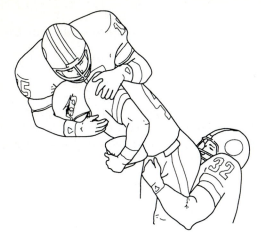

Fig. 5-2 Direct trauma to the forearm, wrist, and hand.

Occasionally, repeated trauma or gross swelling can cause a carpal tunnel syndrome with median nerve compression.

A contusion to the hook of the hamate or pisiform can cause swelling that can compress the ulnar nerve or compress the Tunnel of Guyon (ulnar artery and ulnar nerve). Falling on the palmar surface of the hand is a common mechanism of injury but direct trauma from the handle of a baseball bat or racquet can also be the cause.

HAND AND FINGERS

Repeated direct blows to the hand can cause vascular damage. Contusions often occur to the dorsum of the hand where the blood vessels, nerves, tendons, and bones are relatively superficial and there is little fat or muscle padding. Such injuries occur often in contact sports like football and rugby where the hand is unprotected.

Contusions to the palmar surface of the hand can also cause dorsal hand swelling. Because there is little room for blood to accumulate on the palmar aspect, it moves to the dorsal cavity under the skin. The distal phalanx of the fingers or thumb can be contused (by a direct blow or from being stepped on) causing a subungual hematoma, which is an accumulation of blood under the fingernail.

The fleshy thenar and hypothenar eminences can be contused with a direct blow especially in racquet sports or those that involve catching a ball.

Contusions to the metacarpophalangeal joints are common in contact sports where fights occur or if a fist is used as part of the sport (i.e., boxing, football).

Fractures
FOREARM AND WRIST
Hook of hamate
Styloid process
Pisiform

Most forearm and wrist fractures are a result of a hyperextension mechanism, although, on occasion, direct trauma can cause a fracture. For radius and ulna fractures see Falling on the

ASSESSMENT

INTERPRETATION

Outstretched Arm—Forearm fractures.

The wrist bones most vulnerable to fracture by direct trauma are:

- the hook of hamate
- the radial styloid process
- the ulnar styloid process

A fracture to the hook of hamate or the pisiform bone can occur from repeated trauma to the area. For example, the handle of a baseball bat, a tennis or squash racquet, a hockey stick or a golf club that repeatedly hits the bone can cause this fracture.

HAND—METACARPALS

Base, shaft, neck, or head
Bennett fracture
Roland fracture
Boxer's fracture (Fig. 5-3)

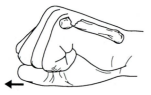

Fig. 5-3 Boxer's fracture. A fracture of the neck of the fifth metacarpal.

Fractures of the metacarpals are more common than phalangeal fractures. Metacarpal fractures are caused by a direct blow to the shaft or to the metacarpal head (with the hand in a fist, which then transmits the force to fracture the shaft) or by a fall on the hand. According to Rettig A et al, metacarpal fractures were evenly divided among the digits in football, whereas most fractures in basketball involved the fourth and fifth metacarpal. These fractures can occur at the base, shaft, neck, or head of the metacarpal. Fractures that are intra-articular (base and head) are the most serious. Often the metacarpal deformity causes the bone to look bowed or can actually cause a shortening of the bone. The metacarpal head depresses while the fracture site elevates (V shape).

A fracture of the proximal end of the first metacarpal is often associated with a subluxation or dislocation of the carpometacarpal joint of the thumb (Bennett fracture). With a Bennett fracture a piece of the base of the thumb metacarpal is often avulsed. As a result, the abductor pollicis longus pulls the large metacarpal fragment radially and proximally while the adductor pollicis pulls the metacarpal ulnarly. This can occur in football or hockey when the player throws a punch at an opposing player, but the player's thumb hits the other player's helmet or padding instead.

A Roland fracture is a proximal T-shaped, intra-articular fracture of the first metacarpal. It is caused by excessive axial pressure through the joint.

A boxer's fracture is a fracture of the neck of the fifth metacarpal and can cause a flexion deformity (see Fig. 5-3). It is usually caused by a "round house" punch with a closed fist where most of the force goes through the fifth metacarpal. This fracture, unfortunately, occurs in contact sports where fights are frequent (e.g., hockey, football, rugby). Such fractures result in a depression of the fifth knuckle with significant swelling in the area. If the finger is angulated under the fourth finger when the fist is closed, there is an associated rotational problem that will require surgical correction. A boxer with proper punching technique will more often fracture the second or third metacarpal.

ASSESSMENT

INTERPRETATION

Fracture and Fracture Dislocation
PHALANGES
PROXIMAL PHALANX

Fractures of the proximal phalanx from a direct blow occur more often than fractures of the middle or distal phalanx. Fractures of the PIP joint include:

- intra-articular fractures (head, shaft, and T fractures that split the condyles)
- base fractures
- comminuted fractures

Fracture dislocations (volar lip and extensor tendon avulsion) can also occur—a V-shaped deformity results, with the midshaft of the phalanx depressed.

Fractures of the proximal phalanges can cause damage to the flexor or extensor tendons; a deformity in the anterior or volar direction usually occurs in proximal fractures.

MIDDLE PHALANX

Fractures of the middle phalanx can also affect the flexor and extensor tendons. If the fracture is distal to both insertions, the stronger flexor sublimus flexes the proximal segment. If the fracture occurs more proximally in the shaft between the central extensor tendon slip and the insertion of the flexor digitorum sublimus, the proximal fragment will be extended and the distal fragment will be flexed.

DISTAL PHALANX

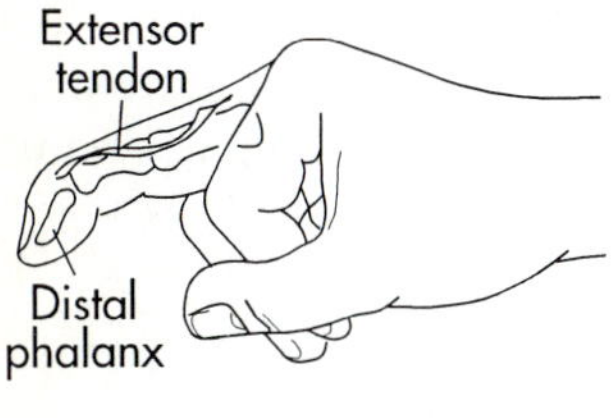

Fig. 5-4 Mallet finger.

The distal phalanx is fractured most often by a crushing mechanism and can have an associated subungual hematoma.

A mallet finger is common in sports where the distal phalanx is forced into flexion (e.g., baseball, volleyball, basketball; Fig. 5-4). The extensor tendon becomes avulsed from its insertion on the distal phalanx with or without a small chip avulsion fracture.

A fracture of the distal phalanx involving one third or more of the articular surface can occur in some cases. This can have a subluxed palmar fragment associated with it.

A child can fracture and dislocate the distal phalanx through the growth plate. Such a fracture is caused by a forced flexion that avulses the central slip of the extensor tendon from its insertion in the middle phalanx or from a direct blow to the proximal PIP joint.

Dislocation
WRIST

A direct blow of significant force to the hand may dislocate the distal carpal bones dorsal to the lunate bone. This perilunate dislocation often also results in a trans-scaphoid fracture.

ASSESSMENT   INTERPRETATION

Indirect Trauma
Falling on the Outstretched Arm (Fig. 5-5)
FOREARM FRACTURES
Distal end of radius
Monteggia fracture
Galeazzi fracture
Colles fracture
Smith fracture
Ulna/radius greenstick fracture
Epiphyseal dislocation
Barton fracture

The distal end of the radius is often fractured when an athlete attempts to break his or her fall by putting a hand down. The force is transmitted up the radius with maximal stress at the distal end of the radius.

Monteggia fracture is a fracture of the proximal half of the ulna and is associated with a radial head dislocation or a rupture of the annular ligament. The ulnar fragments override the fracture site and the posterior interosseous nerve and/or the ulna nerve can be damaged.

Galeazzi fracture is a fracture of the shaft of distal radius accompanied by a dislocation of the distal ulna.

Colles fracture is a fracture of the distal end of the radius (Fig. 5-6), which is angulated dorsally (there may be an associated ulnar fracture) causing a "dinner-fork deformity." This is not a common injury except in the older athlete; it frequently involves the radiocarpal and the distal radioulnar joint.

Smith fracture occurs when the athlete falls on the back of the hand with the wrist flexed, causing a volar angulated distal fragment of the radius.

In the young athlete, the ulna and/or radius can suffer a greenstick fracture. A complete fracture of both bones is difficult to handle, especially because good alignment is difficult to achieve.

The distal radial epiphyseal dislocation is the most common epiphyseal injury in this area. In the adolescent, an epiphyseal separation of the distal radius and ulna can occur.

A Barton fracture is a fracture through the dorsal articular area of the radius with dorsal and proximal displacement.

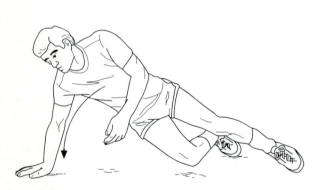

Fig. 5-5 Falling on the outstretched arm.

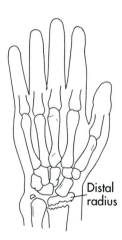

Distal radius

Fig. 5-6 Colles fracture.

ASSESSMENT

INTERPRETATION

Overstretch
Hyperextension
Wrist
FRACTURES (SCAPHOID)

During wrist hyperextension the scaphoid (navicular) may be impinged between the capitate and radius, causing a fracture. The incidence of scaphoid fractures in young athletes is very high, particularly in contact sports. This fracture is often misdiagnosed and thought to be a wrist sprain. An athlete with point tenderness in the anatomical snuffbox and a history of wrist hyperextension should be suspected of having a scaphoid fracture until proven otherwise. There is a high incidence of healing complications because a scaphoid fracture is often unrecognized and the bone heals poorly because of its poor blood supply (only to the distal pole).

The complications from a scaphoid fracture include:

- non-union
- delayed union
- avascular necrosis of the fragments (Preiser disease)
- eventual osteoarthritis

STRAINS

The wrist that is hyperextended can strain any of the flexor tendons anywhere along the muscle but especially where the tendons cross the joint. According to Wright (see Welsh and Shepherd) the tendons most commonly injured are the flexor carpi radialis and the flexor carpi ulnaris. The resulting inflammation can irritate the tendon sheath, causing tenosynovitis, which in turn can lead to a carpal tunnel syndrome.

SPRAINS (FIG. 5-7)

The wrist that is hyperextended and pronated can injure:
- the inferior dorsal radioulnar ligament
- the ulnar collateral ligament
- the fibrous cartilage disc between the ulna and the lunate and triquetral bones
- the interosseous membrane
- the lunate-capitate ligament dorsally
- the radiocarpal ligament palmarly

The more violent the injury, the more of these structures are damaged. In the mild sprain the inferior dorsal radioulnar ligament is usually involved.

The wrist and hand that is hyperextended can also damage the scaphoid-lunate articulation.

DISLOCATION

Dislocations of the distal ulna can occur. Such dislocations often occur with ulnar styloid fractures. For a dislocation to occur, the distal radioulnar ligaments and the triangular fibrocartilage complex must be disrupted.

ASSESSMENT   INTERPRETATION

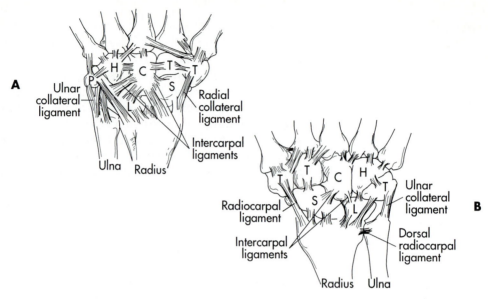

Fig. 5-7 A, Palmar ligaments of the right wrist. **B,** Dorsal ligaments of the right wrist.

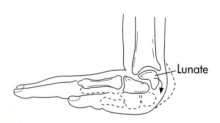

Fig. 5-8 Hyperextended wrist. Lunate dislocation mechanism.

Dislocations of the radiocarpal or midcarpal joints are extremely rare in athletes because these joints are well protected by the ligaments. Dislocations of the entire carpals away from the distal radius and ulna are rare but can occur as fracture-dislocations. In the Barton fracture, the volar lip of the radius fractures and may become displaced with the entire row of carpals. In the reverse Barton fracture the dorsal lip of the radius fractures and may dislocate with the carpals. The radial styloid can fracture with the volar or dorsal lip fracture also.

The carpals themselves can be dislocated or subluxed. With hyperextension, the lunate dislocates anteriorly or it remains stationary and the rest of the carpals dislocate anteriorly (Fig. 5-8). As the hyperextension forces on the wrist increase in magnitude, the following progression of wrist structures become unstable:

- lunate (the central keystone)
- lunate and scaphoid ligaments
- capitate and distal row of carpals
- ligaments between the lunate and triquetrum

The joints themselves may dislocate and spontaneously reduce. The most commonly dislocated carpal is the lunate. It rotates and dislocates anteriorly (volarly) most of the time and tears the posterior radiolunate ligament. Complications of this dislocation can be:

- carpal tunnel syndrome
- median nerve palsy
- flexor tendon constriction

ASSESSMENT

INTERPRETATION

- progressive avascular necrosis of the lunate (Keinboch disease)
- scaphoid fracture (with a proximal displacement with the lunate)

Perilunate dislocation is a ligamentous injury resulting in the distal articular surface of the lunate disengaging from the proximal articular surface of the capitate. If the scapholunate ligament is disrupted, the lunate and triquetrum become unstable and dorsiflex while the scaphoid flexes palmarly. If the scaphoid fractures, the proximal pole of the scaphoid, lunate, and triquetrum become unstable and dorsiflex while the scaphoid distal pole only flexes palmarly. If the triquetrolunate ligament tears, the lunate and scaphoid become unstable and flex dorsally.

Hyperextension or Valgus Stretch
THUMB

First metacarpophalangeal joint sprain to dislocation

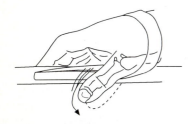

Fig. 5-9 Skier's thumb. Ulnar collateral ligament sprain, tear, or avulsion.

A forceful hyperextension, often combined with abduction, of the first metacarpophalangeal joint is a common injury in athletes ("skier's" thumb; Fig. 5-9). It is commonly seen in people who snow-ski—the pole abducts the thumb when the skier falls.

The thumb is also injured in hockey when the player punches an opposing player and the thumb is forced into hyperextension. It is often injured in sports like baseball, basketball, and volleyball when the catch or volley is misjudged and the thumb is hyperextended.

During thumb hyperextension the following injuries can occur:

- the ulnar collateral ligament can be sprained, torn or even avulsed
- the base of the proximal phalanx on the ulnar side can fracture and be displaced or undisplaced
- the volar plate's membranous insertion may also be sprained, torn, or avulsed from its phalangeal attachment
- the adductor aponeurosis can become trapped between the ends of the completely torn ulnar collateral ligament and it will prevent the ligament from healing (Stenner lesion).

The thumb may also be dislocated posteriorly with a pure hyperextension mechanism. When the thumb is extended and then hit, the collateral ligaments of the metacarpophalangeal joint of the thumb can be sprained. If this happens in the young athlete the growth plate at the base of the proximal phalanx can be damaged.

Chronic laxity of the ulnar collateral ligament of the thumb can develop from repeated trauma. This is described as gamekeeper's thumb because Scottish gamekeepers often sustain this injury by repeatedly wringing the necks of rabbits.

ASSESSMENT

INTERPRETATION

Hyperextension

FINGERS

Second to fifth metacarpophalangeal joint sprain to dislocation
Second to fifth proximal interphalangeal joint sprain to dislocation
Second to fifth distal interphalangeal joint sprain to dislocation
Avulsion of the flexed digitorum profundus
Extensor injury

The second to fifth metacarpophalangeal joints are commonly injured through hyperextension, which usually results in ligament damage.

With violent forces the joint may dislocate volarly. In such a case, the head breaks through a vent in the volar plate and catches between the lumbrical tendon and the flexors—the index finger is most commonly involved. Injuries to the digits are usually caused by a blow on the extended finger (Fig. 5-10).

With hyperextension of the PIP joints the following can be injured:

- joint capsule
- transverse retinacular ligaments
- collateral and accessory collateral ligaments
- volar plate, if subluxation or dislocation occurs

The joint can be sprained, subluxed, or dislocated. If the distal portion of the volar plate of the PIP joint is injured, it may cause a hyperextension deformity or flexion deformity at the PIP joint. If the proximal portion is damaged, it may cause a pseudo "boutonniere" deformity if the extensor tendon remains intact. A true boutonniere deformity with a disruption of the extensor tendon central slip mechanism causes a volar subluxation of the lateral bands and a flexed PIP joint.

Hyperextension of the distal interphalangeal joint is an injury very commonly sustained by those who participate in team sports like basketball and volleyball. The joint is often sprained with anterior capsule damage, ligament damage, and sometimes, volar plate involvement. If the force is significant, the joint can be dislocated. Sometimes the joint is hyperextended so far that the distal phalanx hits the middle phalanx. When this occurs the middle phalanx breaks off a piece of the articular surface on the proximal interphalangeal joint and disrupts the extensor mechanism. This will cause a "drop" or "mallet" finger and the PIP joint surface can also be damaged.

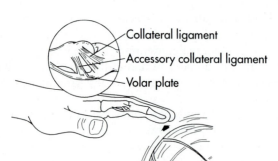

Collateral ligament
Accessory collateral ligament
Volar plate

Fig. 5-10 Proximal interphalangeal joint injury. Direct blow to the extended finger.

ASSESSMENT

INTERPRETATION

A flexed finger that is violently extended can cause the flexor digitorum profundus to rupture or avulse from the insertion on the distal phalanx. In a contact sport such as football or rugby the athlete may grab the opposing teammate's jersey—if the opposing player pulls away forcibly, the athlete's distal phalanx may be extended while the finger is being flexed actively, causing the flexor digitorum profundus to be avulsed from its attachment to the distal phalanx. Such an injury is most common in the ring finger.

Depending on the force, three levels of retraction of the flexor tendon can occur:

- avulsion fracture of the volar lip of the distal phalanx
- avulsion of the flexor tendon that retracts to the level of the flexor digitorum sublimus
- avulsion of the tendon that retracts up into the palm

Any injury to the extensors can upset the balance of all the joints of the finger, resulting in:

- mallet finger
- swan neck deformity
- boutonniere deformity
- claw deformity

Hyperflexion
WRIST

The ligament between the capitate and the third metacarpal can rupture and, as a result, the capitate will not move properly during active wrist flexion. This will lead to wrist joint dysfunction.

FINGERS

The distal interphalangeal joints of the fingers can be forced into flexion and the central slip of the extensor digitorum communis tendon can be ruptured over the proximal interphalangeal joint, producing a boutonniere deformity. This causes the PIP joint to stay in flexion and the DIP joint is extended—the PIP joint cannot be extended actively.

Radial or Ulnar Deviation
WRIST

Forced wrist radial deviation (Fig. 5-11) can:
- sprain or tear the medial ligament of the radiocarpal joint at the ulnar styloid process, the anterior band into the pisiform, or the posterior band into the triquetrum
- fracture the scaphoid or the distal end of the radius
- avulse the ulnar styloid process

Forced wrist ulnar deviation can:
- sprain or tear the lateral ligament of the radiocarpal joint at the radial styloid process, the anterior band into the articular surface of the scaphoid, or the posterior band into the scaphoid tubercle

ASSESSMENT   INTERPRETATION

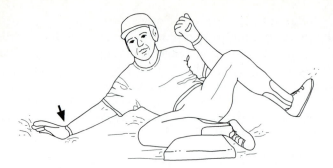

Fig. 5-11 Wrist radial deviation over-stretch.

- strain the extensor carpi radialis longus or the abductor pollicis longus
- avulse the radial styloid process

FINGERS

With forced ulnar deviation of the proximal interphalangeal joint the finger is pushed to the side and the following structures can be damaged:

- radial collateral ligaments can be sprained, torn, or avulsed
- volar plate can be ruptured, depending on the forces involved
- complete dislocation can occur

Hyperpronation
  Radioulnar joint

During a fall causing hyperpronation, dorsal subluxations or dislocations of the distal radioulnar joint can occur.

Hypersupination
  Radioulnar joint

This occurs less commonly during a fall than hyperpronation and can result in a volar radioulnar subluxation or dislocation.

Rotational Force
  Radioulnar joint

The distal radioulnar joint is usually injured with a rotational force around a fixed hand that can result in subluxation or dislocation of the distal ulna dorsally or volarly. The structures that can be damaged are:

- triangular fibrocartilage disc complex
- articular disc (tear)
- dorsal or volar radioulnar ligaments
- ulnar collateral ligaments

Overuse
Carpal Tunnel Syndrome (Median Nerve Entrapment) (Fig. 5-12)

Two overuse mechanisms in baseball that can produce carpal tunnel syndrome are (1) the pitcher repeatedly snapping the wrist when throwing sliders and (2) players using an inadequately padded glove. Repeated trauma to the palm causes thickened carpal ligaments that can put pressure on the nerve.

Flexor tendonitis in sports like rowing and weight lifting can

ASSESSMENT

INTERPRETATION

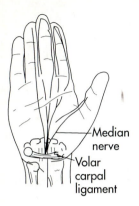

Fig. 5-12 Carpal tunnel syndrome.

also lead to carpal tunnel syndrome. This is a common problem in the wheel chair athlete.

The eight flexor tendons of the fingers, the flexor pollicis longus, and the flexor carpi radialis all pass through the carpal tunnel at the wrist joint. The median nerve also passes through this tunnel.

The tunnel can become constricted if any of the following injuries occur:

- postfracture where there is significant swelling (e.g., Colles or scaphoid fracture). Dysfunction of the median nerve is the most common complication in a Colles fracture
- postlunate, perilunar, or capitate dislocation
- wrist contusion
- flexor tenosynovitis
- synovial hypertrophy or thickening in the synovial covering of the flexor tendons
- ganglia
- endocrine disorders (diabetes, hypothyroidism, menopause)
- tumors
- metabolic disorders (gout)
- body fluid retention (common during pregnancy)

When the tunnel is constricted, the pressure causes numbness or tingling in the hand and fingers that are supplied by the median nerve. Motor weakness can develop from prolonged or severe compression.

de Quervain's Disease (Constrictive Tenosynovitis)

Overuse of the thumb or wrist can lead to a tendonitis of the abductor pollicis longus and extensor pollicis brevis where they pass through the first compartment of the wrist. Inflammation of the tendon sheaths constrict the tendons as they cross the distal end of the radius in the first compartment. Activities where the thumb is overused can cause this problem. It can also develop if the thumb is fixed and the wrist is overstressed (e.g., in paddling, baseball, javelin, hockey). Occasionally, direct trauma can lead to this.

Extensor Intersection Syndrome

Overuse of the thumb or wrist can cause inflammation of abductor pollicis longus and extensor pollicis brevis in the upper forearm where they cross over one another. This is commonly seen in weight lifters and paddlers.

Extensor Pollicis Longus

The extensor pollicis longus is the sole occupant of the third extensor compartment and can become inflamed as it moves around the Lister tubercle of the distal radius—this is a rare condition.

ASSESSMENT   INTERPRETATION

Extensor Digitorum Communis, Extensor Indicis, and Extensor Digiti Minimi

The fourth compartment made up of the extensor digitorum communis and the extensor indicis, or the fifth compartment, made up of the extensor digiti minimi, can become inflamed from overuse as they pass under the extensor retinaculum.

Ulnar Nerve Entrapment or Repeated Trauma

The ulnar nerve can be entrapped or traumatized as it passes around the hook of hamate in the Tunnel of Guyon (Fig. 5-13). It can also be damaged with a scaphoid or pisiform fracture. Chronic overuse of the wrist can affect the ulnar nerve, causing tingling and paresthesia of the hand and fingers (the little finger and the ulnar half of the ring finger). Repeated ulnar trauma from the handle of a baseball bat or hockey stick, or karate blows, can cause ulnar nerve problems here also. Prolonged wrist extension during long-distance cycling can also cause ulnar nerve palsy.

Hand Blisters or Calluses

Overuse friction on the epidermis can lead to blisters or calluses. This occurs in sports that require prolonged or repeated gripping (e.g., gymnastics, rowing, weight lifting, squash).

Pain

Location
Local
Skin
Fascia
Superficial muscle
Superficial ligament
Periosteum

Local point tenderness usually comes from the more superficial structures. The anatomic structures that project localized areas of pain when injured are the:
- skin (i.e., hand blisters)
- fascia (i.e., laceration)
- superficial muscles (i.e., extensor digitorum longus, palmaris longus, and opponens)
- superficial ligaments (i.e., radial and ulnar collateral ligaments of the radiocarpal and interphalangeal joints)
- periosteum (i.e., pisiform, styloid process, and metacarpal heads)

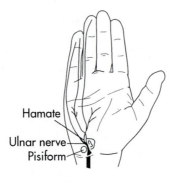

Hamate

Ulnar nerve
Pisiform

Fig. 5-13 Tunnel of Guyon.

ASSESSMENT

INTERPRETATION

Referred
Deep muscle
Deep ligament
Bursa
Bone

Segmental referred pain can come from the following structures:
- deep muscle—myotomal (i.e., pronator teres)
- deep ligament (i.e., inferior radioulnar joint ligament)
- bursa (i.e., radioulnar bursa)
- bone (i.e., scaphoid, radius)

A fracture of the scaphoid bone can be local in the anatomical snuffbox area and can also refer discomfort up the radius (Fig. 5-14).

Type of Pain
Can the athlete describe the pain?

Tingling, Numbness, Shooting Pain

Such pain is usually indicative of a neural problem. It is necessary to determine the exact areas of skin where these sensations are felt.

It could be felt in a specific dermatome if a nerve root irritation exists (cervical problem C6, C7, or C8).

It could be pain along a peripheral nerve (median, ulnar, or radial) from a problem anywhere along the nerve's course (thoracic outlet, cervical rib, Guyon canal).

Carpal tunnel syndrome commonly develops as a result of direct trauma or is secondary to swelling. It causes decreased sensation in the median nerve distribution (thumb, index, third, and half of ring finger).

Tingling or numbness that goes around the entire limb and is not limited to a dermatome or a peripheral nerve supply can be caused by a circulatory problem.

Sharp

Sharp pain can come from:
- skin (e.g., laceration)
- fascia (e.g., palmar fascia)

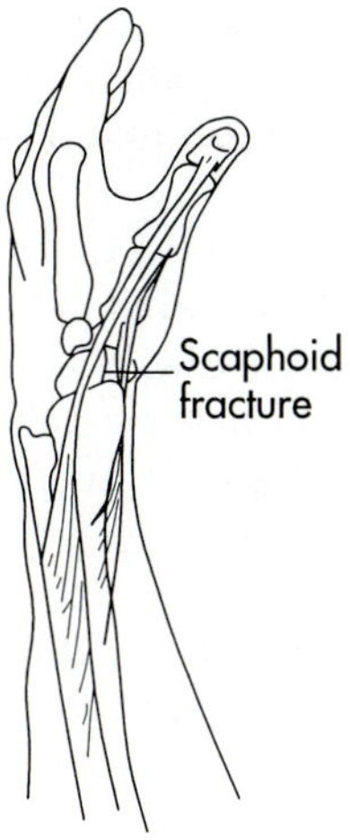

Fig. 5-14 Anatomical snuffbox—location of pain with a scaphoid fracture.

ASSESSMENT

INTERPRETATION

- tendon (e.g., de Quervain's disease)
- superficial muscles (e.g., flexor carpi ulnaris)
- superficial ligaments (e.g., radial collateral ligaments)
- acute bursa (e.g., radioulnar bursa)
- periosteum (e.g., radial styloid process)

Pain that is felt only during specific movements is usually of a ligamentous or muscular origin.

Dull

Dull pain can come from:
- a neural problem (e.g., ulnar neuritis)
- boney injury (e.g., scaphoid fracture)
- a chronic capsular problem (e.g., wrist sprain)
- deep muscle injury (e.g., pronator quadratus)
- a tendon sheath (e.g., extensor intersection syndrome)

Joint Pain or Stiffness

This is often caused by rheumatoid arthritis of the wrist or hand and follows a capsular pattern.

It can also be attributed to reflex sympathetic dystrophy, which causes an abnormal amount of pain, swelling, and stiffness secondary to disease or trauma. It is the result of an increased sympathetic nervous system response to injury.

Ache

Ache can come from:
- the tendon sheath (e.g., flexor tendons)
- a deep ligament (e.g., distal radioulnar ligament)
- a fibrous capsule (e.g., wrist joint capsule)
- deep muscle (e.g., flexor digitorum profundus)

Pins and Needles

These can come from:
- a peripheral nerve (e.g., ulnar nerve)
- dorsal nerve root (e.g., C7 nerve root)
- systemic condition (e.g., diabetes)
- vascular occlusion (e.g., Raynaud's disease)

Severity of Pain

Is the pain mild, moderate, or severe?

The degree of pain is not always a good indicator of the severity of the problem. For example, a ruptured extensor tendon causing a mallet finger may be painless; a cervical disc herniation may only cause painless numbness in the hand, yet a first degree ligament sprain can be very painful. As the severity of the pain increases, it becomes more difficult to localize it. The degree of pain varies with each athlete's emotional state, cultural background, and previous pain experiences.

ASSESSMENT

INTERPRETATION

Time of Pain
When is it painful?
All the time
Only on repeating the mechanism

Acute conditions and long-term chronic injuries can lead to ongoing pain. Some of these conditions are:
- acute ligament sprain
- neoplasm
- osteoarthritis

Ongoing joint pain without a clear mechanism may indicate the presence of rheumatoid arthritis. Ongoing pain in segments of the forearm, wrist, or hand can indicate a cervical nerve root problem.

Pain that occurs only when repeating the mechanism suggests that the joint or joint support structures (muscle, tendon, ligament, or capsule) are injured.

Pain in ligaments, capsule, and muscle increases when these structures are stretched, whereas pain in bursa, synovial membrane, and nerve roots increases when they are pinched or compressed.

Onset of Pain
Immediate
Gradual

Pain that sets in immediately after the injury is sustained is usually indicative of a more severe injury than when pain occurs a few hours later. A gradual onset could indicate an overuse syndrome, a neural lesion, or an arthritic problem.

Swelling

Location
Where is the swelling located?

Local
Wrist ganglion (Fig. 5-15)
Trigger finger
Tendonitis
Nodules (Dupuytren's Contracture)
Bouchard nodes
Heberden nodes
Sprains

The wrist ganglion is a synovial hernia in the tendinous sheath or joint capsule, usually on the dorsum of the wrist (occasionally on the palmar aspect). It is a knotlike mass that is often elevated and about 2 cm in size (see Fig. 5-15). The ganglion fills with fluid and may be very soft or quite firm, depending on its fluid content. This enlargement can occur insidiously or after a wrist sprain or strain.

The trigger finger is a fibrous nodule in the flexor tendon that catches on the annular sheath opposite the metacarpal head; it can occur in the fingers or the thumb.

Inflammation of the tendon or its synovial sheath from overuse or trauma can cause local swelling.

Nodules in the palmar aponeurosis with shortening of the connective tissue occur with Dupuytren contracture. This is a progressive fibrosis of the palmar aponeurosis—the nodules usually appear first on the ring and little fingers.

Swelling and boney enlargement at the PIP joints of the fingers can indicate secondary synovitis from rheumatoid arthritis (Bouchard nodes).

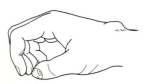

Fig. 5-15 Dorsal wrist ganglion.

ASSESSMENT

INTERPRETATION

Swelling and enlargement around the DIP joints can indicate secondary synovitis from osteoarthritis (Heberden nodes).

Local swelling on the dorsal surface around the DIP and PIP joints is very common with sprains of these joints—the possibility of fracture or damage to the volar plate needs to be determined.

Diffuse
WRIST AND HAND (DORSAL AND PALMER)

In the wrist and hand, diffuse swelling goes to the dorsal surface and radial aspect of the hand where there is more room for fluid accumulation (Fig. 5-16). Less frequently, swelling goes to the palmar aspect where it can enter any of three compartments: the thenar eminence, the hypothenar eminence, or between the thenar and hypothenar eminences.

WRIST JOINT

Swelling in the wrist joint is difficult to observe but will limit most wrist joint movements and can indicate:
- possible carpal fracture
- severe ligament sprain or tear
- arthritic changes

INTERMUSCULAR SWELLING

Swelling from an intermuscular lesion or contusion will often track to the dorsum of the hand because of gravity and the nature of the loose-fitting skin on the dorsum of the hand.

INTRAMUSCULAR SWELLING

Intramuscular swelling will not track and may be palpated within the muscle involved.

Amount of Swelling
Wrist joint
Phalanges or thumb
Reflex sympathetic dystrophy

Swelling around the wrist joint can be dangerous because it can congest the carpal tunnels, resulting in a carpal tunnel syndrome. It can also restrict the extensor tendon compartments. This can occur with:
- scaphoid fracture (carpal fracture)
- Colles fracture (fracture of distal radius displaced posteriorly)

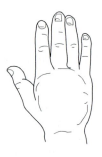

Fig. 5-16 Swelling on the dorsum of the hand.

ASSESSMENT	INTERPRETATION

- Monteggia fracture (fracture of the proximal half of the shaft of the ulna with a dislocation of the head of the radius)
- a dislocated lunate (carpal)
- flexor tenosynovitis
- direct trauma to the carpal area

The phalanges or thumb can also be easily contused—this is often the result of having the hand stepped on accidentally. Swelling in the extremity that seems greater than the preceding injury and is also accompanied by severe burning and constant pain can be reflex sympathetic dystrophy. This occurs secondary to disease state or trauma; it produces increased sympathetic nerve impulses, including:

- "red hand," especially in joints
- pallor or cyanosis in some
- hyperhydrosis
- atrophy of skin and subcutaneous tissue
- increased fibrosis
- joint swelling and stiffness (can last up to 2 years)

Onset of Swelling
Immediate

Immediate swelling in the hand or finger joints suggests a severe injury; gradual swelling suggests a ligament or capsular sprain or subluxation. Immediate joint swelling can be caused by a hemarthrosis or damage to a structure in the joint with a rich blood supply. This is a potentially severe injury and could be:

- carpal fracture in the wrist joint
- dislocated lunate or capitate
- ligament rupture between carpals

6 to 12 Hours Later

Wrist joint swelling 6 to 12 hours postinjury is usually caused by a synovitis or irritation to the joint's synovium. This can be caused by:

- subluxation of the capitate or lunate
- disc lesion between the distal ulna and the lunate or triquetrum
- ligament sprain between the carpals
- capsular sprain

After Activity Only

Swelling in the wrist after activity only suggests that activity aggravates the synovium of the involved joint. This can be caused by:

- Kienboch's disease (progressive necrosis of lunate)
- scaphoid (non-union or necrosis problem)
- bone chip
- arthritic changes in the articular cartilage

ASSESSMENT

INTERPRETATION

- carpal instability

Tendinous swelling after activity or overuse occurs with:
- de Quervain's disease (e.g., paddler's wrist)
- extensor intersection syndrome
- extensor tendonitis (e.g., cross-country skiing)
- flexor tendonitis (e.g., bowling, pitching)

Insidious Onset, Yet Swelling Persists

Swelling with an insidious onset that persists can indicate an arthritic joint problem, systemic disorders, or reflex sympathetic dystrophy.

Immediate Care

Was the injury given immediate care?

If pressure, ice, elevation, and rest were used to treat the injured area immediately after injury, the amount of swelling may be reduced. If heat was applied or activity was allowed to continue, the swelling may be more extensive.

Function

What is the degree of disability?
Could the athlete continue to participate in his or her sport?

Injuries to the hand or fingers are very disabling because they affect daily function a great deal. Problems with the thumb limit daily function even more. If the hand is needed for the sport (e.g., volleyball, baseball, tennis), a wrist, hand, or finger injury will often prevent the athlete's return to play. The athlete may subject other fingers or joints to extra stress to help overcome the functional restrictions imposed by the injury.

Sensations

Ask the athlete to describe the sensations felt at the time of injury and now.

Warmth

Warmth can indicate the presence of inflammation or infection.

Numbness

Numbness can indicate neural involvement, such as the presence of:
- carpal tunnel syndrome at the elbow or wrist
- radial nerve palsy or injury
- cervical nerve root problem
- thoracic outlet syndrome
- local cutaneous nerve injury
- cubital tunnel syndrome at the elbow

Tingling

Tingling can indicate neural involvement (see numbness above) or a circulatory problem (ulnar or radial artery problem, or the presence of Raynaud's disease).

ASSESSMENT	INTERPRETATION

Clicking and Catching

This can indicate a lesion to the intra-articular disc between the radius and the lunate and triquetral carpal bones. The click is usually repeated on wrist rotation. Clicking may be a sign of carpal bone subluxations (i.e., lunate or capitate).

Snapping

Snapping can indicate a "trigger finger or thumb," a form of stenosing tenosynovitis where the thickening catches during finger or thumb flexion to extension.

Popping or Tearing

Popping or tearing at the time of injury can indicate a ligament or muscle tear. This may occur with carpal subluxation or joint dislocation.

Grating

Grating sounds can indicate osteoarthritic changes or articular cartilage deterioration.

Crepitus

The presence of crepitus can indicate a tenosynovitis of the flexor or extensor tendons in their tendon sheaths as the digits move. Crepitus with joint movement can indicate irregularities or degeneration of the joint surface (osteoarthritis).

Particulars

Has this happened before?
Has a family physician, orthopedic specialist, neurologist, physiotherapist, physical therapist, athletic therapist, athletic trainer, or other medical personnel treated the injury this time or previously?
Were x-rays taken?
What were the results?
Was treatment administered previously?
What medications, if any, were prescribed?
Any previous physiotherapy?
What was done?
Was it successful?

Repeated trauma or recurrences of the condition need to be noted, including the dates of injury, mechanism of injury, and length of disability. Common chronic problems of the wrist and hand include:
- scaphoid fractures
- wrist sprains
- DIP and PIP joint sprains

If the athlete has seen a physician or other medical personnel, their diagnosis, treatment, prescriptions, and recommended care should be recorded. All prescriptions and x-ray results should also be noted. It is important to record what treatment methods were effective in the past and which were ineffective.

OBSERVATIONS

The cervical spine, shoulder joint, thoracic outlet area, elbow joint, fore-

ASSESSMENT

INTERPRETATION

arm, wrist, and hand should be exposed as much as possible during the observations.

General Carriage and Movements

Observe the cervical and thoracic spine for problems.

Observe arm carriage during the athlete's gait (Fig. 5-17).

Observe the athlete for limb and hand function during clothing removal and the remainder of the assessment. Compare bilaterally the postural positions.

Excessive cervical lordosis, forward head, or cervical muscle spasm should be looked for and recorded. Any cervical or upper thoracic problems will make it necessary to rule out spinal pathology that might affect the whole quadrant.

During gait, the arm should swing comfortably from the shoulder joint with a relaxed elbow flexion and extension motion. The wrist and hand should be relaxed and move freely. Any injury to the wrist or hand will cause a decrease in the arm swing and, if the injury is severe, the athlete may support the forearm, wrist, and hand with his or her other hand.

Difficulty during fine motor movements while undoing belts or buttons should be noted.

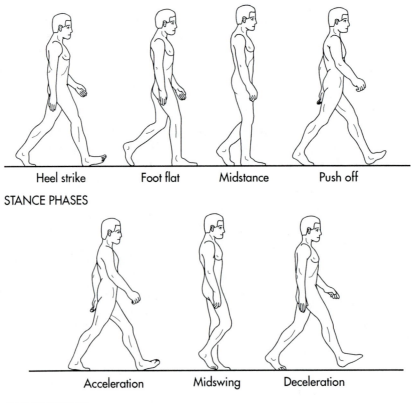

Heel strike   Foot flat   Midstance   Push off

STANCE PHASES

Acceleration   Midswing   Deceleration

SWING PHASES

Fig. 5-17 Gait.

ASSESSMENT

INTERPRETATION

Sitting or Standing

Anterior, Posterior, and Lateral Views
Cranial and Cervical Position
Excessive cervical lordosis—forward head
Cervical spine rotation or side bending

Excessive cervical lordosis in the mid and lower cervical spine with a forward head position leads to problems anywhere along the upper quadrant. This postural position closes the suboccipital space and thoracic outlet and can lead to neural dysfunction with referred or radiating pain into the upper limb, even the forearm, wrist, and hand. Cervical spine rotation and side bend may indicate:

- cervical disc protrusion or herniation
- facet joint dysfunction
- acute or chronic torticollis (wry neck)

A cervical disc protrusion or facet dysfunction can cause sensory and motor changes of the entire upper extremity, including the forearm, wrist, and hand in the involved myotome and/or dermatome.

Glenohumeral Joint Position
Level—Drop Shoulder
Anterior glenohumeral joint

Overdevelopment of one upper extremity due to repetitive overuse of one arm (as in tennis serve, pitching, and javelin throwing) will cause the entire shoulder complex to move forward and drop lower than the opposite extremity (Fig. 5-18). This anterior and drop position can lead to a reduced thoracic outlet and referred neural (brachial plexus) and circulatory (subclavian artery) problems of the involved extremity.

An anterior glenohumeral joint will develop tight adductors and medial rotators that can lead to joint impingement problems (i.e., subacromial bursitis, biceps tendonitis, supraspinatus tendonitis). These impinged structures can refer pain down the extremity into the forearm, wrist, and hand.

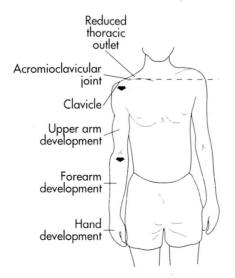

Fig. 5-18 Drop shoulder.

ASSESSMENT   INTERPRETATION

Acromioclavicular and Sternoclavicular Joint Position

Level

These joints should be symmetrical. Any previous acromio-clavicular or sternoclavicular sprains or separation can lead to upper extremity dysfunction, which will have an effect on the entire kinetic chain.

Thoracic Outlet

The thoracic outlet can be reduced by:
- tight pectoral fascia
- an extra scalene muscle
- an anterior and dropped glenohumeral joint
- clavicular callus
- cervical rib

It can cause neural (brachial plexus) or circulatory changes into the extremity (subclavian artery or vein).

Elbow Joint

Any elbow deformity (cubital valgus, cubital varus, or hyper-extension) or dysfunction will affect the humeroradial, humer-oulnar, or proximal radioulnar joints. These joints in turn affect the function of the distal radioulnar joint, the wrist, and the hand.

Forearm

Position
Muscle hypertrophy
Muscle atrophy
Deformity

Any injury to the radioulnar joint will cause it to rest in the midposition or in a position of slight pronation.

The athlete who plays racquet sports or indulges in any activity that requires long periods of gripping with one hand will develop hypertrophy of the forearm musculature and even of the boney development. This overdevelopment may also lead to an imbalance between the muscle groups and can result in epicondylitis or tendonitis in the weaker muscle group.

Any atrophy in the forearm muscle groups can be caused by:
- cervical spine dysfunction (C6, C7, and C8 myotomes)
- thoracic outlet motor involvement
- elbow medial, ulnar, or radial nerve involvement

The boney contour should be observed for deformity (Fig. 5-19); for example, a Colles fracture has a "dinner-fork deformity" (Fig. 5-20).

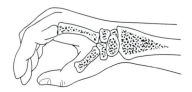

Fig. 5-19 Normal attitude of the hand.

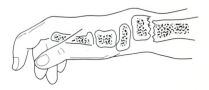

Fig. 5-20 "Dinner fork" deformity.

ASSESSMENT

INTERPRETATION

Wrist Joint
Effusion
Alignment

Any joint effusion will cause the wrist to flex at an angle of about 10°, with slight ulnar deviation. Soft-tissue swelling will be present on the dorsal aspect of the wrist and hand and may fill the anatomical snuffbox (e.g., scaphoid fracture). Problems of boney alignment can be seen with a subluxed lunate or capitate.

Hands
General attitude of the hand (see Fig. 5-19)
Muscle wasting
Thenar or hypothenar eminence
Vasomotor changes
Skin color
Loss of hair
Increased or decreased sweating
Temperature difference

The hands should be observed in their resting position—the dominant hand is usually larger.

Muscle wasting of the thenar eminence can be caused by a C6 nerve root problem; muscle-wasting of the hypothenar eminence can be caused by a C8 nerve root problem.

Wasting of the hypothenar muscles, interossei, and medial lumbricals is due to an ulnar nerve palsy (bishop's deformity). Wasting of the thenar muscles is due to a median nerve palsy (Fig. 5-21) and causes an ape hand appearance—the thumb moves back in line with the other fingers. The extension muscles pull the thumb back and it can not be flexed.

The hand will assume a clawed position if the intrinsic muscle action is lost and it is therefore overpowered by the extrinsic extensor muscles acting on the proximal phalanx of the fingers (Fig. 5-22). The hand will hang with the wrist dropped in the athlete who has a radial nerve palsy ("drop wrist"). The extensor muscles of the wrist are paralyzed and the wrist and fingers cannot be extended (Fig. 5-23).

Dupuytren's contracture is a contracture of the palmar aponeurosis, which pulls the fingers into flexion.

It is important to note any vasomotor changes or differences between the hands. If the hand has areas of redness or blanching, suspect a circulatory problem. Raynaud disease is an idiopathic vascular disorder where the blood vessels of the extremities can spasm, causing the finger(s) to become pale and numb, followed by vasodilation, which causes the part to become red and hot. This can be triggered by cold temperatures or emotions. Rheumatoid disease can cause a warm, wet hand, joint swelling, and ulnar deviation of the joints. Causalgic states can produce a swollen, hot hand. The entire skeleton of the hand enlarges with acromegaly.

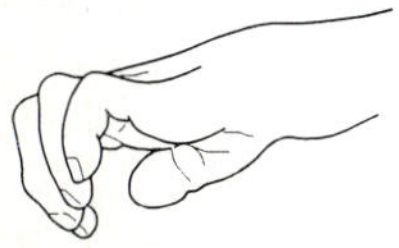

Fig. 5-21 Median nerve palsy. "Ape hand."

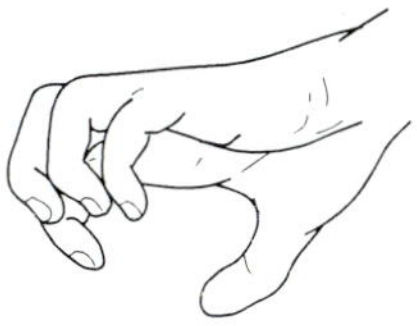

Fig. 5-22 "Claw hand."

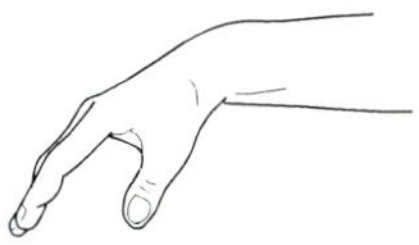

Fig. 5-23 "Drop wrist" radial nerve palsy.

ASSESSMENT   INTERPRETATION

Fingers
Shape, length and joint disturbances

NONTRAUMATIC ABNORMALITIES
Syndactylism
Clubbed fingers
Shortened digits
Spindle fingers
Swelling
Trigger finger
Heberden nodes
Bouchard nodes

Compare the fingers for shape (especially of the distal pha-
lange), length, and joint disturbances:
- Syndactylism (an extra finger) is an inherited trait.
- Clubbed fingers can be caused by pulmonary or coronary
  problems.
- Shortened digits can be caused by hormonal or inherited
  conditions.
- Spindle-like fingers can be caused by systemic disorders
  (e.g., lupus erythematosus, rubella, psoriasis, rheumatoid
  arthritis).
- Swelling of the distal phalanges with radiographic evidence of boney erosion, which occurs in psoriasis.
- Swelling of the finger joints is usually caused by
  osteoarthritis and rheumatoid arthritis.
- Trigger finger, which is thickening of the flexor tendon
  sheath, usually in the third or fourth finger, causes the tendon to stick when the finger is flexed. The tendon snaps
  back when released.
- Enlargement of the distal interphalangeal joints is called
  Heberden nodes and is seen in osteoarthritis.
- Enlargement of the proximal interphalangeal joints is
  called *Bouchard nodes* and is seen in rheumatoid arthritis
  and gastrectasis.

FINGER ABNORMALITIES—TRAUMATIC
Fractures or tendon problems
Mallet finger
Swan neck deformity
Boutonniere deformity

Observe the fingers and thumb for presence of fracture, dislocation, swelling, or discoloration.
- Mallet finger, which is flexion of the distal interphalangeal
  joint (see Fig. 5-4), is caused by an avulsion fracture or a
  tear of the distal extensor tendon from the distal phalanx.
- Swan neck deformity, which is flexion of the metacarpophalangeal joint and the distal interphalangeal joint and
  extension of the proximal interphalangeal joint, is caused
  by trauma with damage to the volar plate or by rheumatoid arthritis.
- Boutonniere deformity, which is extension of the metacarpophalangeal joint and the distal interphalangeal joint and
  flexion of the proximal interphalangeal joint, is usually
  caused by rupture of the central slip of the extensor tendon
  by trauma.

Finger Nails
NONTRAUMATIC ABNORMALITIES
Scaling
Clubbing

- Scaling, ridging, and deformity of the nails can be caused
  by psoriasis.

ASSESSMENT

INTERPRETATION

Ridging
Infection

- Clubbing and cyanosis of the nails is caused by chronic respiratory disorders or congenital heart disorders.
- Ridging and poorly developed nails occur in hyperthyroidism.
- Paronychia is the presence of a local infection beside the nail.

An infection of the nail tuft (felon) is very painful and can be serious.

Finger Nails
TRAUMATIC ABNORMALITIES
Depressions
Discoloration

- Depressions that form ridges in the nails are caused by avitaminosis or chronic alcoholism.
- A direct blow to the nail will cause bleeding under the nail and it will eventually turn black—this is called a subungual hematoma.

Skin
Lesions
Color
Texture
Hair patterns

Trophic changes of the skin are common in peripheral vascular disease, diabetes mellitus, reflex sympathetic dystrophy, and Raynaud disease.

SUMMARY OF TESTS

FUNCTIONAL TESTS

Rule Out
  Cervical spine
  Shoulder joint
  Thoracic outlet
  Brachial Plexus
  Elbow joint
  Systemic conditions
Forearm—Radioulnar joint
  Active radioulnar pronation
  Passive radioulnar pronation
  Resisted radioulnar pronation
  Active radioulnar supination
  Passive radioulnar supination
  Resisted radioulnar supination
Wrist Joint
  Active wrist flexion
  Passive wrist flexion
  Resisted wrist flexion
  Active wrist extension
  Passive wrist extension
  Resisted wrist extension
  Active wrist radial and ulnar deviation

ASSESSMENT   INTERPRETATION

Passive wrist radial and ulnar deviation
Resisted wrist radial and ulnar deviation
Hand
Active metacarpophalangeal flexion and extension
Passive metacarpophalangeal flexion and extension
Resisted metacarpophalangeal flexion and extension
Active DIP and PIP flexion and extension
Passive DIP and PIP flexion and extension
Resisted DIP and PIP flexion and extension
Active finger abduction and adduction
Resisted finger abduction and adduction
Thumb
Active thumb flexion and extension
Passive thumb flexion and extension
Resisted thumb flexion and extension
Active thumb abduction and adduction
Passive thumb abduction and adduction
Resisted thumb abduction and adduction
Active opposition of thumb and fifth finger
Resisted thumb and fifth finger opposition

SPECIAL TESTS

Finkelstein test
Tinel sign—median nerve
Phalen test
Carpal compression test
Sensation testing
Dermatomes
Circulatory testing
Allen test
Digital Allen test
Varus and valgus stresses to PIP and DIP joints
Thumb ulnar collateral ligament laxity test
Bunnel-Littler test
Grip tests
"O" test
Measurements

ACCESSORY MOVEMENT TESTS

Distal radioulnar joint
Dorsal and volar glide
Traction
Radiocarpal joint
Dorsal and volar glide
Ulnar glide
Radial glide

ASSESSMENT

INTERPRETATION

Midcarpal joint
  Traction
  Dorsal and volar glide
Metacarpophalangeal joint
  Distraction
  Dorsal and volar glide
  Side tilt
  Rotation
Interphalangeal joint
  Distraction
  Dorsal-volar glide
  Side tilt
  Rotation

Rule Out

Rule out problems of the cervical spine, shoulder joint, thoracic outlet, brachial plexus, and elbow joint with history taking, observations, and by performing the following functional tests.

Cervical Spine

Have the athlete perform active forward bending, side bending, back bending, and rotation. If these are clear, overpressures can be done.

If any of the active movements or overpressures indicate limitation and/or pain, a full cervical assessment is necessary to clear the cervical spine. There are cervical problems that refer pain to the forearm, wrist, and hand. For example:
- C6 nerve root injury can cause weakness or pain during radioulnar supination and resisted wrist extension
- C7 nerve root injury can cause weakness or pain during resisted wrist flexion
- a trigger point for cervical dysfunction often refers pain to the lateral epicondyle

Shoulder Joint

Have the athlete perform active forward flexion and abduction. Overpressures can then be performed.

If any of the active movements or overpressures indicate limitation and/or pain, a full shoulder assessment is necessary because:
- severe subacromial bursa can refer pain to the elbow or even into the forearm or hand
- injury to the humerus can refer pain along the involved sclerotome and into the elbow joint or forearm

Thoracic Outlet

(See test instructions under Elbow Assessment)

It may be necessary to clear the thoracic outlet with these tests because occluded blood vessels and compressed neural structures can cause pain and tingling down the extremity and often into the forearm and hand.

ASSESSMENT

INTERPRETATION

Adson Maneuver (see Figs. 3-21 and 3-22)

This test determines if a cervical rib or a reduced interscalene triangle is causing compression of the subclavian artery. The compression of the artery is determined by a decrease in or an absence of the radial pulse during the test.

Costoclavicular Syndrome Test

This test causes compression of the subclavian artery and vein by reducing the space between the clavicle and first rib. A modification or absence of the radial pulse indicates that a compression exists. Pain or tingling can also accompany a dampening of the pulse. If this test causes symptoms that are the athlete's major complaints, a compression problem is at fault. A dampening of the pulse may occur even in healthy athletes who do not have symptoms because they do not assume this position repeatedly or for long periods of time.

Hyperabduction Test (see Fig. 3-23)

Repeated or prolonged positions of hyperabduction can compress the structures in the outlet. Such overhead positions are often assumed in sleeping, in certain occupations (painting, chimney sweeping) and certain sports (volleyball spiking, tennis serving). The subclavian vessels can be compressed at two locations: (1) between the pectoralis minor tendon and the coracoid process or (2) between the clavicle and the first rib. Pain or a diminished pulse indicates that a compression exists.

Brachial Plexus

Have the athlete side bend the head away from the involved side, with the shoulder and elbow extended on the involved side (Fig. 5-24). This is intended to stretch the brachial plexus.

It is important to rule out brachial plexus involvement because it serves the entire upper limb and an injury to it can cause neural symptoms in the limb. With this test, the plexus is put on stretch and any brachial nerve damage will elicit discomfort to the involved nerve and sometimes throughout its distribution. Cervical facet joint problems can also refer pain during this test because the facet joints are compressed during side bending; cervical nerve root problems can also cause pain because of the reduction in the vertebral foramen caused by the cervical side bending.

Elbow Joint

Have the athlete perform active flexion and extension and then add overpressures.

If the active tests or overpressures indicate limitations and/or pain, a full elbow assessment is necessary because:
- The humeroradial and humeroulnar joints can cause dysfunction all the way into the radioulnar joints and the wrist.
- Pronator teres, the common flexor tendon, the extensor carpi radialis longus, and the common extensor tendon cross the elbow joint and also function at the forearm, wrist or hand; therefore an injury to these muscles can refer pain

ASSESSMENT

INTERPRETATION

along the myotome, and what might appear to be a wrist problem may originate at the elbow.
- Brachialis and triceps insert on the ulna; the biceps brachii inserts on the radius; therefore these muscles can influence the superior radioulnar joint and secondarily the inferior radioulnar joint or even the wrist and hand.

Systemic Conditions

Systemic disorders that influence the forearm, wrist, and hand must be ruled out with a thorough medical history, injury history, and observations of the athlete. A systemic disorder can exist with any or all of the following responses or findings:
- bilateral forearm, wrist, and hand pain and/or swelling
- several inflamed or painful joints
- the athlete's general health is not good, especially when the injury flares up
- repeated insidious onsets of the problem

The systemic disorders that can affect the forearm, wrist, and hand are the following:

Rheumatoid Arthritis

Rheumatoid arthritis often begins in the metacarpophalangeal joints or proximal interphalangeal joints, usually bilaterally. It never begins in the distal interphalangeal joints but osteoarthritis does, according to Cyriax. There is often involvement of the tendon and tendon sheath as well as joint involvement.

Psoriatic Arthritis

Psoriatic arthritis can cause widening and shortening of the distal phalanx of the thumb because of distal boney absorption.

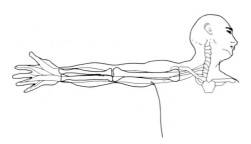

Fig. 5-24 Brachial plexus stretch.

ASSESSMENT

INTERPRETATION

Osteoarthritis

Osteoarthritis most often affects the weight-bearing joints but can also affect the distal interphalangeal joints of the fingers and the carpometacarpal joint of the thumb. Any individual joint of the hand can be effected if there is repeated trauma or stress to it (e.g., in archery, boxing, football). Osteoarthritis of the wrist can follow a severe injury or repeated trauma.

Gout

An acute gouty attack, according to Cyriax, can affect the flexor tendons of the wrist, resulting in a carpal tunnel syndrome. Chronic gout can affect all joints, especially those of the hand.

Neoplasm (Tumors)

Tumors can affect any joint and should be ruled out by x-ray, particularly if the bones themselves are tender.

Infections

Infections of the joints of the forearm and wrist are rare but they can occur more readily in the hand and finger joints. If infection does exist, there will be redness, heat, and often an abraded area nearby.

FOREARM—RADIOULNAR JOINT

Active Radioulnar Pronation (80° to 90°) (Fig. 5-25)

The athlete's forearms should rest on a plinth to prevent humeral movements.

The athlete has the elbow flexed and then turns the palm down from midposition so that the palm faces the floor.

The measurement may be more

Pain, weakness, or limitation of range of motion can come from the radioulnar pronators or their nerve supply.

The prime movers are:
- Pronator teres—median N (C6, C7)
- Pronator quadratus—median N (C7, C8, T1)

Pain may come from the radioulnar joint when there is a fractured radial head or a dislocation of the radius from the annular

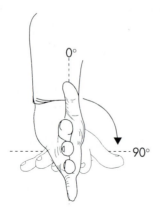

Fig. 5-25 Active radioulnar pronation.

ASSESSMENT

INTERPRETATION

observable if the athlete holds a pencil clasped in the hand parallel to the fingers during the movement and the therapist measures the pencil range.

ligament. Limitation of range of motion can come from dysfunction of the superior, middle, or inferior radioulnar joints. In a capsular pattern, both pronation and supination show pain and limitation at the extremes.

Passive Radioulnar Pronation (90°)

Grasp the athlete's distal forearm above the wrist joint with one hand and stabilize the elbow with the other hand. Pronate the forearm until the athlete's palm faces downward and an end feel is reached.

The end feel should be a tissue stretch. Pain or limitation of range of motion can be caused by:
- dorsal radioulnar ligament sprain or tear
- ulnar collateral ligament sprain or tear
- dorsal radiocarpal ligament sprain or tear
- fracture or osteoarthritis of the radial head
- biceps strain at the tenoperiosteal junction
- quadrate ligament sprain or tear at the proximal radioulnar joint
- interosseous ligament sprain
- triangular ligament sprain or tear (of the distal radioulnar joint)

Resisted Radioulnar Pronation

Stabilize the elbow joint to prevent shoulder abduction and internal rotation.

The resisting hand is placed against the volar surface of the distal end of the radius (use the entire hand and thenar eminence).

The fingers wrap around the ulna.

The athlete is asked to attempt forearm pronation from a midposition so that the palm turns downward.

Weakness or pain can come from the radioulnar pronators or their nerve supply (see Active Radioulnar Pronation).

A common cause of pain is a pronator teres injury at the medial epicondyle. If this is the cause, pain will be felt on resisted wrist flexion.

The pronator teres syndrome is caused by a compression of the median nerve. The nerve can be compressed:
- by the lacertus fibrosis (the band of fascia off the insertion of biceps brachii)
- by a supracondylar process
- between the two heads of pronator teres
- by the proximal arch of the flexor digitorum superficialis
Pronator quadratus is rarely involved.

Active Radioulnar Supination (90°) (Fig. 5-26)

The athlete's forearm should rest on a plinth to eliminate humeral movement.

The athlete has his or her elbow flexed and moves the forearm from midposition until the palm faces up.

Using a pencil to measure the range may be helpful, as described in Active Radioulnar Pronation.

Pain, weakness, or limitation of range of motion can come from the radioulnar supinators or their nerve supply.

The prime movers are the:
- Biceps brachii—musculocutaneous N. (C5, C6)
- Supinator—radial N. (C5, C6, and C7)
The limits of supination are determined by the degree to which the radius can rotate around the ulna. Damage to the radial head or the distal or proximal radioulnar articulation can limit the rotational range.

Passive Radioulnar Supination (90°)

As above, with stabilization at the elbow, supinate the distal forearm until the palm faces upward and an end feel is reached.

The end feel should be tissue stretch.

Pain or limitation of range of motion may be caused by:
- volar radioulnar ligament (the triangular ligament) sprain or tear

ASSESSMENT   INTERPRETATION

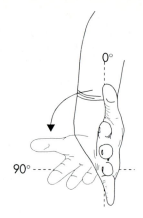

Fig. 5-26 Active radioulnar supination.

- annular ligament sprain or tear
- medial collateral ligament (anterior fibers) sprain or tear
- lateral collateral ligament (anterior fibers) sprain or tear
- pronator muscle strain or tear
- capsule sprain of the distal radioulnar joint

Resisted Radioulnar Supination

Stabilize the elbow at the athlete's side to prevent shoulder adduction and external rotation.

Your thenar eminence of the other hand is placed on the dorsal distal surface of the athlete's radius with the fingers wrapped on the ulna.

The athlete's forearm is in midposition. The athlete is asked to attempt to turn the forearm so that the palm faces upward while you resist the movement.

Pain or weakness can come from the radioulnar supinators or their nerve supply (see Active Radioulnar Supination).

Pain on resisted radioulnar supination and elbow flexion is evidence of a biceps brachii injury.

If supination is painful but elbow flexion is not, the supinator muscle is injured.

To help differentiate between a biceps injury and a supinator injury, you can test supination with the elbow extended, which minimizes involvement of the biceps.

WRIST JOINT

Active Wrist Flexion (80° to 90°) (Fig. 5-27)

The athlete is sitting with hands over the edge of the plinth.

The forearm must be supported and stabilized.

The forearm is in pronation.

The athlete flexes his or her wrist as far as possible.

Pain, weakness, or limitation of range of motion can come from the wrist flexors or from their nerve supply.

The prime movers are:
- Flexor carpi radialis—median N. (C6, C7)
- Flexor carpi ulnaris—ulnar N. (C8, T1)

The capsular pattern for the wrist is about the same limitation of flexion as of extension. Capsular pattern limitation and pain can be caused by:
- acutely sprained joint
- carpal fracture
- rheumatoid arthritis

ASSESSMENT   # INTERPRETATION

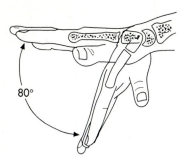

Fig. 5-27 Active wrist flexion.

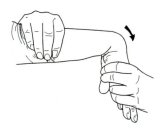

Fig. 5-28 Passive wrist flexion.

* osteoarthritis
* capsulitis

During flexion most movement occurs in the midcarpal joints (50°), while less occurs in the radiocarpal joint (35°).

Passive Wrist Flexion (90°) (Fig. 5-28)

Stabilize the athlete's distal radioulnar joint with one hand while the other hand grasps the metacarpals.

Move the athlete's wrist joint through the full range of wrist flexion until an end feel is reached.

The range of motion can be limited by an injury to the wrist extensors or to the dorsal radiocarpal ligament. If the ligament between the capitate and the third metacarpal ruptures, you can feel a depression at this point on full flexion. If the lunate-capitate ligament is sprained, pain is felt at the dorsum of the hand at the extreme of passive flexion and there is point tenderness over the ligament. Other ligament sprains are:

* radiolunate
* capitate-third metacarpal
* ulnar-triquetral

Point tenderness helps determine which ligament is involved.

Resisted Wrist Flexion

The athlete's forearm is in supination and resting on the plinth.

The athlete's elbow is extended and the fingers are flexed.

Resist at the athlete's hand while your other hand stabilizes the forearm (do not allow the elbow to flex).

The athlete attempts wrist flexion.

Weakness or pain can come from the wrist flexors or their nerve supply (see Active Wrist Flexion).

If the pain is felt in the lower forearm, the flexor tendons of the wrist and fingers can be at fault (resisted finger flexion and resisted radial and ulnar deviation will determine which tendon is involved). There may be point tenderness of the flexor digitorum profundus at 4 cm up from the wrist, the flexor carpi radialis down the whole distal extent of tendon (sometimes to the base of the second metacarpal), or flexor carpi ulnaris both proximal and distal to the pisiform.

Weakness on resisted wrist flexion and elbow extension indicates a C7 nerve root lesion.

A C8 lesion causes weakness in ulnar deviators also, so the hand deviates radially during resisted wrist flexion; thumb extension and abduction will also be weak.

ASSESSMENT

INTERPRETATION

Active Wrist Extension (70° to 90°)

The athlete is positioned in active wrist flexion. The athlete extends his or her wrist as far as possible.

Pain, weakness, or limitation of range of motion can come from the wrist extensors or from their nerve supply. The prime movers are:

- Extensor carpi radialis longus—radial N. (C6, C7)
- Extensor carpi radialis brevis—radial N. (C6, C7)
- Extensor carpi ulnaris—deep radial N. (C6, 7, C8)

An extensor muscle strain or tendonitis can cause pain and weakness. During extension, most movement occurs in the radiocarpal joints (50°) while less occurs in the midcarpal joints (35°).

Passive Wrist Extension (80° to 90°) (Fig. 5-29)

The athlete is positioned as above but you lift the metacarpals and move the wrist joint through the full range of wrist extension until an end feel is reached.

Range of motion can be limited by a wrist flexor lesion or a palmar radiocarpal ligament sprain or tear. Limitation of both passive flexion and extension is a capsular pattern and can suggest:

- carpal fracture
- rheumatoid arthritis
- osteoarthritis
- chronic immobility (from prolonged immobilization or joint effusion)
- synovitis

An acute scaphoid fracture is a common cause of pain and limitation during flexion and extension.

- the entire wrist is swollen
- there is a history of trauma
- the end feel is a hard muscle spasm
- there is pain when the carpals are pushed together or when pressure is put on the end of the thumb
- there is snuffbox pain

This is true of all wrist fractures but there are different locations for point tenderness.

Limitation of extension can be caused by the following:

- capitate subluxation
- Kienböck's disease (aseptic necrosis of lunate)
- ununited fracture (especially of the scaphoid)

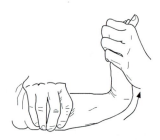

Fig. 5-29 Passive wrist extension.

Resisted Wrist Extension

The athlete's elbow is extended with the forearm pronated.

The wrist is in midposition with the fingers flexed.

Resist on the dorsum of the athlete's hand while the other hand stabilizes the athlete's forearm.

With the fingers flexed the extensor digitorum longus is not at a good mechanical advantage.

Weakness or pain suggests an injury to the wrist extensors or to their nerve supply (see Active Wrist Extension).

Pain with wrist extension usually comes from the wrist, seldom from the fingers (flexing the fingers rules out the finger extensors). Resisted radial and ulnar deviation will indicate which extensor is at fault.

Crepitus during extension can come from extensor digitorum, indicis tendonitis, or tenosynovitis.

There may be point tenderness at the insertion of the muscles. In the extensor carpi radialis longus, it occurs at the base of the

ASSESSMENT

INTERPRETATION

second metacarpal. In the extensor carpi ulnaris, it occurs at the base of the fifth metacarpal, between the triquetrum and the ulna or at the groove in the ulna. In the extensor carpi radialis brevis, it occurs at the base of the third metacarpal (tenoperiosteal).

Painless weakness could be due to the following:
- radial nerve palsy
- C6 cervical nerve root irritation (with elbow flexor weakness)
- C8 nerve root irritation (the extensor and flexor carpi ulnaris become weak, and when resisted wrist extension is tested, the hand deviates radially)

Active Wrist Radial (20°) and Ulnar Deviation (30°) (Fig. 5-30)

The athlete's forearm is supported on the plinth in pronation. The hand is extended.

The athlete is asked to move his or her wrist radially and ulnarly. The forearm must not move.

Ulnar deviation is greater than radial deviation because of the shortness of the ulnar styloid process.

Pain, weakness, or limitation of range of motion can come from the radial or ulnar deviators or from their nerve supply. The prime movers for radial deviation are:
- Flexor carpi radialis longus—median N, C6, C7
- Extensor carpi radialis longus—radial N, C6, C7
- Extensor carpi radialis brevis—radial N, C6, C7

The prime movers for ulnar deviation are:
- Extensor carpi ulnaris—deep radial N, C6, C7, C8
- Flexor carpi ulnaris—ulnar N, C8, T1

Passive Wrist Radial and Ulnar Deviation

The athlete is positioned as for Active Wrist Radial and Ulnar Deviation.

Carry the athlete's hand through full ulnar and radial deviation with one

Radial deviation limitation of range of motion or pain can come from:
- ulnar collateral ligament sprain (tear)
- fracture of styloid process of the ulna
- imperfect reduction of Colles fracture

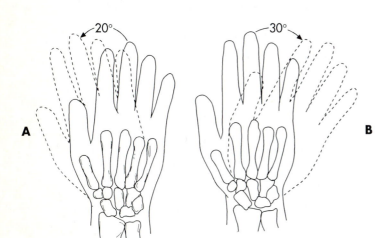

Fig. 5-30 A, Active wrist radial deviation. **B,** Active wrist ulnar deviation.

ASSESSMENT

hand while the athlete's forearm is stabilized with your other hand.

The athlete's hand is moved through the full range of motion until an end feel is reached.

Resisted Wrist Radial and Ulnar Deviation

The athlete's forearm should be supported and in pronation.

For ulnar deviation, resist the athlete's hand just below the ulnar styloid process while your other hand stabilizes the athlete's forearm.

For radial deviation, resist just distal to the radial styloid process of the athlete's hand.

HAND

Pain in the hand is very specific and usually results from local trauma or overuse. The athlete can usually tell if the hand pain is referred or local.

Active Metacarpophalangeal Flexion (90°) and Extension (20° to 30°) (Fig. 5-31)

The athlete's forearm and hand up to the metacarpophalangeal joints must be supported.

The athlete flexes and extends the fingers while keeping the PIP and DIP joints extended.

INTERPRETATION

Ulnar deviation limitation of range of motion or pain can come from:
- radial collateral ligament sprain (tear)
- tenosynovitis of thumb tendons (de Quervain's disease)

This tests the integrity of the radial or ulnar deviators and their nerve supply (see Active Radial and Ulnar Deviation). This test can be performed in combination with resisted flexion and extension to determine the exact muscle causing the problem.

Pain, weakness, or limitation of range of motion can be caused by an injury to the metacarpophalangeal flexors or extensors or to their nerve supply.

The flexion prime movers (90°) are:
- Lumbricals—median N, C6, C7; ulnar N, C8
- Interossei dorsales—ulnar N, C8, T1
- Interossei palmares—ulnar N, C8, T1

The extension prime movers (20° to 30°) are:
- Extensor digitorum communis—deep radial N, C6, C7, C8
- Extensor indicis—deep radial N, C6, C7, C8
- Extensor digiti minimi—deep radial N, C6, C7, C8

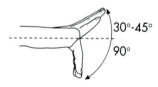

Fig. 5-31 Active metacarpophalangeal flexion and extension.

ASSESSMENT

INTERPRETATION

Passive Metacarpophalangeal Flexion (90°) and Extension (30° to 45°)

To test the metacarpophalangeal joints, the fingers should be tested individually and together.

Stabilize the hand being tested by gripping around the dorsal aspect of the athlete's hand (the athlete's thumb is tucked in).

Passively flex and extend the metacarpophalangeal joint only.

The athlete's fingers should hyperextend beyond their active range.

The athlete's index finger can hyperextend as much as 45°.

Passive flexion may be limited by an injury to the extensor tendons or to the dorsal ligaments. Injury to the collateral ligaments may cause pain during passive flexion also because these ligaments are taut in flexion.

Passive extension may be limited by a capsular injury, flexor tendon lesion, or sprains of the palmar or collateral ligaments. Any swelling within the joint will cause pain during these passive movements.

Resisted Metacarpophalangeal Flexion and Extension

You must stabilize the athlete's wrist in the neutral position. Your other hand resists just distal to the metacarpophalangeal joints for both flexion and extension.

An injury to the metacarpophalangeal flexors or extensors or to their nerve supply will cause weakness or pain (see Active Metacarpophalangeal Flexion and Extension).

Active DIP and PIP Flexion and Extension (Fig. 5-32)

The athlete clenches the fist tightly, then extends the fingers. Each finger should be tested separately if there is a problem with one of these joints.

To test just the flexor digitorum profundus, the proximal interphalangeal joint must be fully blocked from motion.

To test the flexor digitorum superficialis, the metacarpophalangeal joint must be fully blocked or stabilized.

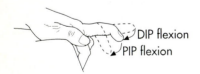

Fig. 5-32 Active distal and proximal interphalangeal flexion.

Flexion DIP (90°) and PIP (100°). Pain, weakness, or limitation of range of motion in active DIP and PIP flexion and extension can come from the DIP or PIP flexors or extensors or from their nerve supply. The prime movers for flexion are:
- Flexor digitorum superficialis—median N, C7, C8, T1
- Flexor digitorum profundus—ulnar N, C8, T1; median N, C8, T1

Extension DIP (0°) and PIP (-10°) with extension of the MP joints.

The prime movers for extension are:
- Extensor digitorum—radial N, C6, C7, C8
- Extensor indicis—radial N, C6, C7, C8
- Extensor digiti minimi—radial N, C6, C7, C8

With the pressure of a capsular pattern in the hands there is limitation of flexion and extension. A capsular pattern can be caused by:
- rheumatoid arthritis, which begins in the DIP joints with stiffness in the morning and progressing as nodules develop. The fingers will ultimately deviate ulnarly
- trauma to the joint from a direct contusion, indirect sprain, chip fracture, or reduced dislocation

If these traumatic injuries are suspected, active, passive, and resisted movements must all be done to rule out the existence of tendinous lesions.

A trigger finger consists of a nodular swelling in the flexor tendon (usually 3 or 4) that forms proximally to the MP joint.

ASSESSMENT

INTERPRETATION

When the finger is fully flexed, the nodule sticks within its sheath and the finger is fixed in that position. The athlete must pull the finger to allow extension again—this can occur to the thumb also.

In the case of a mallet finger the DIP joint remains flexed because the extensor tendon is ruptured at the base of the distal phalanx and the athlete is unable to actively extend the DIP joint.

A ruptured flexor tendon is rare but when it occurs the entire tendon coils into the palm—obviously active flexion is affected.

A flexor tendon laceration of the flexor digitorum profundus will result in the inability to flex the distal interphalangeal joint while the PIP joint is stabilized.

A laceration of the flexor digitorum superficialis will result in the inability to flex the proximal interphalangeal joint. To test for this laceration flexion of the proximal interphalangeal joint, test with the MP joint fully stabilized. If not stabilized adequately the laceration may be missed.

Dupuytren's contracture causes nodules in the palmar aponeurosis that limit finger extension and eventually can cause a flexion deformity, usually in the fourth and/or fifth fingers.

A boutonniere deformity is caused when the central slip of the extensor communis is avulsed from its insertion on the middle phalanx, the PIP joint is flexed, and the DIP joint is extended.

Passive DIP and PIP Flexion and Extension (Fig. 5-33)

You must isolate each joint. When moving the joints through full flexion and extension the surrounding joints must be stabilized.

Stabilize the PIP joint when testing the DIP joint.

Carry the joints through the full range of motion until an end feel is reached.

Be gentle if swelling around the joint is obvious.

The presence of limited passive extension in the PIP joint may mean that there is a tightness of or injury to the lumbricals or interossei. Limited passive PIP flexion or extension may be caused by:

- contracture in the joint capsule
- extensor tendon injury
- capsular swelling
- tightness in the flexors
- joint swelling
- volar plate damage
- collateral ligament sprain

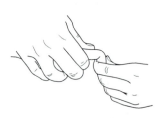

Fig. 5-33 Passive distal interphalangeal flexion.

ASSESSMENT   INTERPRETATION

Resisted DIP and PIP Flexion and Extension
Flexion
Ask the athlete to make a fist curling all fingers at the DIP and PIP joints.

Put your fingers against the athlete's finger pads and resist the flexion.

The athlete's forearm, wrist, and hand should be stabilized by letting them rest on the plinth.

Pain or weakness can originate from the DIP and PIP flexor and extensor muscles or from their nerve supply (see Active DIP and PIP Flexion and Extension).

Extension
Stabilize the athlete's wrist.

The athlete extends the MP joints. Apply resistance against the athlete's DIP and PIP joints (this test can be used to rule out the long finger extensor muscles).

Active Finger Abduction (Fig. 5-34) and Adduction (20°)
The athlete is asked to splay, then close his or her extended fingers. The movement is measured from the axial line of the hand.

The fingers should spread apart equally about 20°.

Pain, weakness, or limitation of range of motion can come from an injury to the finger abductors or adductors or to their nerve supply. The prime movers for abduction are:
- Interossei dorsales—ulnar N, C8, T1
- Abductor digiti minimi—ulnar N, C8, T1

Prime mover for adduction is:
- Interossei palmares—ulnar N, C8, T1

Resisted Finger Abduction (Fig. 5-35) and Adduction
Abduction
With the athlete's forearm supported, the athlete abducts his or her extended fingers.

Attempt to push each pair of fingers together.

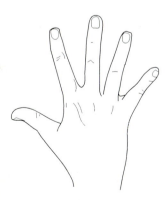

Fig. 5-34 Active finger abduction.

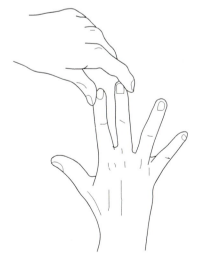

Fig. 5-35 Resisted finger abduction.

ASSESSMENT   INTERPRETATION

Adduction

Attempt to push pairs of fingers apart while the athlete attempts to prevent this.

Weakness and/or pain can come from the finger abductors or adductors or their nerve supply (see Active Finger Abduction and Adduction).

Painless weakness can come from a T1 nerve root irritation.

THUMB

No examination of the wrist is complete without ruling out the thumb. Arthritis, joint effusion, and tendonitis at the thumb can give rise to pain in the wrist.

Active Thumb Flexion and Extension (Fig. 5-36)

The athlete must move the thumb across the palm.

There is active flexion of the MP, IP joints of the thumb.

- MP flexion is 50°
- MP extension is 0°
- IP flexion is 90°
- IP extension is 20°

Pain, weakness, or limitation of range of motion can come from an injury to the thumb flexors or extensors or to their nerve supply. The prime movers for flexion are:

- Flexor pollicis brevis (MP flexion)—median N, C6, C7; ulnar N, C8, T1
- Flexor pollicis longus (MP and IP flexion)—median N, C8, T1

The prime movers for extension are the:

- Extensor pollicis longus (MP and IP extension)—deep radial N, C6, C7, C8
- Extensor pollicis brevis (MP extension)—deep radial N, C6, C7

Joint effusion can cause pain during the active ranges of flexion and extension.

Passive Thumb Flexion and Extension

Move the joint through full flexion and extension until an end feel is reached.

Passive flexion can be limited by the tension of the thumb extensors, joint effusion, or joint sprains (collaterals). Pain may be caused by de Quervain's disease.

Passive extension can be limited and painful because of:

- thumb flexor muscle injury
- damage to the anterior joint capsule
- osteoarthritis or rheumatoid arthritis
- scaphoid fracture

In chronic cases of ulnar collateral ligament sprains, there may be excessive extension at the metacarpophalangeal joint.

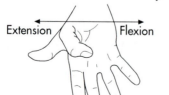

Fig. 5-36 Active thumb flexion and extension.

ASSESSMENT

INTERPRETATION

Resisted Thumb Flexion and Extension
Flexion—MP

The athlete flexes the proximal phalanx against your resistance. Stabilize the base of the first metacarpal with the other hand.

Flexion—IP

The athlete fully flexes the thumb. Hook your thumb around the athlete's thumb and attempt to straighten it.

Pain during thumb MP flexion is usually an injury to flexor pollicis brevis.

Weakness or pain can come from the thumb flexors or from their nerve supply (see Active Thumb Flexion).

Pain during thumb IP flexion is usually located in the flexor pollicis longus.

Trigger thumb is a swelling in the flexor pollicis tendon that may become engaged in the tendon sheath—the thumb has to be manually straightened by the other hand.

Extension—MP

The athlete extends the thumb at its proximal phalanx while you resist. Stabilize the base of the thumb with the other hand.

Extension—IP

The athlete attempts to extend the thumb against your resistance at the distal phalanx. Stabilize the MP joint of the thumb.

Weakness or pain can come from the thumb extensors or from their nerve supply (see Active Thumb Extension).

Pain with resisted extension can come from the extensors if they are strained or partially torn.

Pain can be elicited on extension and abduction if the athlete is suffering from de Quervain disease (abductor pollicis longus and extensor pollicis brevis tenosynovitis). Inflammation for this condition can occur in three places:
- level of the carpals
- insertion point of the abductor pollicis longus—at the base of the first metacarpal
- groove at the base of the radius

Weakness of thumb extension may also characterize a C7 disc herniation—there will also be weakness with ulnar deviation and adduction of the thumb.

Active Thumb Abduction (70°) and Adduction (30°) (Fig. 5-37)

The athlete lifts the thumb off the palm and then returns it to the palm.

Pain, weakness, or limitation of range of motion here can be caused by an injury to the thumb abductors or adductors or to their nerve supply.

The prime movers for abduction are:
- Abductor pollicis longus—deep radial N, C6, C7
- Abductor pollicis brevis—median N, C6, C7

The prime mover for adduction is:
- Adduction pollicis—ulnar N, C8, T1

ASSESSMENT   INTERPRETATION

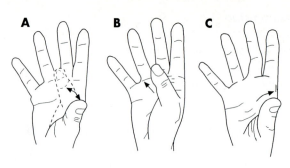

Fig. 5-37 A, Thumb abduction and adduction. **B,** Thumb adduction. **C,** Thumb abduction.

Passive Thumb Abduction (70°) and Adduction (30°)

Stabilize the thumb with one hand at the level of the anatomical snuffbox and the radial styloid process, and the other hand down the length of the first metacarpal. Move the thumb away from the palm and then back to the palm. In each case, the thumb is moved until an end feel is reached.

Passive abduction is limited by:
- first dorsal interossei muscle strain
- thumb capsule sprain
- ligament sprain
- joint involvement (i.e., articular cartilage problem)

These movements occur primarily at the carpometacarpal joint. A sprain, partial tear, or avulsion of the ulnar collateral ligament will cause pain with abduction. Laxity may be present here in the case of chronic ulnar collateral ligament sprains or if a Stenner lesion is present.

Resisted Thumb Abduction and Adduction

Abduction

Stabilize the four metacarpals and the wrist with one hand while the other hand resists the length of the thumb.

Adduction

Stabilize the four metacarpals and the wrist with one hand; the other hand resists the thumb as it adducts.

Any injury to the thumb abductors or adductors or to their nerve supply will elicit pain or weakness (see Active Thumb Abduction and Adduction). Pain could also be caused by de Quervain's disease.

Active Opposition of Thumb and Fifth Finger (Fig. 5-38)

The athlete opposes the thumb and fifth finger so that the pad of the thumb and the fifth finger come together.

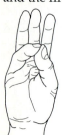

Fig. 5-38 Active thumb and fifth finger opposition.

Pain, weakness, or limitation of range of motion can come from the thumb opposers or from their nerve supply. The prime movers are:
- Opponens pollicis—median N, C6, C7
- Opponens digiti minimi—ulnar N, C8, T1

The abductor pollicis longus and brevis must then be used to return the thumb to its original position.

ASSESSMENT   INTERPRETATION

Resisted Thumb and Fifth Finger Opposition

The athlete opposes the thumb and little finger while you attempt to separate them.

Weakness or pain can come from the thumb opposers or from their nerve supply (see Active Opposition of Thumb and Fifth Finger).

SPECIAL TESTS

Finkelstein Test (de Quervain's Disease—Thumb) (Fig. 5-39)

The athlete makes a fist with the thumb flexed inside the hand. The athlete actively (or you passively) ulnar deviates the wrist. A positive test causes pain.

This tests for the presence of de Quervain's disease or tenosynovitis of the abductor pollicis longus and the extensor pollicis brevis in the first carpal tunnel.

Tinel Sign

Median Nerve

Whenever there are neural signs, you must rule out cervical disc lesion (C6), brachial plexus, and thoracic outlet. The Upper Limb Tension Test may be done to determine the origin of the neural problem along the entire quadrant. (See ULTT in Cervical and Shoulder Joint Assessment Sections)

Tap on the volar carpal ligament (carpal tunnels). A positive test causes tingling that spreads into the thumb, index finger, third finger, and lateral half of the ring finger (median nerve distribution).

This is a test of the median nerve and it is used to confirm that a carpal tunnel syndrome exists. Constriction in this tunnel puts pressure on the median nerve and can affect motor function and sensation in the hand. It can cause:
- thenar atrophy and a weak abductor pollicis brevis muscle
- diminished sweating along the median nerve distribution
- decreased sensation in the thumb, index finger, and half of the long finger palmarly

Some of the causes of carpal tunnel syndrome are:
- anterior dislocation of the lunate
- swelling secondary to Colles fracture (at the distal end of radius)
- synovitis secondary to rheumatoid arthritis (gout, rubella, pregnancy)
- general trauma to the area (sprains, contusions)
- overuse or repeated use of the hand in extension
- repeated trauma to the hand (as in karate, baseball, racquet sports)

Phalen Test (Median Nerve)

The athlete flexes his or her wrists to the maximum degree and holds them together that way for 1 minute. A posi-

This, like the Tinel Sign test, is another test for the carpal tunnel syndrome (or compression of the median nerve) (see Tinel sign for test results and causes).

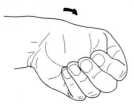

Fig. 5-39 Finkelstein test for de Quervain's disease.

ASSESSMENT   INTERPRETATION

tive test elicits tingling into the median nerve distribution of the hand.

Carpal Compression Test (Fig. 5-40)

Using both thumbs, the therapist applies direct pressure on the carpal tunnel and the underlying median nerve for as long as 30 seconds.

Durkan et al. found this test more accurate than the Tinel or Phalen tests in diagnosing a carpal tunnel syndrome. The onset of median nerve symptoms usually occur with 16 seconds of compression.

Sensation Testing (Neural Problems)

Problems of the cervical nerve roots or peripheral nerves may affect both muscular strength and sensation of the upper extremity. Major peripheral nerves and each neurological level should be tested. Use a sharp object to touch the areas of the skin supplied by the nerve or nerve root while the athlete looks away.

The athlete should comment on the sensation felt. Touch several points in each area. If the athlete does not report feeling a sharp sensation, other sensation tests should be done to test for warmth, cold, and pressure. Test bilaterally.

Peripheral Nerves (Fig. 5-41)
Radial Nerve

Apply pressure with a sharp object to the web between the thumb and index finger on the hand's dorsal sur-

The radial nerve serves the dorsum of the hand on the radial side of the third metacarpal, as well as the dorsum of the lower half of the thumb, index, and middle fingers. The web between

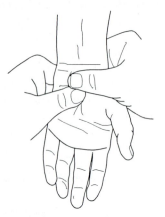

Fig. 5-40 Carpal compression test.

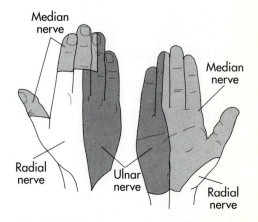

Fig. 5-41 Cutaneous nerves of the hand.

ASSESSMENT

face while the subject looks away. Compare bilaterally. The athlete should report feeling a sharp or dull sensation and report if the sensation is the same bilaterally.

INTERPRETATION

the thumb and index finger is supplied by the radial nerve and therefore a convenient location to test for normal sensation. Damage to this nerve will elicit paresthesia.

Radial nerve compressions can occur at the axilla (called "Saturday night palsy") or in the forearm with compression of the posterior interosseous nerve. The posterior interosseous nerve is the major branch of the radial nerve in the forearm. Impingement of the radial nerve at the axilla can cause:

- wrist drop
- loss of finger and thumb extension
- numbness at the first dorsal interspace

Posterior interosseous nerve compression causes:

- forearm pain (especially at night)
- pain along the nerve length
- aching with repetitive activity
- pain on supination and long finger extension

This impingement is often misdiagnosed as lateral epicondylitis (also called tennis elbow).

Compression of the posterior interosseous nerve can occur:

- as it passes between the two heads of the supinator muscle in the canal of Frohse (a fibrous arch in the supinator muscle)
- because of synovial proliferation from rheumatoid arthritis
- as a result of a radial head dislocation
- from a tumor, fibrous bands, or a ganglion at the humeroradial joint
- as a result of a fracture of the proximal radius
- from the fibrous border of extensor carpi radialis brevis

The radial nerve can also be compressed in the anatomical snuffbox at the wrist following a scaphoid fracture or wrist injury.

Median Nerve

Test the skin on the side of the index finger on the palmar surface with the pinprick method.

The median nerve supplies the radial portion of the palm and the palmar surface of the thumb, index, and middle fingers and may also supply the palmar skin on the tips of the index, middle, and half of the ring fingers.

Median nerve compression syndromes cause numbness and sometimes pain in the median nerve distribution. The compression may cause:

- diminished sudomotor activity (sweating) in its distribution
- a positive Phalen, Carpal Compression Test, and Tinel sign
- weakness and atrophy of the flexor pollicis longus, flexor digitorum profundus, and abductor pollicis brevis muscles

Compression of the median nerve can occur in the cubital fossa or just below by:

- the lacertus fibrosis (also called bicipital aponeurosis)
- the supracondylar process

ASSESSMENT

INTERPRETATION

- the ligament of Struthers (a ligament that runs from an abnormal boney spur on the shaft of the humerus to the medial epicondyle of the humerus)
- the pronator teres
- an arch in the proximal flexor digitorum superficialis

Compression of the median nerve can occur at the carpal tunnel by:

- a Colles fracture
- an anterior lunate dislocation
- tenosynovitis of the flexors
- fluid retention (as in pregnancy, rheumatoid arthritis, gout, and sepsis)
- severe forearm swelling
- overuse of the forearm musculature
- repeated trauma to the hand (as incurred during karate and racquet sports)

Ulnar Nerve

Test the skin on the lateral aspect of the little finger.

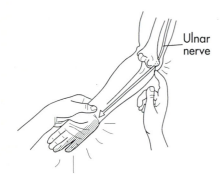

Ulnar nerve

Fig. 5-42 Ulnar nerve Tinel sign.

The ulnar nerve supplies the ulnar side of the hand (both dorsal and palmar aspects), half of the ring finger, and all of the little finger. Its area of purest sensation is the tip of the little finger and therefore is best tested here.

Ulnar nerve compression or overuse can cause pain and numbness along the ulnar nerve distribution. Ulnar nerve compression syndromes can originate at:

- the thoracic outlet
- the cubital tunnel
- the tunnel of Guyon
- between the heads of flexor carpi ulnaris (especially with elbow valgus stress in the throwing athlete)

Compression in the cubital tunnel (called cubital tunnel syndrome) can cause:

- pain and numbness down the forearm and into the hand (small and ring fingers)
- weakness and atrophy of the ulnar instrinsic muscles
- a positive Tinel sign of the ulnar nerve (Fig. 5-42)

Ulnar nerve compression at the tunnel of Guyon can cause:

- numbness of the small and ring fingers
- weakness of the abductor digit quinti
- weakness of the ulnar intrinsics (if the deep motor branch of the ulnar nerve is involved)

Compression in the tunnel of Guyon can occur from:

- repeated ulnar compression (i.e., while gripping bicycle handlebars, while playing baseball or racquet sport where the bat or racquet handle repeatedly hits this area)
- pisiform fracture
- hook of hamate fracture
- pisohamate ligament fibrosis
- a ganglion distal to the hook of hamate

ASSESSMENT

INTERPRETATION

Dermatomes (Fig. 5-43)

The dermatomes are tested. See illustration for dermatome locations.

These areas are affected when there is cervical nerve root impingement and can be verified by muscle testing (myotome testing).

Finger Paresthesia (adapted from Cyriax)

When the athlete explains the sensation of pins and needles or of numbness in the fingers it is important to determine which fingers and what aspect of the fingers are affected. These areas should be tested with a pin and with hot and cold objects to determine sensitivity.

According to Cyriax, paresthesia in the hand or fingers can be caused by a local neural injury or it can be referred from nerve or nerve root problems anywhere from the cervical spine, along any of the neural pathways right down to the hand.

Paresthesia in the thumb can come from:
- pressure on the digital nerve
- contusion of the median nerve—thenar branch as it crosses the trapezio-first metacarpal joint

Paresthesia in the thumb and index finger can come from:
- C5 disc lesion (C6 dermatome)

Paresthesia in the thumb, index, and middle finger can come from:
- C5 disc lesion (C6 dermatomes)
- thoracic outlet
- cervical rib

Paresthesia in the middle finger (volar and dorsal surfaces) can come from:
- C6 disc lesion (C7 dermatome)

Paresthesia in thumb, index, long, and half of ring finger (volar or palmar surface) can come from:
- median nerve compression (usually in carpal tunnel)

Paresthesia in proximal half of the thumb, index, and middle finger (dorsal surface) can come from:
- radial nerve compression

Paresthesia in all five digits (one or both hands) can come from:
- thoracic outlet
- central intervertebral disc protrusion
- circulatory problem

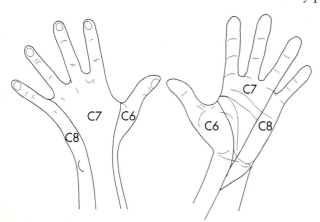

Fig. 5-43 Dermatomes of the hand (*Gray's Anatomy*).

ASSESSMENT   INTERPRETATION

Paresthesia in the ring and little finger (volar and dorsal) can come from:
- ulnar nerve compression (Tunnel of Guyon, cubital tunnel)
- C7 disc lesion (C8 dermatome)
- thoracic outlet

Pins and needles in all four limbs can occur with systemic disorders or disease. These include:
- diabetes
- pernicious anemia
- peripheral neuritis

Circulatory Testing

The radial artery pulse can be palpated proximal to the thumb on the palmar surface of the wrist (Fig. 5-44). The ulnar artery can be palpated proximal to the pisiform bone on the palmar surface of the wrist.

These pulses should be palpated, especially after a forearm or wrist fracture—any signs of a dampened or diminished pulse can indicate a circulatory occlusion or a circulatory problem. This indicates a medical emergency and the athlete should be transported to the nearest medical facility immediately.

Allen Test (Circulatory Problems) (Fig. 5-45)
Wrist

The athlete must open and close the fist quickly several times and then squeeze it tightly so that the venous return is forced out. Place the thumb over the radial artery and the index and middle finger over the ulnar artery and press against them to occlude them. The athlete then opens the hand (the palm should be pale). Release one artery. Arterial filling on the respective side can be observed as pressure is released from one artery at a time. The hand should flush immediately. Both arteries should be tested separately.

This test makes it possible to determine whether or not the radial and ulnar arteries are supplying the hand to their full capacities. When the arteries are released, the hand should flush immediately. If it flushes slowly, the artery is partially or completely occluded.

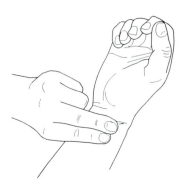

Fig. 5-44 Location for palpation of the radial pulse.

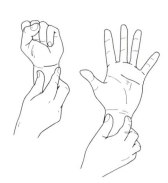

Fig. 5-45 Allen test.

ASSESSMENT

INTERPRETATION

Digital Allen Test

Instruct the patient to open and close the fist several times, then hold it tightly closed. Then occlude the digital arteries at the base of the finger on each side. The athlete then opens the fist (the finger should be pale). Each side of the finger is then released to see how quickly the finger flushes.

This test allows you to test the patency of the digital arteries.

Varus and Valgus Stresses to PIP and DIP Joints

Apply varus and valgus forces to the athlete's extended finger at the PIP and DIP joints.

These tests determine the integrity of the collateral ligaments and the capsule surrounding the joint. Pain will be elicited in the presence of a ligament or capsule sprain, subluxation, or dislocation. It is important to determine the laxity and degree of the opening and to compare bilaterally.

Thumb Ulnar Collateral Ligament Laxity Test (Metacarpophalangeal Joint)

With the athlete's thumb carpometacarpal joint in extension, stabilize the metacarpal by grasping it just proximal to the condyles of the metacarpal head.

Your other hand grasps the proximal phalanx with your thumb on the radial side opposite the joint line and your index finger on the ulnar side of the midshaft of the proximal phalanx.

Then place stress on the ulnar collateral ligament by pushing the athlete's phalanx radially with the index finger.

The joint is retested the same as above but the metacarpophalangeal joint is flexed fully.

According to Palmer and Lewis, when the thumb is fully extended there is normally 6° of laxity in the average joint. If there is as much as 30° of laxity then there is ulnar collateral ligament and volar plate damage.

When the metacarpophalangeal joint is flexed and the joint is still unstable, there is ulnar collateral damage. If there is no instability in full flexion, the ulnar collateral ligament is intact.

If there is no laxity in full flexion and more than 30° of laxity in full extension, there is damage only to the volar plate.

Bunnel-Littler Test

The metacarpophalangeal joint is held in slight extension while you flex the PIP joint. If the PIP joint cannot be flexed, the test is positive. If so, the test should be repeated with the metacarpophalangeal joint flexed.

If the PIP joint cannot be flexed, there is tight intrinsics or a tight joint capsule.

When the test is repeated with the MP joint slightly flexed, the PIP joint will flex fully if the intrinsics are tight, but if the capsule is tight, the PIP will still not flex fully.

Grip Tests (Reid)

Test these if you suspect a problem with the arches or fine-motor control of the hand.

These tests determine the integrity of the intrinsics, coordination of the muscles, and manual dexterity of the athlete. The

ASSESSMENT

INTERPRETATION

Hook grasp (briefcase; no use of thumb; Fig. 5-46)

Cylindrical grasp (bottle; Fig. 5-47)

Fist grasp (use of thumb, as when holding a tennis racquet; Fig. 5-48)

Spherical grasp (around ball; Fig. 5-49)

Palmar prehension—pinch thumb, index, middle finger, pulp to pulp (allows writing hand position; Fig. 5-50)

Lateral prehension (grasp card—with thumb pad against radial border of the first phalanx of index finger; Fig. 5-51)

Tip prehension—thumb and tip of other digit (as when picking up a pin; Fig 5-52)

muscles, ligaments, and joints must work harmoniously to allow these grips.

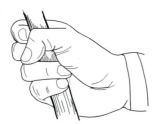

Fig. 5-46 Hook grasp.

Fig. 5-47 Cylindrical grasp.

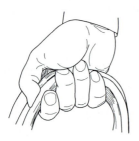

Fig. 5-48 Fist grasp.

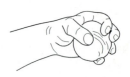

Fig. 5-49 Spherical grasp.

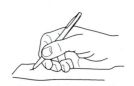

Fig. 5-50 Palmar prehension.

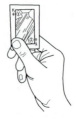

Fig. 5-51 Lateral prehension.

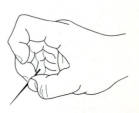

Fig. 5-52 Tip prehension.

ASSESSMENT

INTERPRETATION

"O" Test

The athlete attempts to make an "O" with his or her thumb and index finger.

Inability to make the "O" shape indicates anterior interosseous nerve syndrome. This nerve divides from the median nerve 4 to 6 cm below the cubital fossa and can be impinged by:

- tendinous bands or pronator teres, flexor digitorum superficialis, or flexor carpi radialis
- thrombosis of the ulnar collateral vessels or the aberrant radial artery
- an enlarged bicipital bursa
- forearm fracture

Inability to make the "O" shape is caused by paralysis of flexor pollicis longus, the pronator quadratus, and the flexor digitorum profundus to the index finger.

Measurements (as described by Fess et al.)

Measurements with a tape measure are made:

- 7 cm proximal to the elbow flexion crease (upper arm)
- 11 cm proximal to the distal wrist flexion crease (forearm)
- at the wrist flexion crease (wrist)
- at the distal palmar flexion crease of the hand

These measurements are done to determine if there is any muscle atrophy, hypertrophy, or swelling.

Atrophy can be caused by:
- disuse (e.g., post cast)
- cervical nerve root compression
- local nerve damage
- thoracic outlet syndrome

Hypertrophy can be caused by overuse of the muscles of that area. Swelling can be caused by:
- trauma
- arthritis
- body water retention

ACCESSORY MOVEMENT TESTS

Distal Radioulnar Joint
Dorsal and Volar (Palmar) Glide (Fig. 5-53)

The athlete rests his or her forearm on the plinth in a slightly supinated position. Stabilize the distal radius with your thumb on the palmer surface and your fingers on the dorsal aspect of the radius. Then move the ulna dorsally and volarly.

These dorsal and volar glides are necessary for full pronation and supination.
- dorsal glide increases supination
- volar glide increases pronation

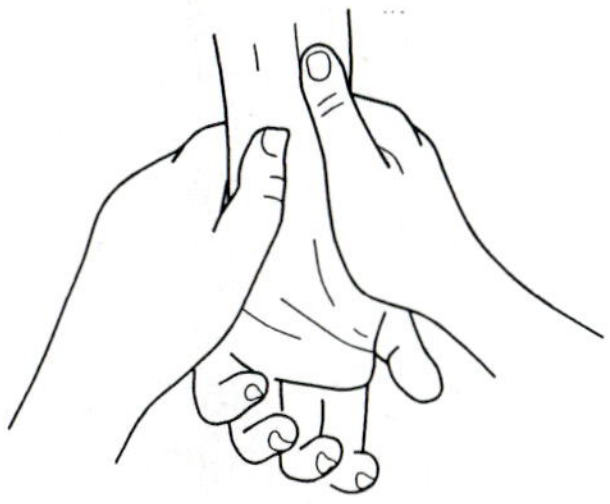

Fig. 5-53 Distal radioulnar joint dorsal glide—volar glide.

ASSESSMENT

INTERPRETATION

Traction (Including Ulnomeniscocarpal Joint) (Fig. 5-54)

The elbow is flexed at an angle of 90°, the forearm is in neutral, and the wrist is in slight ulnar deviation over the edge of the plinth.

A rolled towel can help stabilize the ulna and radius. Place the stabilizing hand over the distal radius and ulna around the styloid process.

Your other hand grasps the athlete's proximal row of carpals distal to the styloid process. Traction is gently applied to the joint to determine the amount of hypomobility or hypermobility that is present.

Hypomobility in the radiocarpal joint will cause a decreased amount of wrist extension.

Hypermobility may indicate radiocarpal joint laxity, which may be due to a ligament or capsular sprain or tear. Traction occurs to the joint naturally with wrist flexion.

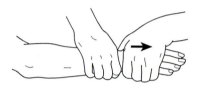

Fig. 5-54 Radiocarpal joint traction.

Radiocarpal Joint

Dorsal and Volar (Palmar) Glide (Fig. 5-55 and 5-56)

The athlete's elbow is flexed with his or her forearm pronated and hand over the edge of the plinth.

Grasp the distal end of the radius and ulna just proximal to the styloid processes.

With slight traction on the joint, gently move the carpals dorsally and volarly to determine the amount of joint play that is present.

Dorsal glide is needed for full wrist flexion and palmar glide is needed for full wrist extension.

Ulnar Guide (Fig. 5-57)

With the athlete's elbow flexed and forearm in neutral with the thumbs upward, place one hand just proximal to the styloid processes. With your other hand, grasp the proximal row of carpals on the volar aspect and glide them gently ulnarly.

Ulnar glide is needed for full radial deviation.

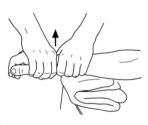

Fig. 5-55 Radiocarpal joint dorsal glide.

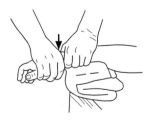

Fig. 5-56 Radiocarpal joint volar glide.

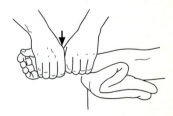

Fig. 5-57 Radiocarpal joint ulnar glide.

ASSESSMENT

INTERPRETATION

Radial Glide (Fig. 5-58)

The athlete should be in the same position as for the radiocarpal joint ulnar glide test but with his or her thumb down. Stabilize with one hand on the forearm proximal to the styloid processes.

The mobilizing hand is on the dorsal aspect of the athlete's hand over the proximal row of carpals. With slight traction, gently glide the carpals radially.

Radial glide is needed for full ulnar deviation.

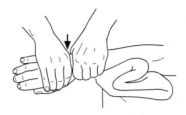

Fig. 5-58 Radiocarpal joint radial glide.

Midcarpal Joint

Traction

This traction is applied with the same hand placements and limb positions as for the radiocarpal joint but you apply traction on the distal row of carpals and stabilize the proximal row of carpals.

Hypomobility in the midcarpal joint will cause a decrease in wrist flexion. Hypermobility may indicate midcarpal joint laxity that may be due to a ligamentous or capsule sprain or tear.

Dorsal and Volar (Palmar) Glide

This technique is similar to the radiocarpal joint glides except you stabilize the proximal row of carpals with one hand and attempt to move the distal row dorsally and volarly.

Dorsal glide is needed for full wrist flexion. Volar (palmar) glide is needed for full wrist extension.

Metacarpophalangeal Joint

Distraction (Fig. 5-59)

Hold the head of the metacarpal bone between your thumb and index finger with one hand while your other hand grasps the shaft of the proximal phalanx with the joint in slight flexion.

Then distract the base of the phalanx away from the head of the metacarpal until an end feel is reached.

Full joint play in the MP joints is necessary for a normal palmar arch and for finger function. Distraction is necessary for full MP extension.

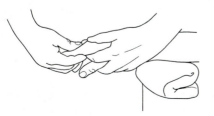

Fig. 5-59 Metacarpophalangeal joint distraction (traction).

ASSESSMENT

INTERPRETATION

Dorsal and Volar Glide (Fig. 5-60)

Grasp the metacarpal head and proximal phalanx as for the previous test. With the finger in slight flexion (10°) the tips of the thumb and index finger hold the base of the proximal phalanx. Stabilize the metacarpal head with one hand while moving the base of the phalanx dorsally and volarly.

Dorsal glide is necessary for full MP joint extension. Volar glide is necessary for full MP flexion.

Side Tilt (Ulnar-Radial Tilt) (Fig. 5-61)

Stabilize the metacarpal head as above and place the thumb and index finger on the medial and lateral sides of the proximal phalanx just distal to its base.

Open the joint ulnarly and radially with pressure from the thumb and index finger respectively.

Ulnar tilt is necessary for full MP joint extension. Radial tilt is necessary for full MP joint flexion.

Rotation (Fig. 5-62)

Stabilize the head of the metacarpal bone with one hand and slightly flex the proximal and distal interphalangeal joints with the other hand.

Your thumb and index finger grasp the proximal phalanx at the distal end and your remaining fingers grasp the semiflexed finger. Then rotate the phalanx clockwise and counterclockwise through its long axis.

Clockwise movement is necessary for full MP flexion and counterclockwise movement is necessary for full MP extension.

Interphalangeal Joint

Distraction, Dorsal-Volar Glide, Side Tilt, and Rotation

All of these joint-play movements occur in the interphalangeal joints as in the metacarpophalangeal joints. The

As above, the joint-play movements are important for full flexion and extension of the interphalangeal joints. Full IP flexion needs volar glide, radial tilt, and rotation. Full IP

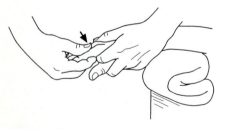

Fig. 5-60 Metacarpophalangeal joint volar glide.

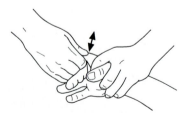

Fig. 5-61 Metacarpophalangeal joint side tilt (ulnar-radial tilt).

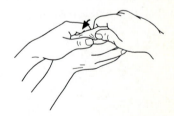

Fig. 5-62 Metacarpophalangeal joint rotation.

ASSESSMENT	INTERPRETATION

only difference in hand placements involve stabilizing the head of the proximal phalanx and moving the distal phalanx.

extension needs joint distraction, dorsal glide, ulnar tilt, and rotation.

PALPATION

Palpate for point tenderness, temperature differences, swelling, adhesion, calcium deposits, muscle spasm, and muscle tears. Palpate for muscle tenderness, lesions, and trigger points.

According to Janet Travell, trigger points in muscle are activated directly by overuse, overload, trauma, or chilling and are activated indirectly by visceral disease, other trigger points, arthritic joints or emotional distress. Myofascial pain is referred from trigger points that have patterns and locations for each muscle. A myofascial trigger point is a hyperactive spot, usually in a skeletal muscle or in the muscle's fascia, that is acutely tender on palpation and evokes a muscle twitch. These points can evoke autonomic responses (e.g., sweating, pilomotor activity, local vasoconstriction).

Dorsal Aspect (with forearm pronated)

Forearm
Boney
RADIAL HEAD

Acute point tenderness is present in the case of radial head fracture or dislocation (pulled elbow).

PROXIMAL (SUPERIOR) RADIOULNAR JOINT

A sprain of the proximal (superior) radioulnar joint would be painful but this is rare.

DISTAL (INFERIOR) RADIOULNAR JOINT

This joint can be sprained, subluxed, or dislocated. Dislocation of the distal ulna occurs dorsally or volarly and causes pain on rotation.

Soft Tissue
BRACHIORADIALIS

The brachioradialis functions largely at the elbow and is not injured very often. There are trigger points in the deep part of the muscle that can evoke pain, primarily to the wrist and to the dorsal web between the thumb and index finger.

COMMON EXTENSOR ORIGIN

Point tenderness from the lateral epicondyle or one of the extensor tendons is very common here (tennis elbow).

EXTENSOR CARPI RADIALIS LONGUS

Overuse tendonitis makes this tendon point-tender just distal to its origin. Trigger points from this muscle can refer pain and

ASSESSMENT

INTERPRETATION

tenderness to the lateral epicondyle and dorsum of the hand (anatomical snuffbox area).

EXTENSOR CARPI RADIALIS BREVIS

This is the most common site for tendonitis or tenoperiosteal problems caused by overuse of the wrist extensors (also called "tennis elbow"). Trigger points in the muscle can refer pain to the back of the hand and wrist.

EXTENSOR CARPI ULNARIS

This muscle is injured less often but can be strained. Its trigger points refer pain to the ulnar side of the wrist.

EXTENSOR DIGITORUM

This muscle is rarely injured—pain can be referred from myofascial trigger points in the muscle down the forearm, back of the hand, and fingers.

EXTENSOR DIGITI MINIMI

This muscle is rarely injured.

EXTENSOR INDICIS

This muscle is rarely injured. Trigger points in the muscle can refer pain along its course distally.

EXTENSOR POLLICIS LONGUS AND BREVIS

These muscles are rarely injured but they are occasionally strained or contused.

ABDUCTOR POLLICIS LONGUS AND EXTENSOR POLLICIS BREVIS

These muscles can be inflamed where their muscle bellies cross (extensor intersection syndrome).

Wrist
Boney
STYLOID PROCESS OF THE RADIUS

The styloid process, which is the attachment for the lateral ligaments, of the radius can be fractured or avulsed.

DORSAL RADIAL TUBERCLE

If the radial dorsal tubercle is abnormal in contour, suspect a Colles fracture.

HEAD OF THE ULNA

The head of the ulna can be contused.

STYLOID PROCESS OF THE ULNA

The styloid process of the ulna can be avulsed or fractured.

ASSESSMENT

INTERPRETATION

CAPITATE CARPAL BONE

The capitate articulates with the base of the third metacarpal and is palpable on the dorsal surface of the wrist. A subluxing capitate allows the bone to shift upward during wrist flexion.

LUNATE CARPAL BONE

The lunate just proximal to the capitate will be tender if it subluxes, dislocates, or if Kienböck's disease is present.

Tissue
ABDUCTOR POLLICUS LONGUS

The abductor pollicis longus and extensor pollicis brevis muscles run through the first compartment of the wrist. A tenosynovitis or trauma to this compartment can cause de Quervain's disease and point tenderness here. This is quite common.

ANATOMICAL SNUFFBOX

Point tenderness in the anatomical snuffbox occurs with a scaphoid (navicular) fracture.

BRACHIORADIALIS

A brachioradialis strain at the insertion will be point tender.

EXTENSOR CARPI RADIALIS LONGUS, BREVIS, AND ULNARIS

The extensor carpi radialis longus, brevis, or ulnaris muscles can be strained or can develop tenosynovitis, although this is rare.

EXTENSOR POLLICIS LONGUS

The extensor pollicis longus can be ruptured from a Colles fracture or inflamed as it passes over the Lister tubercle of the distal radius.

ULNAR COLLATERAL LIGAMENT

The ulnar collateral ligament can be sprained, torn, or avulsed where it inserts into the styloid process.

ARTICULAR DISC

The fibrocartilaginous disc can be torn, causing point tenderness between the head of the ulna, the lunate bone, or the triquetrum. This disc acts as a shock absorber between the lunate and triquetrum, as well as a joint stabilizer. It is torn with overpronation or supination with joint compression.

EXTENSOR TENDONS

The extensor retinaculum can adhere to the extensor tendons following a severe sprain or fracture.

ASSESSMENT

INTERPRETATION

EXTENSOR CARPAL TUNNELS

Deep to the extensor retinaculum are six tunnels for the passage of the extensor tendons, each containing a synovial sheath. Overuse or direct trauma can affect any of these tunnels. The tunnels contain the following tendons:
- Tunnel 1—abductor pollicis longus, extensor pollicis brevis
- Tunnel 2—extensor carpi radialis longus, extensor carpi radialis brevis
- Tunnel 3—extensor pollicis longus
- Tunnel 4—extensor digitorum (Fig. 5-63), extensor indicis
- Tunnel 5—extensor digiti minimi
- Tunnel 6—extensor carpi ulnaris

GANGLION

A ganglion (a pea-sized swelling under the connective tissue) can develop on the dorsum of the wrist and sometimes between the heads of the second and third metacarpal bones. It may be quite firm according to the amount of fluid in it.

Hand
Boney
METACARPALS AND PHALANGES

The metacarpals or phalanges can be fractured—fractures of the head of the fifth metacarpal (boxer's fracture) and the base of the first are common in sports.

Soft Tissue
EXTENSOR DIGITORUM

The extensor digitorum crosses the dorsum of the hand where tendonitis can develop. The extensor tendon can be avulsed from the proximal, middle, or distal phalanx.

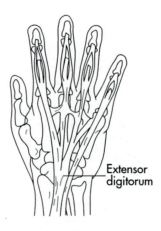

Fig. 5-63 Dorsal aspect of the hand—extensor digitorum muscle.

ASSESSMENT   INTERPRETATION

Palmar (Volar) Aspect (Fig. 5-64)

Forearm
Soft Tissue
PRONATOR TERES

Pronator teres syndrome is an impingement of the median nerve, resulting in sensory and motor loss. The flexor carpi radialis, palmaris longus, and flexor digitorum muscles can be affected. The trigger points refer pain deeply into the forearm and wrist on the radial palmar surface.

FLEXOR CARPI ULNARIS

The flexor carpi ulnaris refers pain and tenderness to the ulnar palmar surface of the wrist with a trigger point at the midbelly location.

FLEXOR DIGITORUM SUPERFICIALIS AND PROFUNDUS

The flexor digitorum superficialis and profundus can refer pain down the muscle fibers that they activate—the trigger points are at the midbelly location.

FLEXOR CARPI RADIALIS

The flexor carpi radialis can refer pain to the radial aspect of the wrist crease and can extend into the hand—its trigger point is also at the midbelly location.

FLEXOR POLLICIS LONGUS

The flexor pollicis longus can refer pain along the palmar aspect of the thumb and has a midbelly trigger point.

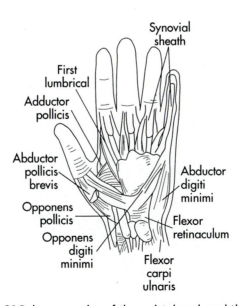

Fig. 5-64 Palmar muscles of the wrist, hand, and thumb.

ASSESSMENT   INTERPRETATION

PALMARIS LONGUS

> The palmaris longus can refer a prickling pain into the palm of the hand mainly, with some pain in the distal forearm. Its trigger point is in the midbelly location.

Wrist
Boney (Fig. 5-65)
TRAPEZOID, TRAPEZIUM, TRIQUETRUM, PISIFORM, AND CAPITATE

> The trapezoid, trapezium, triquetrum, pisiform, and capitate should be gently palpated for fracture, displacement, or point tenderness.

SCAPHOID

> The base of the first metacarpal should be palpated for swelling and point tenderness if a scaphoid fracture or a radial collateral ligament injury is suspected.

HOOK OF HAMATE

> The hook of the hamate forms the lateral border of the tunnel of Guyon, which houses the ulnar nerve and artery. A fracture or severe contusion to the hook can affect the structures in the tunnel.

Soft Tissue
FLEXOR CARPI ULNARIS

> The flexor carpi ulnaris is attached to the pisometacarpal ligament while the abductor digiti minimi and the extensor retinaculum are attached to the pisiform bone. An injury to any of these structures can cause point tenderness in all three.

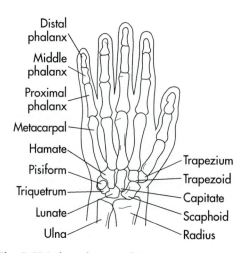

Fig. 5-65 Palmar bones of the wrist and hand.

ASSESSMENT

INTERPRETATION

ULNAR ARTERY

The ulnar artery can be palpated proximal to the pisiform and medial to the flexor carpi ulnaris. Any circulatory problems should be investigated further.

SYNOVIAL SHEATHS

Two synovial sheaths envelop the flexor tendons as they cross the carpal tunnel. One is for the flexor digitorum superficialis and profundus and one is for the flexor pollicis longus. Trauma or inflammation of either sheath can cause tenosynovitis.

PALMARIS LONGUS

The palmaris longus can be strained; it is absent in 7% of the population.

CARPAL TUNNEL

The carpal tunnel lies deep to palmaris longus and is bounded by four boney landmarks (the pisiform, the hook of hamate, the tubercle of scaphoid, and the tubercle of trapezium). The tunnel's upper boundary is the transverse carpal ligament; its lower border is the carpals. If the tunnel space is reduced, the median nerve is compressed and sometimes the flexors are affected.

Some common causes of carpal tunnel problems are:
- direct trauma
- Colles fracture
- lunate anterior dislocation
- synovitis
- rheumatoid arthritis
- systemic disorders, which cause joint swelling

GANGLION

A ganglion may form on the palm distal to the hamate bone; if it enlarges significantly it can compress the ulnar nerve.

Hand (see Fig. 5-65)
Boney
METACARPALS AND PHALANGES

The metacarpals and phalanges can be fractured or dislocated and local point tenderness will indicate the problem site.

Soft Tissue
PALMAR FASCIA

Point tenderness of the palmar fascia associated with tightness or nodules can be caused by Dupuytren's contracture—the ring and little finger are most often involved.

ASSESSMENT

INTERPRETATION

MUSCLES OF THE HAND AND THUMB

A

B

Fig. 5-66 A, Infection of the nail tuft (felon). **B,** Paronychia.

The hand and thumb muscles can be contused or strained and the location of point tenderness will indicate the site of the lesion.

Tenderness and a palpable lump at the level of the metacarpophalangeal joint after a severe ulnar collateral ligament tear can be a Stenner lesion, in which the adductor aponeurosis becomes trapped between the torn ends of the ulnar collateral ligament.

The fingers are very susceptible to injury and infection. In the pulp of the distal phalanx, infection can settle and remain confined to this area by the strong fibrous septa—this is called a felon (Fig. 5-66, *A*). Inflammation or infection will increase the temperature of the skin in the involved area and can spread along the flexor tendons. An infection beside the finger nail (paronychia) is common (Fig. 5-66, *B*).

Infection of the sheath around the thumb or fifth digit is more serious because these digits communicate with the principal sheath around the flexors and may cause the inflammation to extend into the palm or into the flexor retinaculum in the forearm.

BIBLIOGRAPHY

Anderson JE: Grant's Atlas of anatomy, Baltimore, 1983, Williams & Wilkins.

APTA Orthopaedic Section Review for Advanced Orthopaedic Competencies Conference, Carol Waggly, David Labosky. Chicago, Aug 10, 1989.

Booher JM and Thibodeau GA: Athletic injury assessment, Toronto, 1985, Times Mirror/Mosby College Publishing.

Brand WP and Hollister A: Clinical mechanics of the hand, ed 2, St Louis, 1993.

Carr D et al: Upper extremity injuries in skiing, Am J Sports Med 9(6):378, 1981.

Collins K et al: Nerve injuries in athletes, Physician and Sportsmedicine pp. 16(1):92, 1988.

Cyriax J: Textbook of orthopedic medicine: diagnosis of soft tissue lesions, vol 1, London, 1978, Bailliere Tindall.

Dangles C and Bilos Z: Ulnar nerve neuritis in a world champion weightlifter, Am J Sports Med 8(6):443, 1980.

Daniels L and Worthingham C: Muscle testing: techniques of manual examination, Toronto, 1980, WB Saunders.

Degroot H and Mass D: Hand injury patterns in softball players using a 16-inch ball, Am J Sports Med 16(3):260, 1988.

Dobyns J et al: Sports stress syndromes of the hand and wrist, Am J Sports Med 6(5):236, 1978.

Durkan JA: A new diagnostic test for carpal tunnel syndrome, The Journal of Bone and Joint Surgery Vol 73-A, #4, 535 April 1991.

Fess EE et al: Evaluation of the hand by objective measurement: rehabilitation of the hand, St Louis, 1978, The CV Mosby Co.

Gould JA and Davis GJ: Orthopaedic and sports physical therapy, Toronto, 1985, The CV Mosby Co.

Haycock C: Hand, wrist, and forearm injuries in baseball, Physician Sports Med 7(7):67, 1979.

Hoppenfeld S: Physical examination of the spine and extremities, New York, 1976, Appleton-Century Crofts.

Itoh Y et al: Circulatory disturbances in the throwing hand of baseball pitchers, Am J Sports Med 15(3):264, 1987.

Jupiter J: Current concepts review. Fractures of the distal end of the radius, the Journal of Bone and Joint Surgery 73-A, 3, 461, March 1991.

Kaltenborn F: Mobilization of the extremity joints, ed 3, Oslo, 1980, Olaf Norlis Bokhandel.

Kapandji IA: The physiology of the joints, vol 1, Upper limb, New York, 1983, Churchill Livingstone Inc.

Kendall FP and McCreary EK: Muscles testing and function, Baltimore, 1983, Williams & Wilkins.

Kessler RM and Hertling D: Management of common musculo-skeletal disorders, Philadelphia, 1983, Harper and Row.

Kisner C and Colby L: Therapeutic exercise foundations and techniques, Philadelphia, 1987, FA Davis Co.

Klafs CE and Arnheim DD: Modern principles of athletic training, ed 5, St Louis, 1981, The CV Mosby Co.

Kulund D: The injured athlete, Toronto, 1982, JB Lippincott.

Louis D et al: Rupture and displacement of the ulnar collateral ligament of the metacarpophalangeal joint of the thumb, J Bone Joint Surg 68A(9):1320, 1986.

Magee DJ: Orthopaedics conditions, assessment and treatment, vol 2, ed 3, Alberta, 1979, University of Alberta Publishing.

Magee DJ: Orthopaedic physical assessment, Toronto, 1987, WB Saunders Co.

Maitland GD: Peripheral manipulation, Toronto, 1977, Butterworth & Co.

Manzione M and Pizzutillo P: Stress fractures of the scaphoid wrist, Am J Sports Med 9(4):268, 1981.

Mannheimer JS and Lampe GN: Clinical transcutaneous electrical nerve stimulation, Philadelphia, 1986, FA Davis Co.

Mosher J: Current concepts in the diagnosis and treatment of hand and wrist injuries in sports, Med Sci Sports Exerc 17:48, 1985.

Nitz R et al: Nerve injury and grades II and III sprains, Am J Sports Med 13(3):177, 1985.

O'Donaghue D: Treatment of injuries to athletes, Toronto, 1984, WB Saunders Co.

Palmer K and Louis D: Assessing ulnar instability of the metacarpophalangeal joint of the thumb, J Hand Surg 3:545, 1978.

Parker R et al: Hood of hamate fracture in athletes, Am J Sports Med 14(6):517, 1986.

Petersen L and Renstrom P: Sports injuries, their prevention and treatment, Chicago, 1986, Year Book Medical Publishers Inc.

Reid DC: Functional anatomy and joint mobilization, Alberta, 1970, University of Alberta Press.

Rettig A: Stress fracture of the ulna in an adolescent tournament tennis player, Am Sports Med 11(2): 103, 1983.

Rettig A, Ryan R, Shelbourne D, McCarroll J, Johnson F, and Ahlfeld S: Metacarpal fractures in the athlete, Am J Sports Med, Vol 17(4):567, 1989.

Rovere G: How I manage skier's thumb, The Physician and Sportsmedicine 11(11):73, 1983.

Rovers G et al: Treatment of "Gameskeeper's Thumb" in hockey players, J Sports Med 3(4):147, 1975.

Roy S and Irvin R: Sports medicine, prevention, evaluation, management and rehabilitation, New Jersey, 1983, Prentice-Hall.

Ruby L, Stinson J, and Belsky M: The natural history of scaphoid non-union, J Bone Joint Surg 67-A(3):428, 1985.

Shively R and Sundaram M: Ununited fractures of the scaphoid in boxers, Am J Sports Med 8:6, 440, 1980.

Stark H et al: Fracture of the hook of hamate in athletes, Bone Joint Surg 59A:575, 1977.

Stover CN et al: The modern golf swing and stress, Physician Sports Med 9:43, 1976.

Tomberlin JP et al: The use of standardized evaluation forms in physical therapy, J Orthop Sports Physical Therapy, pp 348-354, 1984.

Travell J and Simons D: Myofascial pain and dysfunction—the trigger point manual, New York, 1980, Williams & Wilkins.

Tubiana Raoul: Examination of the hand and upper limb, Toronto, 1984, WB Saunders.

Vetter W: How I manage mallet finger, Physician Sports Med 17:2, 1989.

Wadsworth C: Wrist and hand examination and interpretation, J Orthop Sports Physical Therapy 5(3):108, 1983.

Welsh P and Shepherd R: Current therapy in sports medicine 1985-1986, Toronto, 1985, BC Decker Inc.

Williams PL and Warwick Roger: Gray's Anatomy, New York, 1980, Churchill Livingstone Inc.

Index